Disorders of the Knee

Disorders of the Knee

Arthur J. Helfet

B.SC. (Cape Town), M.D., M.CH. ORTH. (Liverpool),
F.R.C.S. (England), F.A.C.S.

Clinical Professor, late Chairman, Department of Orthopaedic Surgery, Albert Einstein College of Medicine, New York; Consulting Orthopaedic Surgeon, Hospital for Joint Diseases, New York; Formerly Senior Visiting Orthopaedic Surgeon and Senior Lecturer in Orthopaedic Surgery, University of Cape Town and Groote Schuur Hospital. Hunterian Professor, Royal College of Surgeons

With Twelve Guest Authors

J. B. Lippincott Company
Philadelphia · Toronto

C. S

ISBN 0-397-50322-9
Library of Congress Catalog Card Number 73-21998

Printed in the United States of America

3   4   2

Library of Congress Cataloging in Publication Data

Helfet, Arthur J.

   Disorders of the knee.

   Rev., updated, and enl. version of the author's The
management of internal derangements of the knee.

   Includes bibliographies.

   1. Knee—Diseases.   I. Title.   DNLM: 1. Knee.
2. Knee injuries. WE870 H474d 1974

RC951.H43   1974   616.7′2   73-21998

ISBN 0-397-50322-9

Guest Authors

Endre A. Balazs, M.D.
Boston Biomedical Research Institute
Harvard Medical School
Boston, Massachusetts

Victor H. Frankel, M.D.
Professor of Orthopaedic Surgery and
*   Bioengineering*
Director, Biomechanics Laboratory
*   Case Western Reserve University*
Associate Attending Orthopaedic Surgeon
*   University Hospitals, Rainbow Babies' and*
*   Childrens' Hospital, and the Veterans*
*   Administration Hospital*
Cleveland, Ohio

Robert H. Freiberger, M.D.
Professor of Radiology, Cornell University
*   Medical College*
Director, Department of Radiology, Hospital for
*   Special Surgery*
New York, New York

Jerry Goldsmith, M.D.
Staff Physician, Baptist Memorial Hospital
*   LeBanheur Children's Hospital, and*
*   St. Joseph Hospital*
Memphis, Tennessee

John Ellis Handelsman, M.B., B.Ch.,
**   M.Ch.Orth.**
Principal Orthopaedic Surgeon, The
*   Johannesburg General Hospital Group*
Department of Orthopaedic Surgery, University
*   of Witwatersrand, Orthopaedic Surgeon to the*
*   Hemophilia Clinic, Transvaal Memorial*
*   Hospital for Children*
*   Johannesburg, South Africa*

Joseph E. Milgram, M.D., M.S.
Emeritus Director of Orthopaedic Surgery
*   Hospital for Joint Diseases*
Clinical Professor of Orthopaedic Surgery
*   Albert Einstein College of Medicine*
New York, New York

Maurice E. Müller, M.D.
Professor of Orthopaedics, University of Berne
Director, Clinic for Orthopaedics and
*   Traumatology, Inselspital*
Berne, Switzerland

James A. Nicholas, M.D.
Director, Department of Orthopaedic Surgery
*   and Founding Director, Institute of Sports*
*   Medicine and Athletic Trauma, Lenox-Hill*
*   Hospital*
Associate Professor of Clinical Orthopaedics
*   Cornell University Medical College*
Attending Orthopaedic Surgeon, New York
*   Hospital and The Hospital for Special Surgery*
New York, New York

Joseph Schatzker, M.D., B.Sc. (Med.)
Associate, Department of Surgery
*   University of Toronto*
Active Staff, Division of Orthopaedic Surgery
*   Wellesley and Sunnybrook Hospitals*
Toronto, Ontario

Peter S. Walker, Ph.D.
Director of Bioengineering and Associate
*   Scientist, Hospital for Special Surgery*
Affiliated with New York Hospital—
*   Cornell University Medical College*
New York, New York

Masaki Watanabe, M.D.
Director, Department of Orthopaedic Surgery
*   Tokyo Teishin Hospital*
Tokyo, Japan

Charles Weiss, M.D., B.S.
Instructor in Orthopaedic Surgery
*   Harvard Medical School*
Assistant Orthopaedic Surgeon
*   Massachusetts General Hospital*
Boston, Massachusetts

Preface

I must believe in order that I may understand.
ST. ANSELM, 11TH CENTURY.

I must understand in order that I may believe.
PETER ABELARD, 12TH CENTURY.

Orthopaedic surgery has benefited from the century's tremendous progress in scientific understanding and technology; this is manifest even on the limited canvas of a specialised treatise. *The Management of Internal Derangements of the Knee,* published in 1963, had as its theme the clinical implications of the helical character of the mechanics of the knee. The new edition reports progress in the management of traumatic and arthritic derangements. But since knowledge of basic structure, joint biomechanics, and biochemistry has advanced considerably over the past decade, additional chapters by clinical scientists who are among the most distinguished pioneers in these fields are included.

Victor Frankel describes the modern concepts of the kinematics which underlie the importance of helicoid motion of the knee joint in a form simple to understand and, in lucid biomechanical terms, explains their relation to derangements of the meniscus.

Charles Weiss who familiarised himself with the first "patterns of erosion" in the operating rooms and laboratories of the Albert Einstein College of Medicine illuminates the origin and nature of joint tissues in terms of his ultramicroscopic and histochemical studies.

Endre Balazs has unravelled a chain of molecular action in the lubrication of joints and has introduced with his extract of hyaluronic acid a variant of treatment by transplant or replacement of normal tissue.

In osteoarthritis of the hip joint, replacement by prosthetic implant has yielded considerable success. The knee is a more complex joint and the results are not as successful. Although patients with advanced osteoarthritis may be relieved of pain, restoration of function is limited. Nevertheless, though it would be premature to commend a particular device, Peter Walker's critical and constructive review of engineering principles presages promising developments.

Robert Freiberger demonstrates that expert arthrography adds to the precision of clinical diagnosis, as does Masaki Watanabe's brilliant arthroscope and camera, which, without injuring tissues, display the nooks and crannies of the joint and its disorders. Both techniques should aid in obviating the widely practiced and unnecessarily traumatic "house cleaning," when simple meniscectomy and limited removal of osteophytes are all that is basically necessary in early osteoarthritis.

Major knee injuries are a frequent sequel to the gladiatorial collisions which are a feature of modern professional football and other sports. James Nicholas relates a thoughtful and most valuable report of his considerable experience in the surgical management and rehabilitation of these athletes. These injuries are a grosser version of the more usual derangements of the knee and result in wider disruption of tissues.

Maurice Müller is a leader among the Swiss surgeons who have united to promote the principle that internal fixation with compression fosters synthesis of bone. With his colleagues, J. Goldsmith and Joseph Schatzker, he describes the elegant techniques that have streamlined treatment and improved results in fractures and especially in joints where accurate stable reduction permits early movement and return of function.

In elaborating his previous contributions, Joseph Milgram has continued his original and thought provoking interpretation of the mechanism and character of osteochondral fractures. He emphasizes anew the warning that articular cartilage is vulnerable to corticosteroid therapy and that ill may follow its use. To his contribution he adds the gift of a most valued friendship and his unsurpassed command of orthopaedic literature.

The knee is not a hinge joint. The realization that the tibia navigates a helical course on the condyles of the femur, gives clarity to certain features in the diagnosis and treatment of injuries of the knee joint, and as the concept is developed, leads to new physical signs in the diagnosis of derangements of the knee joint and then to the inescapable conviction that *most traumatic arthritis of the knee in middle-aged and elderly people is due to minor derangements of the soft tissues especially the menisci, and that the pain and the discomfort of the condition are usually cured by simple operation.*

No longer is the outlook hopeless for the osteoarthritic, rheumatoid or hemophiliac knee. We know that in early osteoarthritis the process may be arrested with relief of symptoms and restoration of function. In due course radiographs may show reversal of the degenerative process.

A new Chapter is included on the surgery of the rheumatoid knee; and, Jack Handelsman contributes an erudite report on the considerable progress that has altered the management and improved dramatically the prognosis for the hemophiliac.

Precise diagnosis, gentle nontraumatic surgery, and adequate rehabilitation, however, remain the requisites for successful surgery of the knee.

The knee is used to carry and to propel, to comfort and to supplicate, and merits care on every count.

I am deeply indebted to the valued contributors and in writing and editing this volume, am most grateful to Eli Sedlin, who worked with me in the department of Orthopaedic Surgery of the Albert Einstein College of Medicine; to George Sacks, whose use of words is a constant delight; to Alan Apley who combines friendship with apt counsel; and to Stuart Freeman of J. B. Lippincott Company, who has blended understanding and helpfulness.

Arthur J. Helfet, M.D.

Contents

7. Clinical Features of Injuries to the Semilunar Cartilages
Arthur J. Helfet, M.D. 103

8. Differential Diagnosis of Tears of the Semilunar Cartilages
Arthur J. Helfet, M.D. 117

9. Arthrography of the Knee · *R. H. Freiberger, M.D.* 131

To Nathalie and to Anthony, David, Tim and Tess

1

Anatomy and Mechanics of Movement of the Knee Joint

Arthur J. Helfet, M.D.

The key to understanding the knee joint is the realization that its movement is helicoid* or spiral in character.[4] The knee is not a simple hinge joint. The opening and the shutting of the front of the joint in the acts of flexion and extension involve the tibia in a winding course set by the configuration of the medial condyle of the femur (Fig. 1-1). As the tibia glides on the femur from the fully flexed to the fully extended position it descends and then ascends the curves of the medial femoral condyle and at the same time slowly rotates outward. These movements are reversed as the tibia passes back to the fully flexed position. This screw-action gives to any position of the knee joint a stability that would be denied a straight up-and-down hinge joint.

Movement of the tibial tubercle, which is easily observed, demonstrates this spiral action (Fig. 1-2). Moreover, it shows that rotation occurs not only in the last few degrees of flexion and extension, as was thought previously, but throughout the whole range of movement (Figs. 1-3 and 2-3 E to G). The extent of the rotary movement is roughly equivalent to half the width of the patella. When the knee is fully flexed the tubercle points to the inner half (Fig. 1-4, *left*) of the patella; in the extended knee it is in line with the outer half (Fig. 1-4, *right*).

The anatomy of the knee joint facilitates this pattern of movement and at the same time maintains stability in the lower limb during movement while bearing weight.

THE THIGH MUSCLES— THE CONTROL MECHANISM OF THE KNEE JOINT

Quadriceps

The quadriceps group of muscles, of which the medial vastus is the most prominent, runs from without inward and is inserted into the tibia through the patella and the patellar ligament and has a broad fibrous expansion stronger on the medial side (Fig. 1-5). From the direction of their pull and the preponderance of attachment to the medial side of the tibia their purpose is to rotate the tibia outward while extending the knee. Special fibers from the medial vastus to the quadriceps tendon and the patella control synchronous spiral movement of the patella and prevent lateral dislocation.

Medial Hamstrings

The medial hamstrings are directed from the ischial tuberosity downward and, if anything, slightly inward to be inserted into the upper tibia on its anteromedial and posterior surfaces (Fig. 1-6). Their action is to rotate the tibia inwardly while flexing the knee. In addition, the semimembranosus is inserted into the posteromedial aspect of the capsule of the knee joint which has firm connections with the posterior end of the medial menis-

---

* Helicoid—"having the form of a helix; screw-shaped; spiral."—Shorter Oxford Dictionary.

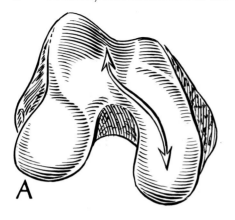

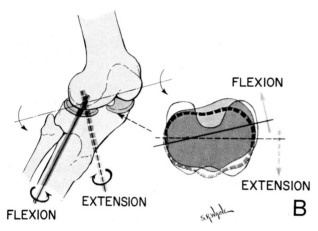

Fig. 1-1. (*A*) The articular surface of the medial condyle of the femur showing the helicoid track followed by the tibia in flexion and extension of the knee. The tibia descends and then ascends the curves of the medial femoral condyle and at the same time slowly rotates outwards. (*B*) Diagrammatic illustration of rotation of the tibia on the femur during flexion and extension of the knee joint. (AAOS Instructional Course Lectures, vol. 19, St. Louis, C. V. Mosby, 1970)

cus in this area. When in action the semimembranosus anchors the posterior end of the meniscus.

Popliteus

The popliteus, which takes origin from the upper end of the posterior surface of the tibia as a fleshy triangular muscle, narrows to a tendon which, synovial-sheathed, winds upward and forward around the posterolateral segment of the knee joint to be inserted in a groove on the lateral femoral epicondyle above the joint line. The tendon crosses and grooves the lateral semilunar cartilage, though separated by a fold of synovium. In turn, it is separated from the fibular collateral ligament by its own sheath and sometimes by a small bursa as well (Fig. 1-16). The popliteus flexes the knee joint and at the same time anchors the femur, while the medial hamstrings rotate the tibia inward. Last points out that en route pos-

terior fibers from the tendon enter the lateral meniscus and so drag the meniscus backward and downward during lateral rotation of the femur.[7] In other words, the posterior end of the lateral meniscus is anchored during flexion of the knee. The muscle also has clinical significance, for synovitis of its tendon sheath causes pain and disability independently of a lesion of the knee joint itself.

The Biceps and the Iliotibial Band

Both are active in stabilizing the fully extended knee. It is suggested also that contraction of these muscles is a preliminary and sometimes a necessary preliminary to strong action by the extensors of the knee. In the initial stages of contraction until the quadriceps group of muscles has shortened sufficiently to exert full power, the position and the stability of the knee must be controlled by the action of the biceps and the iliotibial band. The biceps tendon is inserted into the head of the fibula with the fibular collateral ligament, while the iliotibial band finds insertion into the tibia through the lateral capsule and into the fibula through the lateral ligament. The biceps is also a flexor of the knee, and both play a part in external rotation of the tibia. Indeed, in paralytic contracture of the knee the iliotibial band may be the main contributor to the flexion-external-rotation deformity (Fig. 1-7).[10]

However, their most important function is probably to stabilize the fibular component of the leg in weight-bearing. Through their attachments they exert control on the superior tibiofibular joint. When the knee is fully extended rotation of the tibia on the femur is not possible. Also the weight-bearing knee cannot indulge in any change of its exact ratio of flexion-extension to rotation; but the movements of flexion and extension of the ankle and inversion and eversion of the foot do not take place in isolation in the ankle and the subtaloid and the midtarsal joints. They require a component of rotation in the leg. This necessary movement must take place in the inferior and the superior tibiofibular joints (Fig. 1-8), a factor more easily appreciated when it is realized that the increasing width of the articular surface of the talus posteriorly needs changing accommodation in the ankle mortise. Indeed, one might generalize by saying that most actions of the weight-bearing leg are accomplished

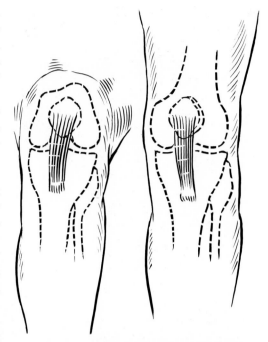

FIG. 1-2. Movement of the tibial tubercle in relation to the patella demonstrates this spiral action. The tibial tubercle of the flexed knee (*left*) is in line with the medial half of the patella. When the knee is extended (*right*) the tubercle rotates toward the outer half of the patella.

by *sinuous adaptatory* movements of all the joints of the leg from the hip downward. "The co-ordination of joints, whether stationary or in motion, is a fundamental part of bodily posture and movement."[1]

FIG. 1-3. The tibial tubercle is in line with the anterior tibial spine and the anterior cruciate ligament which spiral synchronously.

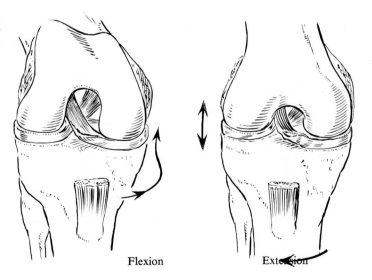

Flexion   Extension

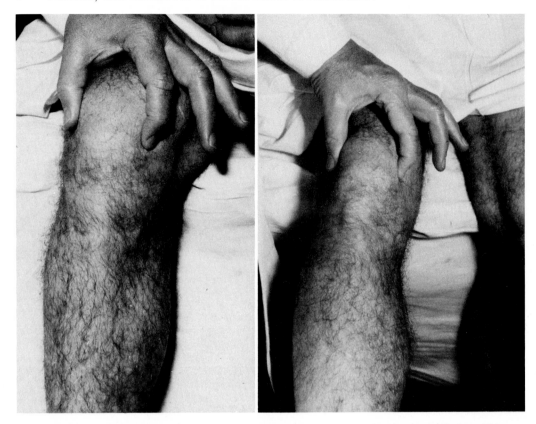

FIG. 1-4. The extent of the rotary movement is roughly equivalent to half the width of the patella. When the knee is fully flexed (*left*) the tubercle points to the inner half of the patella; (*right*) in the extended knee it is in line with the outer half.

The movement of the fibula on the tibia may be confirmed quite simply. With the muscles relaxed and the knee bent, the tibia with the fibula can be rotated quite freely on the femur. With weight taken on the leg, independent rotation of the tibia on the femur is no longer possible. The tibia does not rotate on the femur unless the knee flexes and extends. Different widths of the talus occupy the ankle mortise in flexion and extension. The change in space is accommodated by movement of the fibula on the tibia at the inferior and the superior tibiofibular joints. When weight is taken on the leg as the ankle flexes and extends, the head of the fibula can be felt to move backward and forward on the tibia independently and without rotation of the tibia (Figs. 1-8 and 1-9).

The experiment may be repeated while taking weight on the bent knee. Invert and evert the foot or flex and extend the ankle, and so long as the angle of flexion of the knee does not alter, rotation of the tibia on the femur does not take place. The adjustment is made by independent movement of the superior tibiofibular joint. This is further proof that the helicoid, or spiral, action of the knee joint when controlled by the thigh muscles, as in weight-bearing, demands that flexion and extension be synchronous with inward and outward rotation of the tibia, respectively, and that the stable weight-bearing position for each component is definite and cannot be altered.

In other words, the *normal movement of the knee joint* when bearing weight and under control of the thigh muscles, is a synchrony of extension with lateral rotation of the tibia and of flexion with medial rotation.

FIG. 1-5. The quadriceps group of muscles runs from without inward. (*A* from Quain, J. [ed.]: The Muscles of the Human Body. London, Taylor & Walton, 1836)

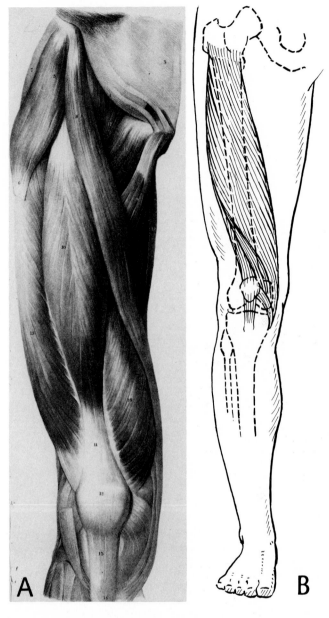

A   B

Only when the thigh muscles are relaxed is it possible to rotate the tibia on the femur freely in both directions, and even in relaxation it is not possible to achieve full extension or full flexion without full lateral or medial rotation, as the case may be. When the slack tibia moves from full extension to flexion the range of free rotation increases. But it should be emphasized again that when the quadriceps and the hamstrings are active, only synchronous movement in each direction is normally possible: when the knee straightens, the tibia must rotate laterally; and as it flexes, the tibia must rotate medially.

The *superior tibiofibular joint,* in the past, has not been accorded proper clinical respect; for injury, as will be shown later, may result in appreciable disability. It is important to recognize the symptoms of this disorder, which must be differentiated from those of injury to the lateral semilunar cartilage.

FUNCTIONS OF MUSCLES ACTING ON THE KNEE

A rough classification of the actions of the muscles acting on the knee joint would be:

1. **Quadriceps group**—mainly extensors and outward rotators of tibia.

2. **Medial hamstrings**—mainly flexors and inward rotators of tibia.

3. **Stabilizers**—popliteus, biceps, tensor fascia femoris and iliotibial band.

CRUCIATE LIGAMENTS AND SEMILUNAR CARTILAGES— THE GUIDE MECHANISM OF THE KNEE JOINT

The spiral movement of the knee is guided by a mechanism of cruciate ligaments and semilunar cartilages (Fig. 1-10). The cruci-

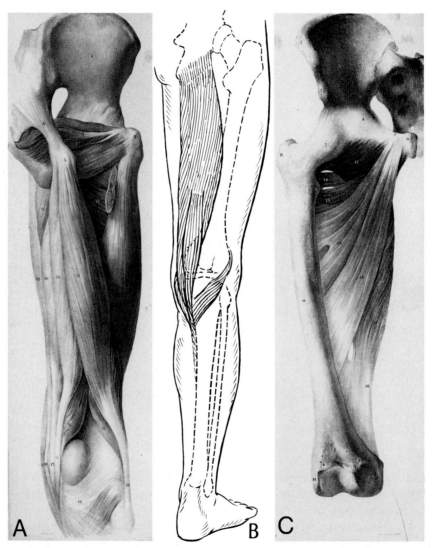

Fɪɢ. 1-6. *(A, B)* The medial hamstrings rotate the tibia inward while flexing the knee. The popliteus anchors the femur and the posterior capsule of the knee joint and so acts as a stabilizer while the medial hamstrings rotate the tibia inward. *(C)* The adductor muscles stabilize the thigh from the inner side. (A & C from Quain, J. [ed.]: The Muscles of the Human Body. London, Taylor and Walton, 1836)

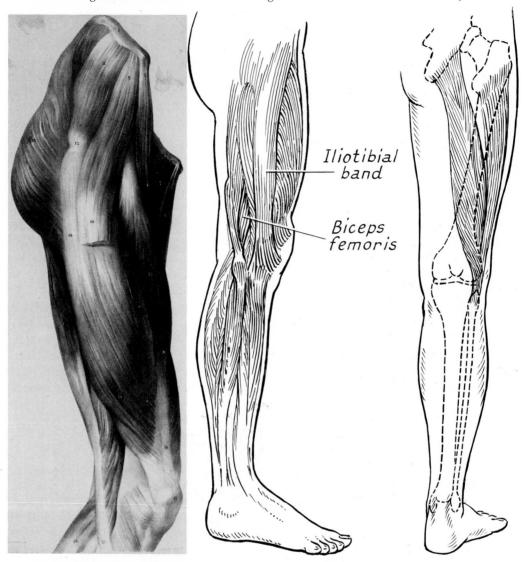

FIG. 1-7. The biceps and the iliotibial band are active in stabilizing the leg on the thigh.

ates do not act as stays to prevent antero-posterior displacement of the tibia on the femur but as guide ropes to keep the tibia on its winding path when the knee extends and flexes. It would be reasonable to expect that the cruciates develop in support of such normal action, rather than as potential obstructions to unnatural anteroposterior displacement.

The anatomic arrangement and continuity of the cruciates with the semilunar cartilages suggest that the function of guiding rotation

of the tibia on the femur is shared in the manner presented diagrammatically in Figure 1-11. It is probable, too, that both the cruciate ligaments and the semilunar cartilages are of similar origin, for the cartilages are differentiated from the same embryologic layer in continuity with the cruciate ligaments and are not truly cartilaginous.[5]

The continuity of the ligamentous and cartilaginous structures, in what Sir Harry Platt aptly termed "figure-of-eight" anatomy, was described accurately by Galeazzi in

1927.[3] Three of his illustrations, reproduced here, emphasize this characteristic. Figure 1-12 shows the strong fibrous band, sometimes a centimeter wide, connecting the posterior horn of the lateral cartilage to the femoral attachment of the anterior cruciate ligament. Figure 1-13 (*left*) shows the fibrous bands which connect the anterior cruciate ligament with the anterior horn of the medial and with the anterior horn of the lateral cartilage.

Figure 1-13 (*right*) shows Barkow's ligament connecting the posterior horn of the lateral cartilage and the anterior horn of the medial cartilage. Galeazzi also referred to the transverse ligament of the knee (Winslow) which joins the anterior horns of the two cartilages, and he emphasized particularly the firm attachments between the anterior cruciate ligament and medial cartilage.

Besides their links with the cruciates, the menisci have attachment to the tibia and move with it. There is play between them and the tibia, especially in the anterior half of the medial and the anterior two thirds of the lateral meniscus, where the attachments through a coronary ligament are lax. The posterior half of the medial meniscus is firmly attached to the deep part of the tibial collateral ligament and the posteromedial capsule. The lateral meniscus is attached equally firmly to the posterior capsule where the popliteus muscle takes part of its insertion.

These arrangements are significant. The medial part of the capsule which is concerned with the quadriceps expansion, in outward rotation of the tibia has, as one would expect, intimate attachments to its pilot, the medial semilunar cartilage. But the lateral ligament, which is designed to stabilize the tibiofibular joint, does not take part in rotating the tibia and therefore is independent of the lateral meniscus, from which it is separated by the tendon of the popliteus and a fold of synovium. Should it become adherent, rotation of the tibia is affected, and flexion of the knee is hampered

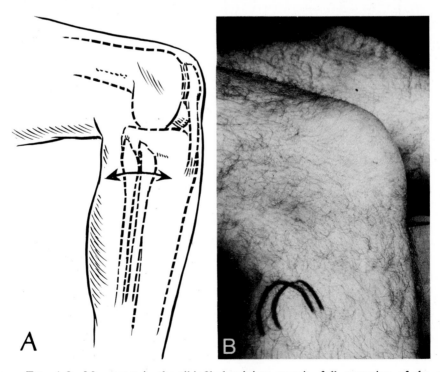

FIG. 1-8. Movement in the tibiofibular joints permits full excursion of the talus in the ankle mortise.

Fig. 1-9. The changing position of the head of the fibula when the ankle or the foot is moved is obvious.

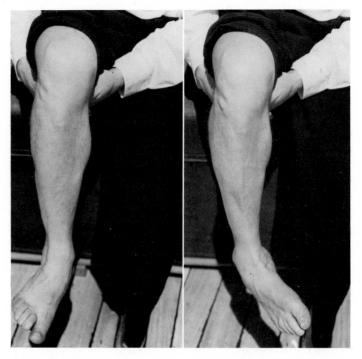

—a feature to consider in the stiff knee after injury or infection.

The insertion of the popliteus into the posterior capsule and the back end of the lateral meniscus means that, as the muscle contracts to flex the knee and to act as anchor for the femur, it also holds the cartilage to the posterior edge of the tibia, so providing a stable axis of pivot while the tibia rotates inwardly on the femur.

An effect of the firm attachment of the posterior ends of both menisci, compared with the loose capsular attachments of both anterior halves, suggests the explanation for another clinical finding. The "retracted" or detached anterior horn occurs frequently (see Fig. 6-10). The main injury is a rupture of the bands binding the anterior horn to the cruciate ligaments and to each other. The loose posterior horn is usually associ-

Fig. 1-10. The cruciate ligaments and the semilunar cartilages act as guide ropes to keep the tibia on its helical path as the knee extends and flexes.

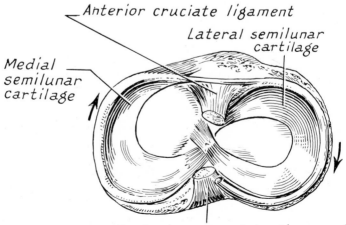

Anterior cruciate ligament

Lateral semilunar cartilage

Medial semilunar cartilage

Posterior cruciate ligament

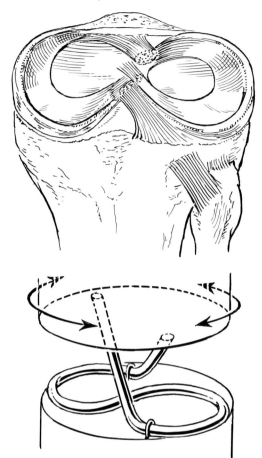

FIG. 1-11. The anatomic arrangement and continuity of the cruciates with the semilunar cartilages suggest that the function of guiding rotation is shared in this figure-of-eight manner.

ated with rupture of the cartilage itself, implying that the meniscus itself is more vulnerable than the extensive and firm capsular attachments.

Watson-Jones drew attention to the part played by the semilunar cartilages in the rotator mechanism, when he described what might be called the *retreating cartilage*.[9]

Place one finger over the joint line on the knee in front of the medial ligament where the curved margin of the medial femoral condyle approaches the tibial tuberosity. Now rotate the foot and leg laterally. It is easy to feel the medial semilunar cartilage disappearing from the surface, leaving a sulcus between the bones.

This sign is present only when the knee is bent and the muscles relaxed and is an expression of the independence of the figure-of-eight mechanism, of which the cartilage is only a part, when rotation is not accompanied by synchronous extension of the knee. The cartilage maintains its relationship to the margin of the tibia in all normal movements and therefore does so when the leg is bearing weight.

On the other hand, when, as will be shown, rupture of the cartilage blocks lateral rotation of the tibia, *absence* of the "retreating" cartilage sign in the flexed knee may be used diagnostically.

In the young the semilunar cartilages, which are not true cartilage, are smooth and firm but yet resilient. With age the cartilage becomes yellowish in color, firmer and fibrotic in consistency and less resilient. In the aged, the free edge retracts, and the cartilage as a whole is harder and narrower and triangular on section (see Fig. 12-4).

The substance of the cartilage is avascular. Blood vessels course only in capsular

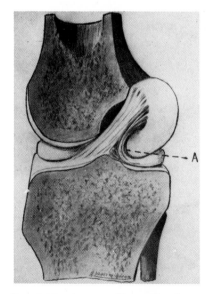

FIG. 1-12. A strong fibrous band, sometimes a centimeter wide, connects the posterior horn of the lateral cartilage to the femoral attachment of the anterior cruciate ligament. (Galeazzi, R.: J. Bone Joint Surg., *9*:515, 1927)

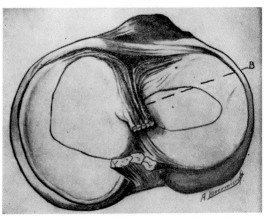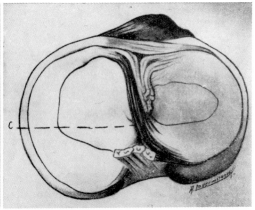

FIG. 1-13. (*Left*) Fibrous bands connect the anterior cruciate ligament with the anterior horn of the medial cartilage, and (B) with the anterior horn of the lateral cartilage. (*Right*) Barkow's ligament connects the posterior horn of the lateral cartilage to the anterior horn of the medial cartilage. (Galeazzi, R.: J. Bone Joint Surg. *9*:515, 1927)

and ligamentous attachments. Consequently, repair will occur in peripheral lesions, but no tear of the substance of the cartilage will heal.

On the other hand, if this is kept in mind, surgery of the semilunar cartilages may be relatively bloodless both during and after operation. The vascular synovium should be sutured hemostatically, and the meniscus excised by incision into the substance only and not through the peripheral attachments.

Regenerated Cartilages

I do not propose to enter the controversial speculation on the manner and frequency of regeneration of semilunar cartilages. One may open a knee in which previously a meniscus had been excised and find practically no evidence of regeneration. In most instances one does find a shape resembling most or part of the meniscus but not of pristine smooth shiny cartilage. Microscopically fibrous tissue in various stages of maturity, but without true cartilage cells may be demonstrated (see Plate 1-1). In some instances at least, the regenerated shape is no more than organized and fibrosed blood clot, duly shaped and nourished by the joint —in the same way as an erosion of articular cartilage fills and smooths and shines with-

out apparent vascular nourishment. These regenerated cartilages seem to occur more frequently when special meniscectomy knives, used blindly to free the back end of the meniscus, take their toll on vascular synovial membrane with consequent postoperative hemarthrosis. In the early days of the Middle East Campaign during World War II, when a large number of relatively inexperienced surgeons were operating on knees, the incidence of postoperative hemarthrosis in some units was as high as 60 to 80 per cent. At operation each incision should be visualized properly and made into the cartilage itself.

CAPSULAR LIGAMENTS

Medial Ligament

The medial ligament is the main strut of the capular tissues of the knee. The deep portion is a thickened part of the capsule itself and is adherent to the medial meniscus. The superficial part forms a strong broad strap of triangular shape. Taking origin just distal to the adductor tubercle, the ligament keeps free of the meniscus and the joint margins and has an extensive insertion into the medial surface of the tibia, at least 1½ inches below joint level. But the pos-

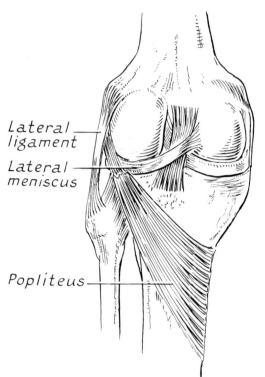

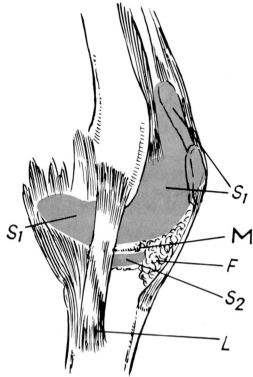

FIG. 1-14. The medial ligament and related anatomy of the knee joint. (*L*) Medial ligament; (*F*) infrapatellar pad of fat embracing the anterior horn of the meniscus; (*M*) medial meniscus; (S_1, S_2) synovial cavities; (S_2) fold of synovium between meniscus and articular cartilage of tibia. The meniscus is extrasynovial as is the fat pad.

FIG. 1-15. The lateral ligament does not take part in rotating the tibia and therefore is independent of the lateral meniscus from which it is separated by the popliteus tendon and a fold of synovium.

terior border has continuity with the strong posterior capsule of the knee joint, and anteriorly there are fibrous connections with the quadriceps expansion and the patellar ligament. Therefore, the whole medial capsule with its ligament is adequately designed to take strong control of the tibia in all movements of the knee, both by its structure and its intimate connections with the anterior and the posterior muscles of the thigh (Fig. 1-14).

Lateral Ligament

The lateral ligament extends in two layers from the lateral epicondyle of the femur to the head of the fibula where it finds inser-

tion in intimate relationship with the biceps tendon. The tendon of the popliteus and frequently a bursa separate it from the knee joint and the lateral meniscus (Fig. 1-15). The only connection with the fibrous capsule is at its posterior border, which is continuous with the fascia covering the popliteus and therefore with that muscle's attachments to the posterior horn of the lateral meniscus. Through the superior tibiofibular joint it plays its part in stability of the leg on the thigh and is independent of rotary movements of the tibia. As observed previously, were it attached to the lateral meniscus, rotation would be prevented, and flexion of the knee curbed. Understandably, for it plays a minor role in the stability of the knee joint, the whole lateral capsule is thinner and weaker than the medial side (Fig. 1-16).

PATELLA

The patella is a pulley, and its excursion is controlled by the direction of action of the quadriceps group of muscles and the position of the tibial tubercle which carries the patellar ligament (Fig. 1-2).

The articular surface of the patella is divided into a large lateral and a smaller medial area. These areas are separated by a vertical rounded ridge (Fig. 1-17). In full extension its shape fits comfortably and evenly into the trochlear surface of the femur (Fig. 1-18). The ridge then lies in

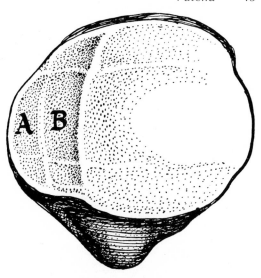

FIG. 1-17. The articular surface of the patella is divided into a large lateral and a smaller medial slope with vertical division into two planes (*A* and *B*). (Frazer, J. B.: Anatomy of the Human Skeleton. London, Churchill, 1933)

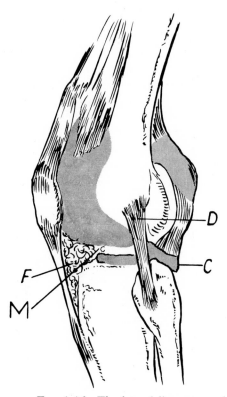

FIG. 1-16. The lateral ligament and its relationships to the knee joint. (*F*) Infrapatellar pad of fat; (*M*) lateral meniscus separated by fold of synovium from articular cartilage of tibia; (*C*) popliteus tendon in synovial sheath; (*D*) lateral ligament separated from meniscus by tendon and fold of synovium.

the hollow or trough of the trochlear surface. When the knee is bent the patella is carried downward and backward on the under aspect of the femur where the trochlear surface is prolonged onto the inner condyle (Fig. 1-19). In flexion the patella tilts away from the lateral condyle, so that only the inner part of its articular surface rests against the medial condyle.[2]

So long as the tibial tubercle rotates smoothly the patella travels its short course smoothly and under even tension. However, any derangement of the joint which prevents lateral rotation of the tibia during extension of the knee would affect normal tension, because contraction of the quadriceps would force the inner border of the patella against the medial condyle of the femur (Figs. 1-20 and 6-28). This explains the patellar symptoms and signs produced by certain cartilage injuries—such as retropatellar pain on climbing and descending stairs, tenderness of the medial border of the patella, and the pattern of cartilage erosion that develops only on the medial surfaces of the patella and the femur. This pattern differs from

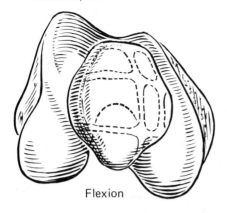

Flexion

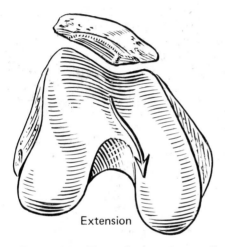

Extension

FIG. 1-18. From flexion the patella ascends a sinuous course from the undersurface of the medial condyle to the trochlear surface of the femur. In full extension its shape fits comfortably and evenly into the trochlear groove.

that produced by retropatellar arthritis complicating recurring dislocation when it is the lateral surface of the patellar cartilage that undergoes fibrillation.[6] Later, the medial surface is damaged from repeated drag over the lateral condyle of the femur during reduction, with consequent erosion of articular cartilage. By this time both sides of the patella are tender (Fig. 1-20).

Dislocation of the patella is encouraged by the angle between the line of action of the quadriceps and the patellar ligament (Fig. 1-5). The muscles act from without inward, whereas the ligament is vertical. As the late Arthur Steindler pointed out, this intro-

duces a lateral-directed horizontal component which tends to force the patella out of its groove.[8] Stability is maintained by the transverse strength of the medial capsule plus the attachments of medial vastus to the quadriceps tendon and the patella and the depth of the lateral trochlear surface of the femur. But should the latter be shallow or short, or the angle be increased, as in genu valgum or external rotation deformity from any cause, or the attachments of medial vastus be divided by injury or ill-repaired parapatellar incision, the propensity to subluxation is greater. Acute traumatic dislocation occurs at the expense of the medical capsule (see Chap. 16).

Infrapatellar Pad of Fat

The infrapatellar pad of fat extends from the lower pole of the patella to the level of the tibia, behind and on each side of the patellar ligament (Figs. 1-14 and 1-16). The pliable fat is a mobile structure and acts as a true cushion as the front of the joint is closed in straightening the knee. Alar folds of the synovium, which cover the joint surface, are so disposed as to maneuver vulnerable lobes of fat away from injury. The fat pad also contains a high proportion of adipose elastic tissue which helps it to regain

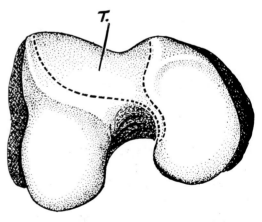

FIG. 1-19. Lower end of right femur showing trochlear surface (T) for patella, extending along inner condyle as an area with which patella articulates in flexion. (Frazer, J. B.: Anatomy of the Human Skeleton. London, Churchill, 1933)

Fig. 1-20. Pattern of erosion expected after recurrent dislocation of the patella, associated in this specimen with genu valgum. The condyles of the femur are relatively unscarred, but the trochlear groove and the patellar articular surfaces are extensively abraded—more on the lateral than on the medial side (*arrows*).

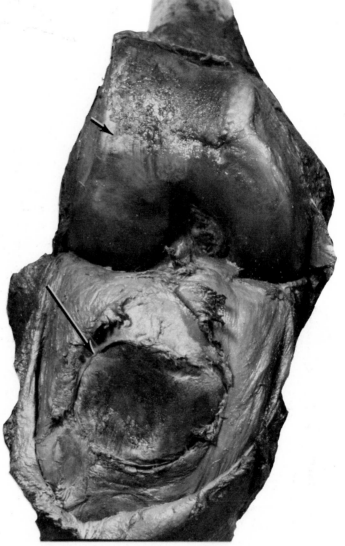

its shape. The pad has connections with the front ends of the semilunar cartilages which are attached and which it overlaps.

It is important to note that the fat pad is a mobile structure in the knee joint and that interference with its free movement results in pain and disability. Care must be taken not to injure the fat pad when operating on the knee, for many discomforts after contusions or rough surgery are due to fibrous scars or adherence to surrounding structures, which affect its mobility. A swollen fat pad, from any cause, may also result in pain as the pad is compressed when

straightening the knee. A vicious circle is created, for the impingement increases the swelling, which aggravates the pain.

TENSION IN CAPSULE AND LIGAMENTS

The tension in the capsule and the ligaments of the knee joint during all normal movements, i.e., with proper synchrony of rotation with flexion and extension, remains unchanged. This may be confirmed by observing the anterior cruciate ligament during operation on the knee. Bend and straighten the leg. The cruciate keeps the

arc of movement into extension is blocked. In the attempt to force it, the anterior cruciate is tensed over the edge of the medial femoral condyle.

It would seem that any crowding of the anteromedial joint space blocks outward rotation of the tibia. Through the usual medial incision, with the knee bent over the table the free rotation of the tibia shows very well. Place a sterile rubber catheter across the joint toward the cruciate notch. The tibia can no longer rotate outward. We now have a so-called locked knee.

Experiments on cadaver knees that purport to show changes in ligamentous tension are misleading.[3] The forces applied produce abnormal straight up-and-down movements without the requisite degree of rotation. Such movements would be expected to produce abnormal tensions.

REFERENCES

1. Barnett, C. H., Davies, D. V., and MacConaill, M. A.: Synovial Joints; Their Structure and Mechanics. New York, Longmans Green, 1961.

2. Frazer, J. B.: Anatomy of the Human Skeleton. ed. 5. edited by A. S. Breathnach, London, Churchill, 1958.

3. Galeazzi, R.: Clinical and experimental study of lesions of the semilunar cartilages of the knee joint. J. Bone Joint Surg., 9:515, 1927.

4. Helfet, A. J.: Mechanism of derangements of the medial semilunar cartilage and their management. J. Bone Joint Surg., *41-B*: 319, 1959.

5. Kaplan, E. B.: The embryology of the menisci of the knee joint. Bull. Hosp. Joint Dis., *16*:3, 1955.

6. Langston, H. H.: Dislocation of the patella and its relation to chondromalacia patellae. Brit. Med. J., *1*:155, 1958.

7. Last, R. J.: The popliteus muscle and the lateral meniscus. J. Bone Joint Surg., *32-B*: 93, 1950.

8. Steindler, Arthur: Mechanics of Normal and Pathological Locomotion in Man. Springfield, Ill., Charles C Thomas, 1935.

9. Watson-Jones, Sir Reginald: Fractures and Joint Injuries. ed. 4. vol 2. Baltimore, Williams & Wilkins, 1955.

10. Yount, C. C.: The role of the tensor fasciae femoris in certain deformities of the lower extremities. J. Bone Joint Surg., *8*:171, 1926.

2

Mechanical Efficiency of the Knee Joint

Arthur J. Helfet, M.D.

Muscles acting on a weight-bearing joint such as the knee have three functions. The first is to maintain posture by stabilizing the leg when standing. The second is kinetic—to move the joint to the limits allowed by its configuration. The third is propulsive—to move the leg on the thigh against resistance. The knee, like other joints in the human body, is wonderfully designed to accomplish these functions with a maximum economy of muscle power. Barnett, Davies and Mac Conaill in their comprehensive review of synovial joints, indicate the considerable achievement in conservation of muscle energy by the evolutionary conversion of multiaxial into biaxial joints.[1] In addition, there are the advantages in economy of effort in maintaining posture, in lifting and in propulsion provided by a helicoid as compared with a hinge joint.

The postural function of muscles is to act as stabilizers. The newborn infant crumples to the ground. Barnett et al. demonstrate through comparative anatomy how the evolutionary trend toward uniaxial joints makes for economy of muscle energy. The multiaxial joint requires much greater muscle power for stability in standing than does the biaxial joint. This is evidenced in the bulky muscles of the multiaxial shoulder joint compared with the leaner arm muscles, in most animals, for the biaxial elbow joint. In the animal's total economy the energy required for standing is wasteful. Muscle energy should be expended in moving the animal, especially in searching for food, and not dissipated in maintaining posture at rest. They cite the example of the members of the cat family which sit or lie down as soon as a burst of activity has ended. This avoids wasteful contraction of these postural muscles. Incidentally, the observation is made that

the almost complete inactivity of most of the muscles of the human body during standing, is one of the most striking ways in which a man is a more efficient machine than the great majority of mammals.[1]

A case in point is the muscle requirements of the elbow region of the spiny anteater compared with those of a dog. The anteater's elbow is capable of multiaxial movements, and, accordingly, its arm and forearm bulge with muscles whose function is largely postural. The shape of the articular surfaces and the tension in the ligaments of the dog's elbow, in which only flexion and extension are possible, permit a more slender upper arm with flexor and extensor muscles only. The configuration of the knee joint in man and the pattern of the capsular ligaments are perfectly designed to permit stability in standing with a minimum of muscle effort.

However, if the knee joint were a pure hinge joint, the effort to lift or propel the leg on the thigh against gravity would be enormous, many times as much as is needed

Fig. 2-1. A child can produce a greater volume of water by pushing the shaft of a waterwheel than a strong man can bring up by pulling a full bucket of water out of a well.

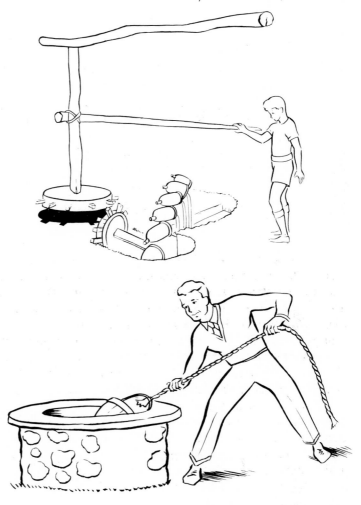

to pull it up the helicoid planes of the knee joint. One may compare the strength and the energy required to pull a fish straight out of the water compared with playing it obliquely to the bank—or the strength required to lift the axle of an automobile compared with that required to lift it by pumping the handle of a jack. A child can push the shaft of a waterwheel (Fig. 2-1, *top*), but it takes a strong man to pull a full bucket of water out of the well (Fig. 2-1, *bottom*).

An engineer (Helfet, 1961) explains it as follows:

From the engineering point of view, the construction of the knee joint is brilliantly conceived. Muscle action is nothing more than contraction and mechanically can be considered only as tension—a "pulling force." To illustrate the effect of this, imagine trying to close a door—against a draft—by hooking a finger around the handle and pulling toward the hinge.

In the plan view shown in Figure 2-2, the effective action is a turning movement equal to the force *F* multiplied by the lever arm *A*, which is the distance from the point of application of the force to the center line of the hinge. As *A* is very small, a strong pull is required if there is to be any appreciable effect.

A similar position would apply to the knee—if it were a plain hinge operated by muscular pull—the lever arm being measured from the attachment point of the muscle to a line from the center of the hinge down the middle of the bone (approximately the length of the patellar ligament). An enormous muscular pull would be required to straighten the knee when weight-bearing, for instance from the position of sitting on the haunches.

However, the actual construction of the joint, results in a screw action. The femoral condyles with the tibia form a bicondylar joint that can rotate in bending, allowing partial rotation of the calf. The lateral condyle forms a ball joint with the tibia, while the medial tibial tuberosity follows the helical track provided for it on the medial condyle. The quadriceps muscles are attached in such a way that the tension they apply tends to rotate the calf, i.e., they produce a torque that forces the tibia to screw itself up, thereby straightening the knee.

The mechanical advantage, or, in other words, the effectiveness of the force applied by the muscles, is increased greatly by this helical action. An illustration of this effect is the ease with which a heavy vehicle can be lifted by means of a screw-jack, whereas it would require a great deal of effort to raise it by a straight pull.

Figure 2-3 shows a model constructed to demonstrate the mechanical action of the knee joint. An eccentric ball-and-socket joint which represents the action of the tibia on the lateral femoral condyle is shown. The curved track represents the medial femoral condyle along which the tibia winds itself in extension and flexion. The rods simulating the femur and the tibia are a dark color on one half and a light color on the opposite half. When the knee is

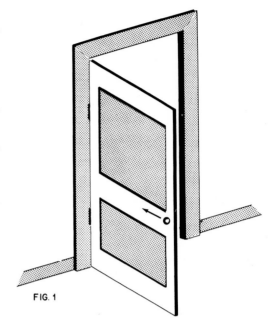

FIG. 1

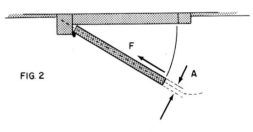

FIG. 2

FIGURE 2-2

straight, the midlines of both are in continuity, but as the joint is flexed, they rotate on each other, and the proportions change.

REFERENCE

Barnett, C. H., Davies, D. V., and MacConaill, M. A.: Synovial Joints; Their Structure and Mechanics. New York, Longmans Green, 1961.

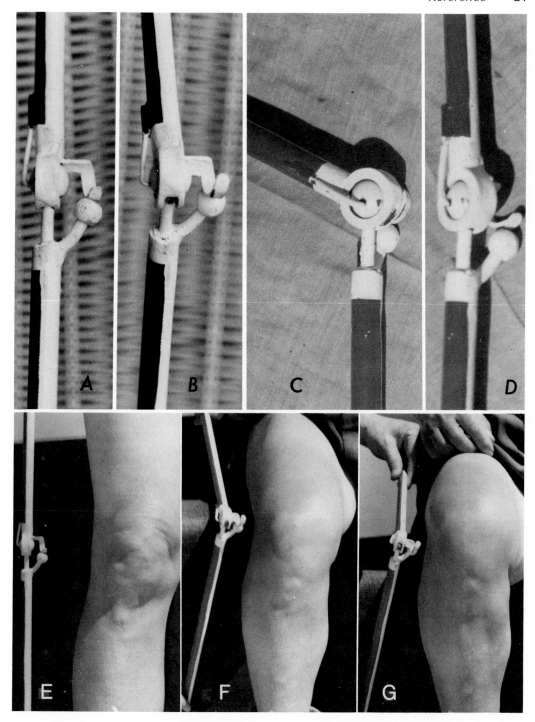

FIG. 2-3. An eccentric ball-and-socket joint represents the action of the tibia on the lateral femoral condyle. The curved part represents the medial femoral condyle along which the tibia winds itself in flexion and extension. (*A, B*) When the joint is extended, the colored strips are in alignment; as it bends and rotates, the proportions change. *C* and *D* are lateral oblique views of the model. The comparable rotation of the tibia on the femur is shown with leg straight (*E*), with the knee partly flexed (*F*), and completely flexed (*G*). Note the relationship between the tibial tubercle and the outer border of the patella.

3

Biomechanics of the Knee

Victor H. Frankel, M.D.

INTRODUCTION

The knee joint transmits loads, participates in kinematic functions, aids in momentum conservation and provides a force couple for purposeful activities involving the foot. The surgeon is frequently called upon to diagnose and treat disorders arising from a pathomechanical state. The assessment of altered function is classically performed by collecting subjective patient data and clinical evaluation. Biomechanics provides the tools for a precise scientific evaluation of the disorders of function.

The science of biomechanics as applied to the musculoskeletal system relates force and motion. Statics and dynamics are used to describe forces acting on a body and are useful engineering tools in biomechanics. In a static situation, there is a state of equilibrium and there are no accelerations acting on the part. In a dynamic situation, such as walking, jumping, or running, there are accelerations acting on a part. Solid mechanics is the engineering science that describes the internal effects of forces acting on a body. These internal effects cause a state of strain, which results in deformation in the object. This state of strain is associated with an internal force system or a stress, which is a force per unit area in a plane. Kinematics is the engineering science that describes the relative motion between two segments of a body and the velocities of the contacting surface particles.

How these various engineering disciplines are used to solve problems in human biomechanics is the subject of this chapter. Although much fine work has been done in the past in the area of knee biomechanics, it is only lately, during the past generation and through the use of more sophisticated engineering measuring techniques, that meaningful work on the mechanics of the knee joint could be performed. It is our purpose here to present several examples of general interest so that the reader will have some orientation in looking at clinical situations that come under his care from the standpoint of biomechanics. (Basic engineering material that applies to the study of the musculoskeletal system is presented in publications by Frankel and Burstein[5] and Williams and Lissner.[19])

In analyzing physical dysfunctions that have as their etiology pathomechanics of some segment of the locomotor system, it is necessary to constantly keep in mind the relationship between force and motion. Abnormal motion is usually easily perceived and measured either with the protractor or in dynamic situations with cinematography or stroboscopic photography, television scanning, or electrogoniometric methods. The forces associated with this motion are more difficult to determine because they must be measured by indirect means until such time as a force transducer is built that

This report was supported by the Social and Rehabilitation Service, Grant Number RD-2516-M.

can be inserted into a knee joint to measure force directly. The techniques of statics and dynamics are utilized to determine the forces. The distribution of the force over the joint surface is even more difficult to determine, for it is necessary to know the contact area and the distribution of force over the contact area. The joint pressure has not been determined for any joint, and only approximations have been attempted.

The relationship of force and motion is expressed by the two well known equations, force = mass × acceleration and torque = area moment of inertia × angular acceleration. The first equation refers to linear motion, the second to angular motion. In the case of the first equation, if the force is to be determined, it is necessary to know the mass of the limb, which can be obtained from tables, and the acceleration, which can be obtained by any of the foregoing kinematic methods. In the case of the second equation, for angular motion, the torque about a joint can be determined if the angular acceleration is found and the mass moment of inertia of the limb is known. The mass moment of inertia can be obtained from tables or from direct calculation. The mass moment of inertia is important because it is not only how much mass is present but the distribution of the mass in the limb. For instance, putting on a heavy shoe may increase the mass of the lower limb by 5 per cent, but the mass moment of inertia by 30 per cent. The relationship between torque, mass moment

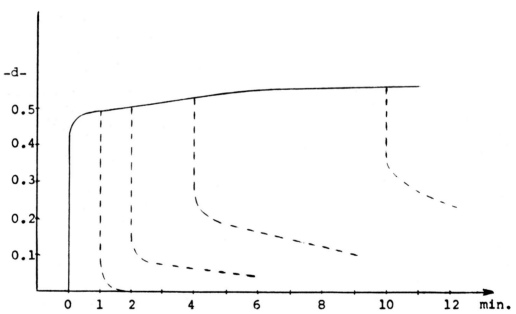

FIG. 3-1. Deformation time diagram for articular cartilage of patella. At zero time, a probe 10.57 mm. square in diameter was placed on the articular cartilage. There was an immediate deformation to 0.46 mm. When the weight was left on, continued deformation of the cartilage occurred. At the end of 1 minute, the deformation was 0.5 mm. The weight was removed, and the compressed cartilage expanded back to its original position but did not reach its total original position until an additional minute of time had gone by. When the weight was left on for longer periods of time, continued compression of the cartilage was noted. The recovery period was also lengthened, and after the weight had been on for 2 minutes, the original geometry was not attained during the experiment. (From Hirsch, C.: The pathogenesis of chondromalacia of the patella. Acta Chir. Scand., vol. *90* [Suppl.]: 83, 1944)

of inertia, and acceleration can be intuitively grasped if one thinks about an ice skater who is spinning on one skate. It is obvious that as she moves at a certain angular velocity, she accelerates by folding her arms tightly across her chest. This in effect decreases her mass moment of inertia so that for the same torque, which was applied originally to the skate, there is an acceleration.

The forces due to gravitational effects or to accelerations that exist on the joint will have internal effects in the joint structure. A study of the stress and strains in the joint tissues is made difficult by the fact that the mechanical response of the tissues is time dependent, viscoelastic, anisotropic, and heterogeneous. This means that a simple analysis of the material, as one would analyze a piece of stainless steel, is inadequate. If a small piece of material is removed from the joint and subjected to a loading test to determine a stress-strain curve, it is necessary to specify the rate at which it is loaded. All the biological tissues made up of collagenous tissue exhibit viscoelastic behavior. This type of behavior is seen to a marked degree in taffy or "silly putty." If the material is pulled slowly, it does not take much stress for a great deal of strain to develop. If, however, the material is pulled rapidly, a large amount of stress is developed for only a small strain.

In addition, joint materials exhibit viscoelasticity, as demonstrated by Hirsch,[9] by placing small loads on articular cartilage and then removing the load (Fig. 3-1). When the load is placed on the cartilage there will be an immediate deformation. As the load is left on it will continue to deform. When the load is taken off, the material will snap back toward its original shape but will not really regain its original shape until a period of time has gone by. Cartilage exhibits an elastic deformation that occurs immediately and an anelastic deformation that occurs as the load is left on. Data for the soft collagenous tissues involving joint structure have been summarized by Viidik and coworkers.[18] The

physical properties of the bony tissues have been summarized by Currey.[2]

Since the study of material properties of the tissues is in its infancy, for the purposes of this paper it is only necessary to understand that the mechanical responses of tissues are time dependent, as far as deformation under load is concerned. They are heterogeneous. Their anisotropy makes it very important to state in what direction the specimen has been taken for the loading experiment. There are regional differences in the physical properties of the joint structures. In the case of the dog tibial plateau, Moskowitz has demonstrated differences in histological structure between the medial and lateral condyles.* Kempson and coworkers[10] have demonstrated regional differences in elasticity of the cartilage in the femoral head. Among the areas that need elucidation are the menisci, the joint cartilage, the effects of aging on ligament strength and stiffness.

STATICS AND DYNAMICS

In the static situation, advantage can be taken of the fact that to establish equilibrium, the forces acting on a free body must be concurrent (absence of couples); that is, all forces acting on the surface of the free body will intersect at a point if continued. In the case of a person who stands on a step with his knee flexed it is possible to calculate the force acting against the tibial plateau by finding the forces acting on the free body of the lower limb. In the free body demonstrated in Figure 3-2, the force W (the ground reaction force) has a known magnitude, line of application, sense, and point of application. The force P (the patellar tendon force) has a known line of application, sense, and point of application. It has an unknown magnitude. There is, in addition, another force J (the joint reaction force) with a known point of application on the surface of the tibia and an unknown

---

* Personal communication.

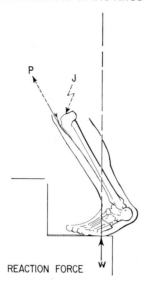

FIG. 3-2. Static analysis of knee joint. P is the patella tendon force with known direction and point of application. J is the unknown reactive force against the tibial condyle. W is the ground reaction force. (Adapted from Frankel, V. H., and Burstein, A. H.: Orthopaedic Biomechanics. Philadelphia, Lea & Febiger, 1970)

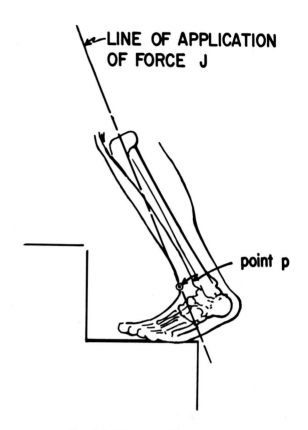

FIG. 3-3. The line of application of force J (the joint reactive force) can now be determined. This force intersects the joint surface and point p. (Adapted from Frankel, V. H., and Burstein, A. H.: Orthopaedic Biomechanics. Philadelphia, Lea & Febiger, 1970)

line of application, sense, and magnitude. When force lines P and W are continued, they will meet at point p (Fig. 3-3). Any other force acting on this free body will also meet this point. Thus, the direction of force J can be found by connecting its contact point on the surface of the upper tibia to the intersecting point of forces W and P.

With the line of application of force J determined, it is now possible to construct the triangle of forces (Fig. 3-4). First, force W is drawn with the proper line of application and sense. Next a vector representing force P is added to W. The line of application and sense of P are known, but the vector cannot be determined since the magnitude is unknown. It is known, however, that when force vector J is added to the sum of W and P, the triangle must close for equilibrium to exist. That is, the head of vector P must touch the original

of vector W and the vector sum of the forces is zero. Therefore, starting at the origin of W, a line is drawn parallel to the line of application of force J. This line intersects vector P at point g. Point g must be the head of vector P and the origin of vector J. The magnitude of forces P and J can now be scaled from the drawings (Fig. 3-5). This technique can be applied to any static equilibrium situation utilizing available anatomical landmarks and geometry.

To find the loads occurring during more usual activities, it is necessary to apply a dynamic analysis instead of a static one. Newton's Second Law of Motion, used to find the loads during nonequilibrium conditions, is given by:

$$F = MA$$

where F is force measured in kilograms, M is measured in kilograms per second squared divided by millimeters, and A is acceleration measured in millimeters per second squared.

The Second Law, expressed for angular motion, is given by:

$$T = I\alpha$$

where T is the torque or moment,
I is the mass moment of inertia, and
α is the angular acceleration.

For instance, during kicking of a football, what is the force acting on the joint (Fig. 3-6)? The maximal angular acceleration that occurs during the act of kicking a football was measured in one example from stroboscopic photos at 453 radians/second² in the athletic male. This acceleration occurs when the lower leg is almost vertical. The mass moment of inertia about the knee joint center is found to be 3.5×10^3 grams cm. seconds² in this subject from data presented by Drillis, Contini, and Bluestein.[4] The torque necessary to produce this angular acceleration can be calculated from the equation:

Torque = $(3.5 \times 10^3$ grams cm. seconds²)
$\times$ 453 radians/second² or
Torque = 15.9×10^5 grams cm.

The only force that can exert a torque about the center of rotation in the knee joint is the tension force in the patellar tendon. Since the perpendicular distance from this force vector to the center of rotation is 5.0 cm. in the subject measured, the force on the patellar tendon can be found from the relationship: force $\times$ distance = moment (or torque).

Force = $\frac{\text{moment}}{\text{distance}}$ or 1590 kilograms cm. divided by 5.0 cm. or 318 kg.

This amount of force is necessary to produce the acceleration needed to kick the football

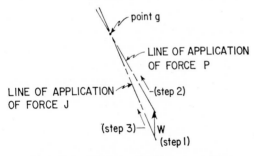

FIG. 3-4. Vector solution to problem of unknown force. Step 1: Force W drawn; this has known direction, line of application, and magnitude. The magnitude is equal to 1 W. Step 2: The direction of force P is drawn in. Step 3: The direction of force J is found by noting that force J must also go through point p, starting at the tibial condyle and extending downward through point p for an unknown length. This direction of force J is transferred to the vector solution, starting at the base of W and continuing until the line intersects the line for force P at point g. The length of the lines for P and J are now known and they can be measured in terms of W. (From Frankel, V. H., and Burstein, A. H.: Orthopaedic Biomechanics. Philadelphia, Lea & Febiger, 1970)

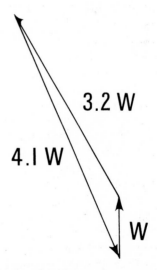

FIG. 3-5. Solution of vector diagram. The patella tendon force is equal to 3.2 times the body weight. The reactive force against the joint is equal to 4.1 times body weight.

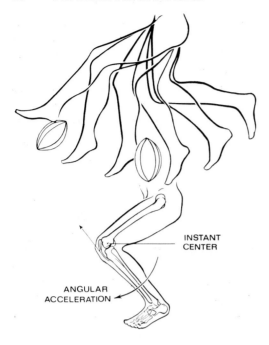

FIG. 3-6. Dynamics problem: A football is propelled through the air by the foot because of the pull of the quadriceps tendon, which imparts an angular acceleration about the knee joint. The angular acceleration can be measured from the stroboscopic photographs. The length of the lever arm is the perpendicular distance between the line of the patella tendon and the instant center. (From Frankel, V. H., and Burstein, A. H.: Orthopaedic Biomechanics. Philadelphia, Lea & Febiger, 1970)

at a particular instant in time. In order to find the force on the joint during this instant of time, it is necessary to subtract the weight of the lower limb, which is 5 kg., from the tendon force of 318 kg. This is done because the radial acceleration is almost zero at the instant when the leg is vertical. These simple examples give the reader an idea of the magnitude of forces that can result in a knee joint from common activities.

Walking is perhaps the commonest activity in which the knee joint participates. Morrison[13] describes the force acting on the knee joint during walking. In his studies it was first necessary to find the accelerations about the knee joint and the external forces acting on the knee joint for a gait cycle and identify by means of electromyography the muscles that were contracting. This permitted a determination of a total muscle force associated with the gait.

From the example given previously, it was demonstrated that the forces that produce a load on the knee joint, the muscle forces, are by far the largest component. In Figure 3-7, after Morrison's paper, the joint forces vertical direction are shown. The peak force during the stance phase is two to four times the body weight, depending on the individual tested. This occurs in the late stance phase and is associated with gastrocnemius contraction. A force equal to body weight is present in the late swing phase as the hamstrings act to decelerate the knee. Morrison noted that during the gait cycle in the stance phase the joint load was shifted to the medial tibial condyle and in the swing phase the load acted mainly on the lateral condyle. The forces acting in the medial-lateral direction were generally small, being approximately one-fourth the body weight. The greatest muscle force was calculated to be 400 pounds. This occurred in the gastrocnemius. There was no significant difference between the joint forces calculated for male and female subjects when the forces were normalized by dividing by the body weight.

Both the phasic activity and the force developed by the muscle are of importance, as pointed out by Close.[1] Tendon transplantations do not always work because the tendon may not be pulling in the proper phase. An attempt to control motion about the knee joint by tendon transplantation must also take into account the large forces that are required if the normal gait cycle is to be reproduced.

The joint force will be greatly modified during exercise. If, for instance, a 10-kg. weight were placed in the weight boot and raised from a position of 90 degrees to full extension of the knee, the quadriceps force required to raise the 10-kg. weight would be approximately 100 kg. For any weight-

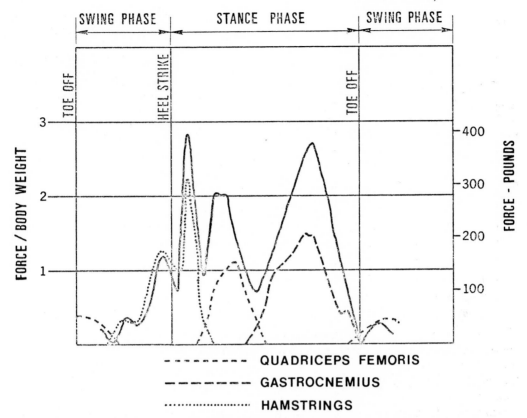

Fig. 3-7. Vertical joint force at the knee, level walking. Superimposed on the joint force curve are the calculated muscle force curves. Each peak in the joint force curve is due to the effect of a specific muscle group. (After Morrison, J. B.: Bio-engineering analysis of force actions transmitted by the knee joint. J. Biomechanics, *3*:164, 1968)

lifting exercise involving flexion and extension, the minimal force multiplier will be 10. That is, raising a 10-kg. weight will require the quadriceps to pull with a force of 100 kg. If this activity is done quickly, there will be additional force required to produce the acceleration needed.

Figures 3-8, through 3-10 from Reilly and Martens[15] show the quadriceps muscle force and the patellofemoral joint reaction force plotted against angle of flexion for the various activities investigated. The ranges shown for the forces represent the influence that the errors in measurement (made from the stroboscopic photographs) have on the calculated values. No range is shown in Figure 3-8 for the leg raising exercise, since these results were obtained from a mathematical analysis.

The lowest values for the QF force and PFJR forces were obtained for level walking. This is to be expected, since an efficient mechanism for walking would be developed so as to minimize energy expenditure and the forces that the skeletal structure would have to bear.

The patellofemoral joint reaction force has a different pattern and different values during level walking than the tibiofemoral joint reaction force.

The highest calculated value for the PFJR force is 35 kg. or 0.5 body weight. The patellofemoral joint reaction force is not only dependent upon the quadriceps muscle force, but also upon the angle of knee flexion. Since the angles of flexion are kept quite low during the activity, the PFJR force is always smaller than the QF muscle force.

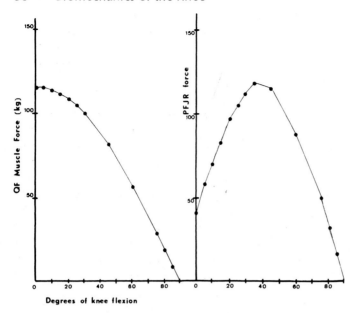

Fig. 3-8. Effect of knee flexion on quadriceps force and patellofemoral joint force. Leg-raising quadriceps exercise against resistance (9 kg. boot). QF = quadriceps force. PFJR = patellofemoral joint force. (Reilly, D. T., and Martens, M.: Acta Orthop. Scand., *43*: 126, 1972)

The opposite is true for an activity during which the knee is flexed to larger angles, such as deep knee bends (Fig. 3-10). Here, the larger angles of flexion yield a higher value for the vector sum of the QF force and the patellar tendon force, which the PFJR force must equilibrate. The maximum value calculated for the PFJR force during this activity was 650 kg. The subject's body weight was 85 kg., and this joint reaction force represents a force which is 7.6 times body weight.

For the stair climbing and descending activities, the PF reaction force attained a level of 3.3 body weight. This value is almost seven times the PF joint reaction

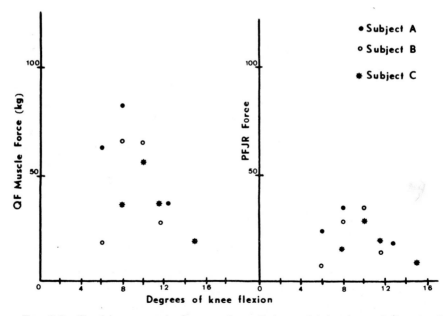

Fig. 3-9. Quadriceps muscle force and patellofemoral joint force during level walking. (Reilly, D. T., and Martens, M.: Acta Orthop. Scand., *43*:126, 1972)

force obtained during level walking. This figure explains why the patients with patello-femoral joint derangements experience more pain while climbing and descending stairs. Patients with PF joint derangements adapt their gait pattern in stair walking by assisting with the uninvolved side in order to decrease the muscle force. The push-off with un-affected leg helps considerably in decreasing the muscle force when climbing stairs.

The patients with derangements of the patellofemoral joint have most difficulties while descending stairs because the only effective adaptation in order to prevent high PFJR forces is a lowering of the body with a controlled knee flexion at the unaffected side while keeping the involved knee straight.

When these patients are treated conserva-tively with quadriceps exercises against re-sistance, by extending the knee from 90 degrees to full extention with a lead boot, most of them are unable to accomplish this exercise because of retropatellar pain. They are able, however, to do straight leg raising against the same resistance.

The explanation is given in Figure 3-8 where a maximum PFJR force of 1.4 body weight is found at 36 degrees of knee flexion when using a 9-kg. boot. If a heavier boot is used, the general shape of the curve obtained remains the same, while the force dimension is proportionally scaled upwards.

Figure 3-8 also illustrates that the PFJR can be kept at a significantly lower level by doing the straight leg raising exercise. When the knee is extended, the line of action of the patellar ligament and quadriceps muscle forces are almost parallel, and because of the small angle between those two forces their vector sum represents a lower value.

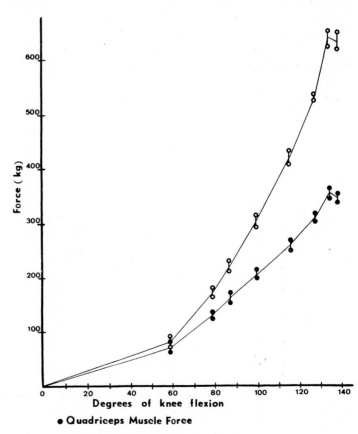

FIG. 3-10. The quadriceps force and patellofemoral joint force during deep knee bends. (Reilly, D. T., and Martens, M.: Acta Orthop. Scand., *43*: 126, 1972)

● Quadriceps Muscle Force

○ P.F. Joint Reaction Force

KINEMATICS

The kinematic data that are used to describe normal gait and that are useful in determining the forces acting in the knee joint have been summarized by Murray.[14] In Figure 3-11, the sagittal rotation of the knee for free speed walking in normal men is illustrated. Maximal flexion in the stance phase is approximately 18 degrees. Maximal flexion in the swing phase is 75 degrees. The knee joint that does not have this degree of mobility will produce a visible limp. The knee requires full extension, both in the beginning of the stance phase at heel strike and at the end of stance phase during toe-off. Kettelkamp[11] found that the knee reached maximal extension just before heel strike in over 60 per cent of the knees, at heel strike in 34 per cent, and between heel off and toe off in 2 per cent.

Rotation of the knee joint in a horizontal plane has been described by Saunders et al.[17] and Kettelkamp.[11] This transverse rotation of the tibia on the femur is difficult to measure. Most authors have based their data on passive motion. Levens et al.[12] studied transverse rotation with skeletal pins and

photographs. Rotation ranged from 4 to 13 degrees with a mean of 8.7 degrees. Kettelkamp in his studies utilized an electrogoniometer and found a range of 5.7 to 25.2 degrees with a mean of approximately 13 degrees. External rotation of the tibia was found to be variable but usually occurred during extension of the knee and reached a peak value just before heel strike. This is the so-called screw home mechanism, which indicates that as the knee goes into extension the tibia externally rotates on the femur. Helfet[8] has demonstrated the clinical importance of this mechanism. Kettelkamp found that maximal abduction of the tibia was associated with the initiation of the stance phase and that the tibia reached its greatest abduction during the swing phase. The electrogoniographic method of analyzing knee function has been extended by Kettelkamp and his associates to studying patients with pathological lesions of the knee. They found that in the sagittal plane, the average knee motion used for climbing stairs in a normal manner is 83 degrees, 93 degrees for sitting, 106 degrees for tying a shoe, 71 degrees for lifting an object without

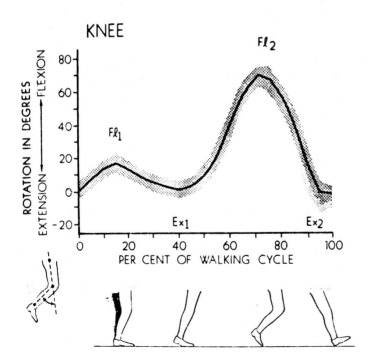

FIG. 3-11. Motion of knee joint in sagittal plane. Zero time corresponds to initiation of stance phase. (After Murray, M. P.: Gait as a total pattern of movement. Amer. J. Phys. Med., *46*:290, 1967)

FIG. 3-12. (*A*, *B*) Lateral roentgenograms of the knee joint used to find the centrode. The femoral shaft is bisected. The intersection of the femoral shaft bisector with the medial femoral condyle is one point. The second point is found by measuring 3 inches upward. (*C*) Superimposition of the roentgenograms A and B. Note displacement of the two points. The instant center is found by connecting the perpendicular bisectors of the displacement lines. (Frankel, V., Burstein, A., and Brooks, D.: J. Bone Joint Surg., *53A*:945, 1971)

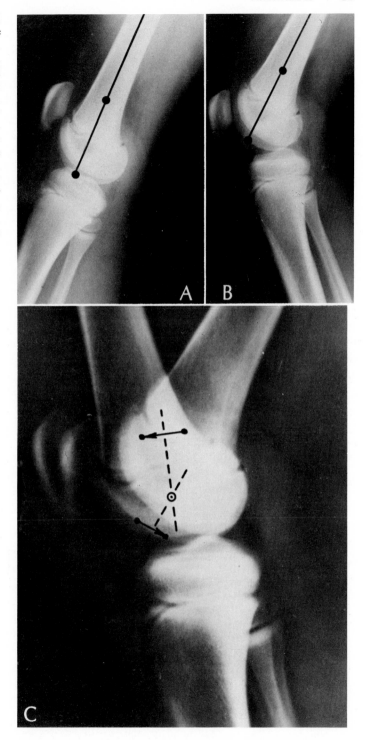

instructions, and 117 degrees for lifting an object with instructions. The average motion in the coronal and transverse planes was less than 25 degrees during these activities. They noted a significant relationship exists between the tibial-foot segment length and knee motion for most of the activities.

Kinematics also describes the motion of particles that are attached to the moving limbs. Kinematics is the study of the relative motion that can exist between rigid bodies; the bodies are called links. In the case of human joints, the bones are the links. As one of the links rotates about the other, there exists in an instant in time a point that has a zero velocity and constitutes the instantaneous center of motion or centrode. The instant center or centrodes for knee motion can be obtained by the method of Reuleaux.[16] The centrode is found by identifying displacement of two points on the link as the link moves from one position to another (Fig. 3-12). A line is drawn con-

necting the displaced pair of points, and the perpendicular bisector of this line is drawn. The intersection of the perpendicular bisectors locates the centrode. This technique has been used by Dempster to identify the hinge point of the knee joint.

These studies may be performed by using multiple x-ray exposures, cineradiography, or by attaching mechanical devices to the bone. The procedure is to expose six or eight lateral roentgenograms of the knee taken at increments of motion from full extension to 90 degrees of flexion. The patient is positioned with the leg resting on the table and the opposite leg in front of or behind the body. The ankle is supported by a small foam rubber pad so that the tibia is horizontal. An attempt is made to take a lateral film of the knee joint at full extension; the joint is then moved approximately 10 degrees to the next position, care being taken to keep the tibia parallel to the table and allowing any rotation to occur about the femur. A film is exposed and the leg again moved. In the case of a patient with a limitation in flexion and extension, the knee joint is placed in the maximal tolerated position and held in this position actively.

Next the films are superimposed in pairs, placing one tibia above the other. Points can be identified on these films that will move in space as the joint moves. Films with marked differences in tibial positions are not utilized. A line is drawn on each film bisecting the femoral shaft and crossing one of the femoral condyles, as is illustrated in Figure 3-12A. The point at which the line crosses the condyle is one point used in analysis; the second point is found by measuring up 3 inches from the first point along the femoral axis. When the films are superimposed, the displacements of the points are found. The centrodes are found by constructing the perpendicular bisectors of the displacements (Fig. 3-12C).

An examination of the instant center leads to a more complete understanding of the mechanics of joint motion. In Figure 3-13 the instant center together with the relative

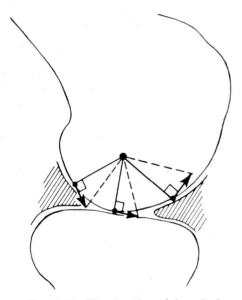

Fig. 3-13. The direction of the velocity of any point on the femoral link may be found by connecting that point to the instant center and constructing a perpendicular to the connecting line at the point in question. (Frankel, V.; Burstein, A., and Brooks, D.: J. Bone Joint Surg., *53A*: 945, 1971)

position of a femur and tibia is shown. Superimposed on the figures are the directions of the velocities of three points on the femur. The directions of the velocities are obtained by drawing perpendiculars to the lines from the instant center to the point in question. The velocity of the point in contact with the tibial plateau is tangential to the contact surface. A normal knee slides with the contact surface particles as they move tangentially over each other, as can be seen in Figure 3-14 when successive knee positions are taken. If the instant center were to be found on the surface, the joint would have a rolling motion and there would be no sliding friction. In 25 normal knees analyzed in our laboratory the instant center was located in all positions from 90 degrees of flexion to full extension. In all cases tangential sliding was noted.

Studies have been performed on knees having internal derangements.[6] The same kinematic technique was utilized, exposing multiple films with the knee in successive positions from 90 degrees of flexion to as much extension as could be obtained. In many cases it was found that for some range of extension-flexion the centrode was located in a position displaced from the normal position. If the joint is extended and flexed about this position, the joint surface particles do not slide tangentially to the surface but are forced into or away from the surface. This would be analogous to bending a door hinge and then opening and closing the door,

and finding that the door now did not fit into the door jam.

If there are displaced structures between the femoral condyles and tibial plateaus with the result that motion occurs about abnormally placed centrodes, the moving structures are forced together, producing local lesions in the articular cartilage at the sites of compression. Under these circumstances the joint may accommodate to localized high pressures by capsular or ligamentous stretching which relieves the pressure. This articular wear may occur at a distance from the primary joint lesion. For example, a medial meniscal rupture may be present with wear of the lateral femoral condyle. Cases of this type demonstrate that when there are kinematic disturbances of the type under consideration here, contact with the displaced structure is not the only mechanism by which wear is produced. Abnormal surface velocities may cause high local surface stresses at a distance from the primary pathologic lesion.

The centrode technique determines whether the surface velocities of the femoral and tibial articulating surfaces produce efficient sliding or not. The technique does not help to localize articular changes to either the medial or the lateral side of the joint, nor does it identify, prior to surgery, the structure responsible for the abnormally located centrode. A kinematic study does allow one to assess the mechanics of the articular surfaces at any degree of flexion. Since most

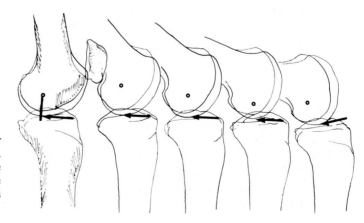

FIG. 3-14. Instant center study for normal knee joint. The velocity of the surface particles is tangential to the joint surface as the joint goes from flexion to extension.

pathologic changes in the joint surfaces are located in the extension-contact areas, roentgenograms made with the knee in more than 90 degrees of flexion were not included in the study. If the direction of the velocity at the joint surface tends to compress the two surfaces together, blocking of further extension or flexion may occur. It is possible to correlate the site of wear of the joint surface cartilage with the findings in the centrode study. When the direction of the velocity tended to drive the joint surfaces together, wear can be identified on the joint surface in the joint motion range where this abnormal compression occurred. The longer that motion about an abnormal centrode has been present, the greater was the chance of finding wear at arthrotomy. The cartilage lesions are similar to those produced by compression studies of animal joints.

The instant center technique elucidates a mechanism for the development of traumatic degenerative joint disease secondary to some remote trauma producing an internal derangement of the knee joint. The centrode technique demonstrates the interrelationship between mechanical alterations and biological response. The following scheme, based on the observations made in our case material, is proposed to explain this relationship:

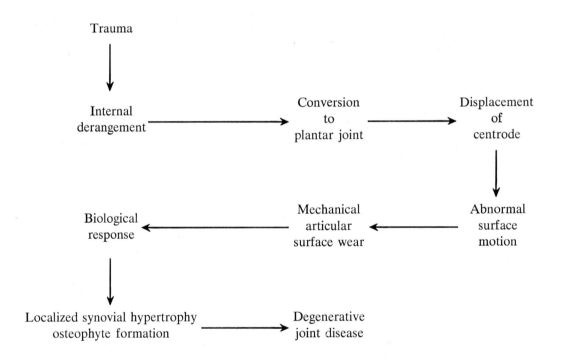

In Figure 3-15 the instant centers for an abnormal knee joint are shown. In the extension range the instant center is displaced so that as the knee joint is extended the joint is compressed. Figure 3-16 is a photograph from this case in which an area in the medial femoral condyle was compressed in a 12-year-old boy who had been walking for 1½ years while the knee joint was forced to rotate about an abnormally located instant center. Other cases demonstrate wear and early degenerative arthritis in the knee joint because the joint had abnormal kinematics so that the surfaces were sliding together in an abnormal manner, causing surface damage.

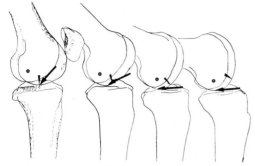

FIG. 3-15. Instant center study from abnormal joint. In the extension range the instant center has been displaced so that when the instant center is connected to the contact surface and a perpendicular is drawn, the perpendicular is not tangential to the surface but directed into the surface. As the knee joint flexes and extends in the particular range, the surfaces are either pulling apart or grinding together. In the flexion zones, the instant center is normally located so that the surface particles have a velocity tangential to the surface. The small triangle indicates the center of a compressed lesion.

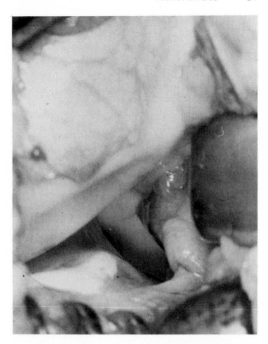

FIG. 3-16. Operative photograph of knee joint. The joint has been extending about an abnormally located instant center. There is a compressed faceted area on both the medial and lateral femoral condyles. There is an area of synovial hyperplasia growing toward the center of this compressed area in the margin of the joint.

REFERENCES

1. Close, J. R.: Motor Function in the Lower Extremity. Springfield, Illinois, Charles C Thomas, 1964.
2. Currey, J. D.: The mechanical properties of bone. Clin. Orthop. *73*:72, 1970.
3. Dempster, W. T.: Study of Hinge Points of Human Body. Wright Air Development Center, USAF Contract No. AF 18(600)-43, 1953.
4. Drillis, R., Contini, R., and Bluestein, M.: Body segment parameters; a survey of measurement techniques. Artif. Limbs, 8:44, 1964.
5. Frankel, V. H., and Burstein, A. H.: Orthopaedic Biomechanics. Philadelphia, Lea & Febiger, 1970.
6. Frankel, V. H., Burstein, A. H., and Brooks, D. B.: Biomechanics of internal derangement of the knee. J. Bone Joint Surg., *53-A*:945, 1971.
7. Frisen, M., Magi, M., Sonnerup, L., and Uukik, A.: Rheological analysis of soft collagenous tissue. J. Biomech., *2*:13, 1969.
8. Helfet, A. J.: The Management of Internal Derangements of the Knee. Philadelphia, J. B. Lippincott, 1963.
9. Hirsch, C.: The pathogenesis of chondromalacia of the patella. Acta Chir. Scandinav., *90* [Suppl.]:83, 1944.
10. Kempson, G., Spivey, C., Freeman, M., and Swanson, A.: Indentation stiffness in articular cartilage in normal and osteoarthritic femoral heads. *In* Wright, V. (ed.): Lubrication and Wear in Joints. Philadelphia, J. B. Lippincott, 1969.
11. Kettelkamp, D. B., Johnson, R. J., Smidt, G. L., Chao, E. Y. S., and Walker, M.: An electrogoniometeric study of knee motion in normal gait. J. Bone Joint Surg., *52-A*: 775, 1970.
12. Levens, A. S., Inman, V. T., and Blosser, J. A.: Transverse rotation of the segments

of the lower extremity in locomotion. J. Bone Joint Surg., *30-A*:859, 1948.

13. Morrison, J. B.: Bioengineering analysis of force actions transmitted by the knee joint. Bio-Med. Eng., *3*:164, 1968.

14. Murray, M. P.: Gait as a total pattern of movement. Including a bibliography on gait. Am. J. Phys. Med., *46*:290, 1967.

15. Reilly, D. T., and Martens, M.: Experimental analysis of the quadriceps muscle force and patello-femoral joint reaction force for various activities. Acta Orthop. Scandinav., *43*:126, 1972.

16. Reuleaux, F.: The Kinematics of Machinery: Outline of a Theory of Machines. London, Macmillan, 1876.

17. Saunders, J. B. DeC. M., Inman, V., and Eberhart, H. D.: The major determinants in normal and pathological gait. J. Bone Joint Surg., *35-A*:543, 1953.

18. Viidik, A.: Biomechanics and functional adaptations of tendons and joint ligaments. *In* Evans, F. G. (ed.): Studies on the Anatomy and Function of Bones and Joints. Berlin, Springer-Verlag, 1966.

19. Williams, M., and Lissner, H. R.: Biomechanics of Human Motion. Philadelphia, W. B. Saunders, 1962.

4

The Structure and Composition of Articular Cartilage

Charles Weiss, M.D.

The primary functions of the knee joints are to provide for weight bearing and movement. The compression forces of weight bearing and the shearing forces of movement are brought to bear upon a specialized form of hyalin cartilage that covers the articulating surfaces of those bones that comprise the knee joint. This opalescent covering, which appears homogeneous and inert, being devoid of both nerves and vessels and containing but a sparse number of cells embedded in a gel-like matrix, has only recently been shown to be chemically complex, structurally heterogeneous and metabotically extremely active. The emphasis in this chapter will be placed upon the structure, physical properties, cellular and chemical composition, metabolism, and nutrition of normal young adult human articular cartilage and how these parameters are altered in osteoarthritis. Developmental and aging processes will be discussed briefly and only in so far as they relate directly to an understanding of normal and osteoarthritic cartilage.

THE ARTICULAR SURFACE

Upon arthrotomy, joint surfaces wet with synovial fluid appear smooth and regular. However, examination under indirect light with only a hand lens shows them to be irregular and undulating. These undulations, which are present in the drawings of the 19th century microscopists[56] have recently received widespread attention, owing in part to the increasing interest in joint mechanics particularly lubrication, brought on by the advent of total joint replacement.

Studies on a wide variety of mammalian species, by incident light microscopy,[55] Linnik interference photomicrography,[58] tally-surf tracings,[178] and scanning electromicroscopy[31,32,57,177] have described three orders of surface irregularities: the primary joint contours; secondary irregularities (0.4 to 0.5 mm. in diameter); and tertiary undulations (20 to 30 μm. in diameter and approximately 2.5 μm. in height with a pitch of 25 μm.). Under conditions of static loading and presumably during periods of simultaneous weight bearing and movement, the elasticity of cartilage permits flattening of the bearing surface and bulging of the non-bearing surfaces.[58] However, while the primary joint contours are altered, the tertiary undulations remain intact.[58]

Under the light microscope a birefringent line is apparent on the articular surface. MacConnaill[86] named this structure the lamina splendens. Scanning[33] and transmission[184] electronmicroscopic studies have demonstrated a layer of fine fibrils (4 to 10 nm. in diameter), occurring in random fashion and up to several micra in height, that covers and appears adsorbed to the intact surfaces (Figs. 4-1, 4-7). One cannot determine the composition of these fibrils by their ultrastructural appearance alone. Bio-

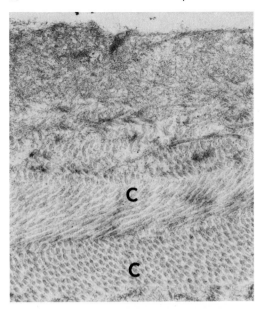

FIG. 4-1. An oblique section through the surface of normal articular cartilage. The surface is covered by a layer of fine fibers 4 to 10 nm. in diameter corresponding to the lamina splendens. Collagen fibers (~32 nm. diameter) of the tangential zone are arranged in tightly packed bundles (C) oriented at right angles to each other and running parallel to the articular surface. (30,000X)

chemical analysis suggests that they are probably hyaluronic acid[8] or other proteoglycans[136] derived from the synovial fluid.

JOINT LUBRICATION

Synovial joints are remarkably efficient in carrying out the dual functions of weight bearing and movement, having a coefficient of friction as low as 0.002.[88] To date the precise mechanism of this lubrication remains incompletely understood, it is apparent, however, that the special properties of the synovial fluid, the macromolecular covering of the cartilage surface, the primary, secondary and tertiary surface contours, and the physical properties of articular cartilage play significant roles in joint lubrication.

The presence of synovial fluid, slimy to touch and with the capacity to decrease in viscosity with increasing joint movement and resultant sheer forces[46,89] led early investi-

gators to postulate a classic hydrodynamic concept of joint lubrication[12]: a wedge of fluid develops between rapidly rotating surfaces and pressure created in this wedge keeps the surfaces apart. In 1960 Charnley[27] demonstrated that fluid wedges are inconsistent with the reciprocating movement of animal joints. The high rate of shear created by the loads that joints support during movement would excessively thin the normally viscous synovial fluid; thus a hydrodynamic system could function only under low loads and at high speeds. Boundary lubrication, as advanced by Charnley, depends upon the affinity of synovial fluid for the articular surface (the lamina spendens). The low coefficient of friction in this system is due to a molecular film which is physiochemically bound to each of the articulating surfaces and keeps them apart. This system while effective at low speeds is ineffective at high loads.

The classic hydrodynamic theory has been modified in two important ways: McCutchen[87] advanced the concept of "weeping" lubrication, a form of hydrostatic lubrication that occurs when, as a result of loading, fluid passes from within the articular cartilage to the joint surface. Secondly the elastic deformation of cartilage increases the contact area between surfaces, thereby decreasing the pressure in the lubricating fluid, and thus permitting the film thickness to be independent of load.[43,51,158,159] These two modifications of the hydrodynamic theory have been termed elastohydrodynamic and allow effective lubrication under high load.[10,43,46,136,137,138] Under lesser loads the concept of boundary lubrication appears valid when one adds to it the concept of "boosted lubrication."[177-179] Synovial fluid subjected to rapid increases in pressure transforms from a viscous liquid to a gel as a result of water being squeezed out and aggregates of macromolecules forming a tangled network. This gel can serve as a boundary lubricant and may increase cartilage resiliency. Pools of this "enriched" gel or concentrate of synovial fluid have been

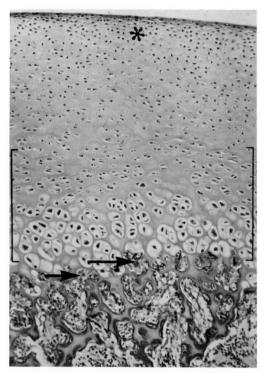

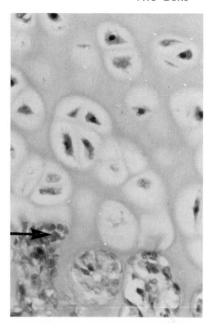

FIG. 4-3. Photomicrograph at higher power showing vascular invasion (*arrows*) of basilar portion of cartilage. (H≃E: 400X)

FIG. 4-2. Photomicrograph of articular cartilage from immature animal. The superficial zone consists of flattened cells. Beneath this zone is the growth zone for the articular cartilage (*). The basilar portion of the articular cartilage consists of an epiphyseal plate for the underlying epiphysis (*area in brackets*). A rich vasculature invades the basilar portion of the cartilage (*arrows*). No well defined radial bone and no calcified bone is present. (H≃E; 100X)

shown under the scanning electron microscope to be trapped in tertiary undulations when the articular surface is placed under load; in this manner they keep the actual cartilagenous surfaces apart.[43,177,178,179]

THE CELLS

The morphology and disposition of cells in normal adult articular cartilage has allowed microscopists to define four distinct zones (Plates 4-1, 4-2). The zone closest to the articular surface is the tangential or gliding zone (often referred to as the "skin" of cartilage) which contains several layers of flattened or oval shaped cells whose long axes run parallel to the joint surface. Deep to the tangential zone lies the transitional zone, a much wider area (accounting for almost half the thickness of cartilage) which contains larger, rounded, randomly arranged cells. Below this region, slightly smaller, rounded cells (often in pairs) lie in short irregular columns; this zone is called the radial zone. Beneath the radial zone lies an area that contains few cells (often with pyknotic nuclei), arranged in short columns and surrounded by a calcified matrix: the calcified zone. In material stained with both hematoxylin and eosin, a thin (about 5 mμ) basophilic irregular line separates the radial from the calcified zone. This structure has been designated by Collins[34] as the "tide mark"; its significance and composition are, as yet, unknown. The calcified zone in turn rests on a dense layer of cortical bone, the bony or subchondral end plate.

Immature articular cartilage differs significantly from that of the adult in being more cellular and having a less distinct zonal pattern (Figs. 4-2, 4-3). By the eighth em-

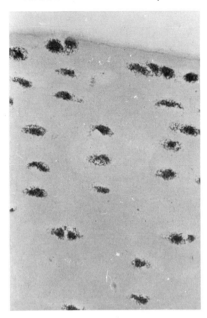

Fig. 4-4. Autoradiograph of tangential zone of normal human articular cartilage. This specimen was incubated in H³ glycine for 2 hours and shows extensive incorporation of the labeled amino acid. Small amounts are starting to appear extracellularly.

bryonic week the developing joint contains cartilage which consists of two separate cell populations: several layers of elongated and tightly packed superficial cells and more loosely arranged, rounded deeper cells. No radial zone, tide mark, calcified zone, or bony end plate is present. Autoradiographic techniques have demonstrated two zones of cellular proliferation: one immediately below the tangential zone, which, presumably, accounts for the growth of the articular cartilage, and a second zone in the basilar portion, which acts as a microepiphyseal plate for endochondral ossification of the underlying epiphysis.[92,95,97,98,135] With termination of epiphyseal growth and the formation of a well defined calcified zone and tide mark, mitotic activity ceases.[98,99] This would appear to suggest that cartilage is unable to compensate for cell death due to attrition or normal aging, and, indeed, studies in cattle[143,176] and rabbits[100] have demonstrated

a decrease in cell count with aging. Studies of human cartilage have indicated that during the period of rapid growth there is a decrease in the number of cells per fixed volume of cartilage. However, once maturity is reached there is little decrease in the cell count despite advancing age.[119,163] It is conceivable that a very low level of mitotic activity is present in aging human articular cartilage since a significant decrease in the number of cells in the tangential zone and a corresponding increase in the number of cells in the transitional and radial zones has been reported.[163] Recent studies have demonstrated that laceration,[94,101] compression,[39,40] enzymatic[185] and arthritic[104,105] insults are capable of initiating mitotic activity in mature cartilage.

In the past decade, the ultrastructure of cells in articular cartilage has been studied in man and other species during growth,[42,152] maturation,[11,152,156] aging,[11,117,124,147,153,156,182] arthritis,[116,117,120,147,183] and under a variety of experimental conditions.[144,145,152,154] These studies have demonstrated considerable and consistent differences among cells of the various zones and have also shown that these cells are capable of rapid ultrastructural changes in response to environmental alterations. Although early histological and metabolic studies of chondrocyte activity indicated that cells of the tangential zone were effete,[37,90] recent autoradiographic investigations[180] have shown them to be active in protein and glycoaminoglycan synthesis (Fig. 4-4). Under the electron microscope these elongated cells appear similar in structure to fibrocytes,[42,155,184] the nuclei are elongated, irregular in shape, contain a dense nucleoplasm with chromatin clumping and an intact nuclear membrane. The groundplasm is moderately dense and contains short, dilated cisternae, of rough endoplasmic reticulum,[129,184] a small Golgi apparatus (consisting of flattened, frequently empty, vacuoles),[42,129,152,184] and dense rounded mitochondria (Fig. 4-5). Large lipid droplets, glycogen deposits, and matrix containing vacuoles are rare. The cell membrane contains numerous pinocytotic vesicles and forms short cytoplasmic processes on the deep surface.

The rounded cells of the transitional zone are metabolically the most active cells of articular cartilage; this activity is reflected by their ultrastructural appearance (Fig. 4-b).[11, 42,116,129,146,153,156,184] They have a large, eccentric, finely granular nucleus which often contains one or more nucleoli and is bounded by well defined internal and external nuclear membranes with regularly spaced nucleopores.[129] The groundplasm is of moderately low electron density. It contains aggregates of glycogen particles and a small number of intracytoplasmic filaments 7 to 10 nm. in diameter.[184] Many oval mitochondria are present adjacent to which large lipid droplets may be found.[35] An extensive rough endoplasmic reticulum is present.[11,42,129,152,184] The rough surface endoplasmic reticulum, Golgi apparatus and large secretory vacuoles contain fibrillar material similar in electron density to that of the extracellular matrix.[129,188] The juxtanuclear Golgi apparatus is especially well developed and consists of closely packed agranular lamellae with small vesicles and larger vacuoles (up to 2.5 μ in diameter).[42,124,152,153,155,184] Ultrastructural autoradiographic studies have shown that these vacuoles migrate from the region of the Golgi apparatus to the periphery of the cytoplasm, where they fuse with the cell membrane and finally rupture to discharge their contents outside the cell.[61] This process occurring all along the cell membrane results in the formation of large invaginations, or "bays," that give the cell a scalloped appearance.

In the deeper portions of the radial zone, cells that appear "normal" under the light microscope frequently contain increased numbers of intracytoplasmic filaments whose function is unknown but is considered a degenerative change,[11,121,129,146,152,153,184] poorly developed rough endoplasmic reticulum, sparse Golgi apparatus, and small dense

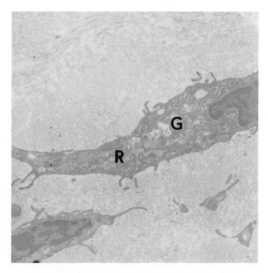

FIG. 4-5. Elongated cell in tangential zone of normal human articular cartilage. Bundles of collagen fibers are arranged at right angles to each other. The elongated cell contains a dense nuclear and cytoplasmic groundplasm. The Golgi apparatus consists of low density lamellae (G) and the rough endoplasmic reticulum (R) is sparse. (5,000X)

mitochondria.[184] Metabolic studies of cells in the basilar portions of articular cartilage have revealed them to be either dead or in an inert phase as they do not take up cytidine-H³, an indicator of RNA synthesis.[96]

THE MATRIX

The matrix of articular cartilage consists of a network of collagen fibers embedded in a gel-like ground substance composed of polyanionic proteoglycans (protein polysaccharides) and water. For a relatively hard tissue cartilage matrix contains an unusually high water content—in the vicinity of 75 to 80 per cent.[7,18,49,78,79,176] This high percentage is relatively unchanged during growth, aging and osteoarthritis.[16,18,79] Although the pericellular areas appear to have an especially high water content,[20] unlike bone, the water of articular cartilage is not highly bound to matrix constituents and may be easily removed by drying or mild heating.[92] It has been postulated that the ease

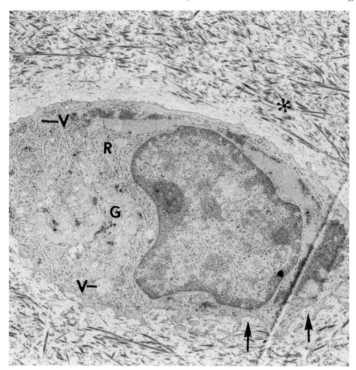

FIG. 4-6. Cell in transitional zone of normal human articular cartilage. The fibrous capsule consists of fibers arranged concentrically around the cell (*). Fine fibers are adjacent to the cell membrane. The cell is rounded and numerous "bays" give it a scalloped appearance (*arrow*). An extensive rough endoplasmic reticulum (*R*), large Golgi apparatus (*G*) and many vacuoles (*V*) containing material similar in electron density to the extracellular matrix are present. (10,000X)

with which water may be driven from and returned to cartilage provides in part not only for the elasticity of cartilage but also for the "weeping" phase of joint lubrication. The concentration of electrolytes in cartilage has been shown to be the same as in the extracellular fluid compartment with two exceptions, sodium and sulfate, both of which are elevated.[49,123] Sodium serves as the principal cation for the polyanionic matrix.[63,150] Sulfate concentration is elevated owing to the high content of sulfated glycoaminoglycans.[7,106,157] Small quantities of other organic materials have also been found in the matrix of articular cartilage. Neutral fats, phospholipids, cholesterol, triglycerides, and glycolipids have been seen in articular cartilage matrix at both the light- and electron microscopic levels.[35,59,119,164,166] The concentration of these extracellular lipids increases with aging, possibly secondary to cellular degeneration.[117,164,166] The frequent proximity of these lipids to degenerating cells and membranous cell remnants sup-

ports this hypothesis. Sialic acid is also present in small amounts probably bound to keratin sulfate.[5,66,173]

Collagen

Collagen constitutes the major organic component of articular cartilage accounting for approximately 60 per cent of the dry weight of and containing 90 per cent of the protein content of the tissue.[7,17,25,26,66,105,123,125] The stability of collagen in cartilage is remarkable. The proportion of collagen protein remains constant throughout life; it has a very slow turnover time; it is virtually insoluble in water or dilute acid; and less than 2 per cent can be extracted by solutions of 5M guanidine hydrochloride.[125] To understand the contribution of collagen to this complex tissue some idea of its composition, structure, assembly, and properties must be understood.

Collagen is a protein. Its constituent amino acids are assembled on the ribosomes of connective tissue cells to form a protocollagen molecule:[38,133] approximately one third of its amino acid residues being glycine and one quarter being proline.[125] This protocollagen molecule has a molecular weight of approximately 100,000 and is arranged in the form of a flexible, left-handed helix. The amino acid composition of all protocollagen molecules is not identical, and these variations have been termed $\alpha1$, $\alpha2$, and $\alpha3$ chains.[132] Enzymatic hydroxylation (a process that requires oxygen, ascorbic acid, ferrous ion and α-keto-glutarate) of some of the proline and lysine residues results in the formation of hydroxyproline and hydroxylysine, amino acids that are not found to any appreciable extent in animal proteins other than collagen.[72,133] At about the time of hydroxylation two hexoses, glucose and galactose, are attached by an 0-glycoside linkage to the hydroxyl group of hydroxylysine as the disaccharide glycosylgalactose.[22] Three protocollagen chains are then assembled intracellularly into a right-handed triple helix held together by easily soluble (salt) hydrogen bonds forming a stiff macromolecule approximately 300 nm. in length, 1.5 nm. in diameter called tropocollagen.[133] The intracellular site of hydroxylation, glycolization, tropocollagen assembly, and the mechanism of secretion into the extracellular matrix has not been completely defined, and considerable controversy exists as to the role of the Golgi apparatus in tropocollagen synthesis and secretion.[38]

It is in the extracellular matrix that these salt soluble tropocollagen molecules begin to assume less readily soluble forms resulting from cross linkages between adjacent $\alpha1$ chains in the same tropocollagen molecule (these chain pairs are called β chains[60]), and by progressive cross linking between chains of adjacent tropocollagen molecules. Very stable cross links may result from aldol type condensations, however it is probable that other cross linking mechanisms exist as well.[162] The typical collagen fiber with 64 nm. periodicity and sub-banding is assembled in the extracellular matrix at a distance from the cell by a linear arrangement of the tropocollagen molecules. These molecules line up in head-to-tail fashion to form long linear polymers. Adjacent polymers are "off set" by approximately 25 per cent of their length, and it is this quarter stagger that produces the characteristic collagen periodicity.[60]

The collagen of articular cartilage differs in a number of important ways from the collagen of skin and bone. Collagen fibers in articular cartilage do not stain with the usual anionic collagen stains, owing, in part, to competitive inhibition by the polyanionic matrix in which the fibers are embedded and in part to the specific composition of the collagen fibers. Miller et al. have demonstrated that two forms of the $\alpha1$ protocollagen chain exist: $\alpha1$ (I), which is found in skin and bone, and $\alpha1$ (II), which accounts for more than 90 per cent of the collagen extracted from cartilage.[124-126]

In addition to quantitative differences in several amino acids the $\alpha1$ (II) chain differs from the $\alpha1$ (I) chain by having two-thirds of its lysine residues hydroxylated (a five-fold increase) and in having an unusually high content of protein-bound hexose (containing 16 to 18 hexose residues per chain or 3 per cent by weight compared to about 2 residues per chain or 0.4 per cent by weight found in the $\alpha1$ (I) chains.[126] Forty per cent of the hydroxylysine residues are substituted in this fasion. Since more than 90 per cent of extracted collagen consists of $\alpha1$ (II) chains, the vast majority of tropocollagen molecules in articular cartilage have the structure $[\alpha1 \text{ (II)}]_3$. These molecules are less heat stable than the molecules of skin and bone. It has been postulated that the hexose coat on the collagen molecule hinders the formation of intermolecular cross links, permits sliding required for cartilage elasticity, obscures the distinct periodicity and banding of the individual collagen fibers observed under the electron microscope, repels anionic collagen dyes, and may by interaction with the glycoaminoglycan side

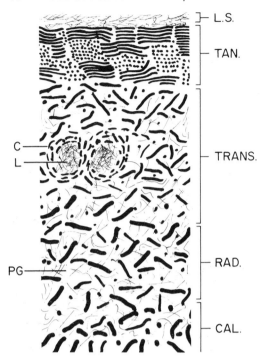

FIG. 4-7. Diagram of the fibrous architecture of normal adult human articular cartilage. The articular surface is covered by a layer of fine fibers (4 to 10 nm. in diameter): the lamina splendens (*L.S.*). The tangential zone (*TAN*) consists of tightly packed bundles of mature collagen fibers (~30 nm. diameter). These bundles lie parallel to the articular surface and frequently at right angles to each other. In the transitional zone (*TRANS*) collagen fibers (~60 nm. diameter) are randomly arranged and spaced farther apart. Fine fibers thought to be proteoglycan macromolecules (*PG*) fill the interfibrillar space and frequently appear attached to the collagen fibers. The area between the cell membrane and the perilacunar rim (which contains a high concentration of proteoglycan molecules) appears as a dense network of fine fibers (4 to 10 nm. diameters) (*L*). Mature collagen fibers sweep in capsular fashion (*C*) about the lacunae. Collagen fibers of the radial zone (*RAD*) are larger (~800 nm. diameter) and also arranged in a random fashion. In the calcified zone (*CAL*) mature collagen fibers often appear to lie perpendicular to the joint surface especially in older specimens.

chains of the proteoglycan molecules play a role in maintaining the structural integrity and properties of cartilage.[112,114,126]

The Fibrous Architecture of Cartilage

The arrangement of the collagen fibers in adult human articular cartilage has been extensively studied, however, their precise disposition still remains controversial. Benninghoff[15] concluded that collagen fibers were arranged in arcades which were anchored in the calcified zone, ran vertically in the radial zone, turned obliquely in the transitional zone, and ran tangential or parallel to the articular surface in the superficial or tangential zone. X-ray diffraction studies,[80] on the other hand, demonstrated that collagen fibers in the tangential zone ran tangential to the articular surface and in the deeper zones were arranged in a random fashion except in the calcified zone of old cartilage where they were arranged perpendicular to the articular surface.

Recent transmission[184] and scanning[33] electron microscopic studies have further elucidated the fibrous architecture of cartilage (Figs. 4-1, 4-5, 4-7, 4-8). The surface of adult human cartilage is covered by a layer of fine fibers 4 to 12 nm. in diameter and several micra deep. This layer probably corresponds to the lamina splendens, consisting of either a hyaluronic acid or other proteoglycan from the synovial fluid which is adsorbed to the articular surface.

The tangential zone of normal young adult human articular cartilage (Figs. 4-1, 4-5, 4-7) consists of tightly packed bundles of collagen fibers (30 to 32 nm. in diameter with 64 nm. periodicity) arranged tangential or parallel to the articular surface and at right angles to each other.[122,184] Little ground substance separates the individual collagen fibers or fiber bundles. Collagen fibers in the vicinity of the elongated superficial cells sweep in capsular fashion about their periphery. At the summit of the medial femoral condyle this zone is approximately 200 micra deep and it reaches 600 micra in depth at the periphery of the joint. The tight

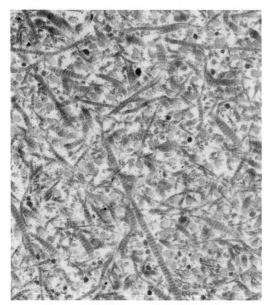

FIG. 4-8. Electronmicrograph of transitional zone from elderly individual showing random arrangement of mature collagen fibers. These fibers have a typical 64 nm. periodicity and vary in diameter from 30 to 200 nm. (15,000X)

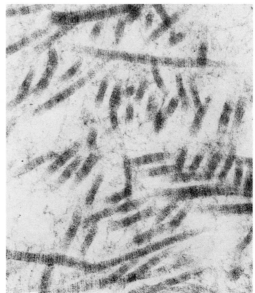

FIG. 4-9. Electronmicrograph of fibrillar matrix in transitional zone. Fibers 4 to 10 nm. in diameter occupy the spaces between individual collagen fibers and frequently appear attached to adjacent collagen fibers. (60,000X)

bundle arrangement of collagen fibers is loosened in the transitional zone, and increased interfibrillar ground substance is present. The individual fibers in this zone are 40 to 80 nm. in diameter, and appear randomly arranged[23,42,80,152,184] (Fig. 4-8) except at the periphery of the lacuna (the perilacunar rim) where fibers are packed closely together and run concentrically about the cells.[23,42,80,152,184] The space between the perilacunar rim and the cell membrane is filled with fine fibers (4 to 10 nm. in diameter), which lack typical collagen periodicity.[23,116,152,184] Fibers of similar appearance are found in the interfibrillar matrix and often appear attached to one or more collagen fibers frequently obscuring their periodicity (Fig. 4-9). These fine fibers, by virtue of their location in areas of high metachromasia and in areas which stain with cationic dyes such as safranin O, are thought to be proteoglycan molecules. Collagen fibers of the deep and calcified zones are large in diameter and in old cartilage

are frequently arranged perpendicular to the joint surface.[80,184]

With aging a number of changes occur in collagen fibers of human articular cartilage.[117,182] Fibers in all zones are increased in diameter, often appear fragmented, and in the vicinity of degenerating cells often contain neucloi of calcification. In the superficial zone collagen fibers frequently lose their bundle arrangement but remain arranged tangential to the articular surface. The lamina splendens in older tissue is often replaced by an accumulation of amorphous debris.[182]

The Proteoglycans

The gel-like ground substance of articular cartilage accounts for approximately 35 per cent of its dry weight and consists of large proteoglycan molecules (protein polysaccaride).[7,13,18,24-26,28,49,63,66,105,112,123,141,157] These macromolecular complexes are composed of a protein core and numerous attached glycoaminoglycans (repeating dimeric units of a hexose and hexosamine (Fig. 4-10).[70] The protein core is approximately 400 nm. in length and contains seventeen amino acids of which glycine (approximately 126 residues per thousand) proline, leucine, alanine, valine, aspartic acid, and glutamic acid constitute the major residues.[9,19,63,127,149,150] To this protein core 50-100 glycoaminoglycans are linked by an 0-glycoside linkage to either serine in the case of chondroitin sulfate or threonine in the case of keratan sulfate.[6,139,151]

Three types of glycoaminoglycan (polysaccharides) have been found in articular cartilage: chondroitin-4 sulfate (chondroitin sulfate A), chondroitin-6 sulfate (chondroitin sulfate C) and keratan sulfate (Fig. 4-11). The chondroitin sulfates are composed of regularly alternating units of N-acetylgalactosamine and glucouronic acid. The galactosamine carries a sulfate group in the fourth or sixth carbon, and there are two anionic charges per period. The chain weight of chondroitin sulfate is 30,000 to 40,000; thus there are 50 to 70 periods, or dimeric units per chain.[18,19,26,63,127,130,141,149,150] In immature cartilage there is a 1:1 ratio of chondroitin-4 sulfate (CSA) to chondroitin-6 sulfate (CSC); with aging this ratio decreases to about 1:4.[115] A smaller molecule, keratan sulfate, which has a chain length of 15 to 30 and consists of repeating units of galactose and N-acetyl glucosamine with an ester sulfate on the C-6 position, increases in concentration with aging.[63,127,149-151] By middle age the concentrations of keratan and chondroitin-6 sulfate (CSC) are about equal and account for over 90 per cent of the total glycoaminoglycan content.[13,19,74,81,82,115,165,167]

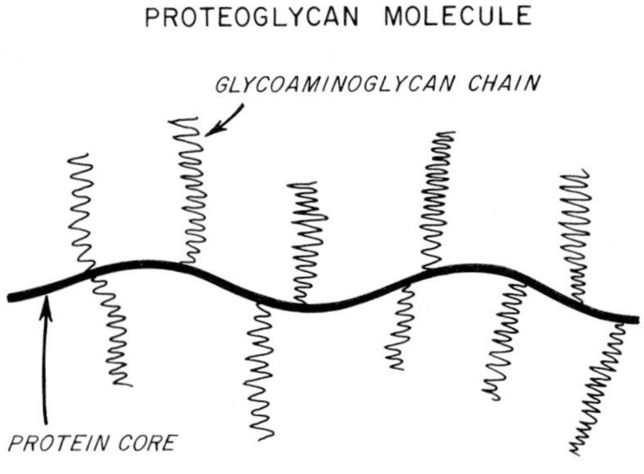

CHONDROITIN-4 SULFATE

CHONDROITIN-6 SULFATE

PROTEOGLYCAN MOLECULE

GLYCOAMINOGLYCAN CHAIN

PROTEIN CORE

FIG. 4-10. Diagrammatic representation of the proteoglycan molecule. The protein core is about 400 nm. in length, 1.5 nm. diameter and to it 50 to 100 glycoaminoglycan chains are attached. The negative charges on the glycoaminoglycan side chains keep the protein core from assuming a coiled shape.

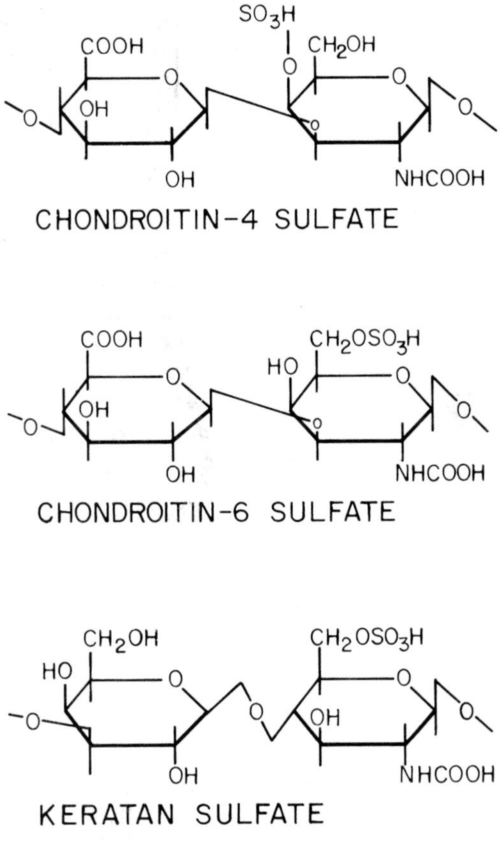

KERATAN SULFATE

FIG. 4-11. The chemical structure of the repeating dimeric units that comprise the three glycoaminoglycans of articular cartilage are outlined above. Chondroitin-4 sulfate consists of a glucuronic acid molecule linked by a 1-3 ester linkage to N-acetyl galactosamine with a sulfate at the C-4 position. Chondroitin-6 sulfate is similar in structure but with a sulfate at the C-6 position. Keratan sulfate consists of galactose linked by a 1-4 ester linkage to N-acetyl glucosamine with a sulfate at the C-6 position.

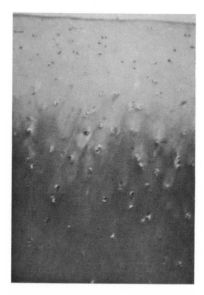

Plate 4-1. Photomicrograph of tangential and transitional zones of normal adult human articular cartilage stained with safranin-O and counterstained with hematoxylin. The tangential zone is characterized by a lack of safranin-O-staining. Cells in the tangential zone are elongated with their long axes parallel to the articular surface; those of the transitional zone are randomly arranged. (100X)

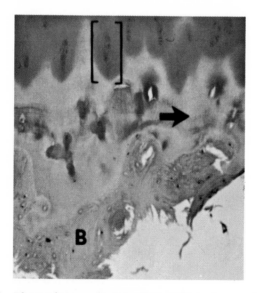

Plate 4-2. Photomicrograph of basilar portion of normal human articular cartilage stained with safranin-O and counterstained with hematoxylin. Cells of the radial zone are arranged in columns. These cell columns are surrounded by "halos" (brackets) indicating areas of increased concentration of glycoaminoglycans. The "tide mark"[34] (*arrow*) separates the radial from the calcified zone. The calcified zone rests upon the subchondral bony (B) end plate. (100X).

A number of investigators have attempted to define the basic subunit of the proteoglycan macromolecule. Schubert and others utilized mechanical fractionation procedures and separated the proteoglycans into heavy (PPH) and a series of light (PPL) macromolecular species.[63,128,141,142,144,150] Nonmechanical methods of extraction using 4M guanidium chloride followed by cesium chloride gradient separation have yielded a subunit which exists in monomeric and dimeric forms (200 nm. in length and containing approximately 20 glycoaminoglycan side chains[142,148]). Another small molecule called glycoprotein link (GPL) is thought to link the basic proteoglycan subunits into their aggregate macromolecular forms.[65] The physiochemical properties of the glycoaminoglycans determine, to a great extent, the properties of elasticity, stiffness, theoretical pore size and the staining characteristics of articular cartilage. The glycoaminoglycans being attached to elongated protein molecules are relatively fixed in position. The mutually repulsive charges on the glycoaminoglycans (chondroitin sulfate has approximately 120 negatively charged groups per chain) tend not only to keep these chains apart but also to elongate the protein core preventing it from assuming a coiled or folded shape. Thus this macromolecular complex occupies a maximum volume.[63,112] It has been postulated that this spatial configuration is capable of entraining large amounts of water and also plays a role in determining the disposition of the collagen fiber network. The metachromatic staining of cartilage is due to the binding of the cationic dye with the polyanionic glycoaminoglycan molecule. Crowding of the molecules of dye results in its polymerization, or stacking, and assumption of the metachromatic spectrum.[63,71,134,150,161,168] Safranin-O is a recently rediscovered dye that binds in its orthochromatic state on a one-to-one basis to the anions of the glycoaminoglycan molecules and can therefore serve as a semiquantitative histochemical measure of glycoaminoglycan concentration.[140]

THE METABOLISM OF CARTILAGE

The absence of a vascular supply and the preponderance of extracellular matrix suggests that this tissue is relatively stable and metabolically inert; however, the respiratory rate and energy production on a per-cell basis is quite high.[44,143] While aerobic, anaerobic, and hexose monophosphate shunts have been demonstrated in cartilage, the tolerance of chondrocytes to potassium cyanide and to oxygen deprivation coupled with their sensitivity to monoiodoacetate, as well as the presence of high lactate concentrations, suggests that the anaerobic pathway is preferentially used.[73,85,107]

The synthesis of the protein core of the proteoglycan molecule is similar to the synthesis of the protocollagen molecule described above; however, the synthesis, sulfation, and polymerization of the glycoaminoglycan molecule is a bit more complex requiring a number of enzymes including nucleoside diphosphokinase, UDP-glucose phosphorylase, UDP-glucose dehydrogenase, and a number of transferases and isomerases.[170] In very brief outline glucose-1-P and N-acetyl-glucosamine-1-P are converted by UTP to UDP glucuronic acid and to UDP-N-acetyl-glucosamine. These are then united by an ether link to form chondroitin.[48,132,159,177] These steps are probably carried out on or near the ribosome. The addition of sulfate to the glycoaminoglycan unit is rapid,[41] occurs in the region of the Golgi apparatus,[61] and involves the addition of ATP to the sulfate to form 3-phosphoadenosine-5-phosphosulfate or "active sulfate," a high-energy molecule from which sulfate can be added to the C-4 or C-6 position of the N-acetyl-galactosamine.[41,131] There is evidence to suggest that the entire glycoaminoglycan molecule is synthesized almost simultaneously by the cell.[1,92,99]

Qualitative and quantitative radioactive tracer techniques (i.e., autoradiography and scintillation counting) utilizing H^3 or C^{14} labeled amino acids, hexoses or $S^{35}O_4$ have been utilized to determine the rate and distribution of matrix synthesis and degradation. Studies on the rate of incorporation of Glycine-H³ and S³⁵O₄ have shown that glycoaminoglycan synthesis is rapid and linear with time,[107] that synthesis is most rapid in immature animals, and that after an initial decline it remains constant despite aging,[100,101] that cortisol,[102,103] antimetabolites,[92] and nitrogen mustard[92] decrease matrix synthesis and that following lacerative injury[101] and in certain phases of osteoarthritis synthesis is increased.[16,37,104,105] The same isotopic techniques have been used to study matrix degradation and have shown that while collagen is relatively stable, a large proportion of the proteoglycans are quite labile.[106] More than 25 per cent of the proteoglycans in adult cartilage behave as a "fast fraction," having a half-life of approximately 8 days.[106] This rate of degradation would appear to be far in excess of that necessary to compensate for normal attrition and suggests that this rapid synthetic and degradative activity is part of an extremely active enzyme-dependent internal remodeling system.[99,106]

Several enzymes are capable of breaking down the proteoglycan molecule: papain,[53,171,172] hyaluronidase,[16,127,150] and a number of intracellular enzymes.[45,52,53,83,171,172] Ali,[2,3] Wossner,[186] and others[29,48,54,62,75,83,156,185] have found a family of lysosomal acid proteases (cathepsin D) which can act to degrade cartilage matrix, and recent studies by Wossner[187] have defined in cartilage a cathepsin D capable of degrading proteoglycans at a neutral pH. This enzyme may be active in osteoarthritis as well as in normal cartilage remodeling.

Nutrition Cartilage

Articular cartilage is avascular except embryonically and for a short time postnatally when vascularized canals extend from the metaphysis and periosteum into the epiphysis and basilar portions of the articular cartilage.[77,84] The source and mechanism by which nutrients reach chondrocytes fascinated investigators for centuries beginning with the microscopic and injection studies of Hunter in 1743.[68] During the 19th century cartilage was thought to be nourished primarily by diffusion from the underlying vasculature,[174] although several authors felt that synovial fluid also played a role.[76,137] More than 50 years ago Strangeways[169] suggested that nutrition was principally derived by diffusion from the synovial fluid. More recent studies have supported this view[21,34,111] or suggested that both synovial fluid and subchondral vasculature provide nutrition to the articular cartilage.[50,69,91] Radioactive tracer studies have confirmed the opinion that in the immature animal with open epiphyseal plates a significant portion of the articular cartilage derives its nutritional support from the underlying vasculature of the epiphysis; however, with maturation, closure of the epiphyseal plate, formation of the subchondral bony end plate, establishment of the calcified zone, and tide mark, almost all the nutrition is derived by diffusion from the synovial fluid.[67]

Early studies revealed that cartilage is completely permeable to cationic dyes, less permeable to neutral, and only slightly permeable to anionic dyes.[21,71] There are, however, a number of physical and chemical factors that influence the type, size, and rate of diffusion of various substances into this tissue. Maroudas has developed the concept that the articular surface acts as a membrane (with a pore size of 62 Å as determined by McCutchen[88]) and that Donnan equilibrium and ion exchange theories are applicable in articular cartilage.[108,109,110,111,112] The fixed charge density of the matrix (due to the polyanionic glycoanioglycans) controls in large measure the diffusion characteristics of cartilage: as the fixed charge density increases with increasing depth of the cartilage, the permeability to fluid flow decreases.[108] The diffusion coefficients for NaCl, K, and SO, have been shown to be approximately 40 per cent of their value in aqueous solution and that for glucose about 30 per cent.[109] Toward smaller molecules the water in cartilage appears to behave as

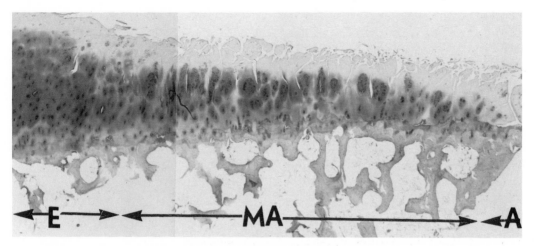

FIG. 4-12. Photomicrograph of .osteoarthritic distal femoral condyle stained with safranin-O and counterstained with hematoxylin, showing areas of early (*E*), moderately advanced (*MA*) and advanced (*A*) disease within an area of several millimeters. Early osteoarthritis has superficial fibrillation, slight hypercellularity and loss of glycoamino-glycans extending into transitional zone. Moderately advanced lesions have a decreased cartilage height, clefts extending into the radial zone, hypercellularity in the form of chondrocyte clones in the superficial zone (no halo) and in the deeper zones (intense halos), loss of glycoaminoglycans extends deeper into the cartilage. Areas of advanced disease are further decreased in height, contain clefts that extend full thickness through the cartilage, the tissue is hypocellular and almost completely devoid of glycoaminogly-cans. (50X)

solvent water; but with large molecules some water becomes inaccessible due to steric exclusion effects exerted by the proteoglycan molecules. Therefore the distribution of small molecules such as glucose is only slightly affected, but as the weight of the solute increases the distribution and diffusion coefficients decrease significantly.[109] Hemoglobin is the largest molecule capable of penetrating into cartilage. Solute agitation (joint movement) appears to increase the rate of diffusion of a number of small molecules.[111] Although most investigators have felt that no active cellular transport system exists in articular cartilage, and this view is not unreasonable in view of the high matrix-to-cell ratio, recent studies have demonstrated that the diffusion of nutrients (amino acids, sugars, and sulfate) into articular cartilage is extremely rapid (within seconds) and dependent in part upon the presence of viable cells.[181]

To summarize, then, the articular surface acts as a membrane having a pore size of 62 Å, and the diffusion of molecules into articular cartilage depends upon agitation, molecular size, steric configuration, and the charge of the solute and upon the pore size tortuosity, fixed charge density, and (possibly) cellular composition of the cartilage matrix.

OSTEOARTHRITIS

The etiology and pathophysiology of osteoarthritis has been the subject of much scientific investigation during the past two centuries.[160] One of the problems inherent in studying this disease is its focal nature. A single joint may contain the entire histologic and chemical spectrum from normal to far advanced disease; furthermore, areas of cartilage separated by no more than 100 micra may differ markedly in physical properties, histologic appearance, and metabolic activity (Fig. 4-12). During the 19th and early 20th century histologic studies established the anatomic pattern,[14,34,64,160] and

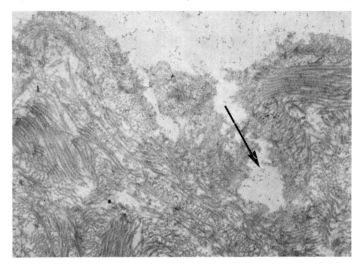

Fig. 4-13. Articular surface from moderately advanced osteoarthritic lesion. Bundles of mature collagen fibers run parallel to the surface of the clefts (*arrow*). (20,000X)

recent technological advances have enabled scientists to correlate the anatomic, metabolic, and chemical alterations which occur in osteoarthritic cartilage.[104] Mankin has devised a histologic-histochemical grading system for the osteoarthritic lesion that correlates very closely with the metabolic and chemical analysis of this tissue.[104] For purposes of this discussion we will divide the cartilage changes in osteoarthritis into early, moderately advanced, and advanced stages (Fig. 4-12).[183] The first two stages are characterized by anabolic and catabolic cell function and will be considered together. Advanced disease consists primarily of catabolic cellular function and will be discussed separately.

The changes in early osteoarthritis consists of: fibrillation of the articular surface which extends into but not through the tangential zone; slight increase of the number of cells per unit volume of tissue; and loss of glycoaminoglycans (or alteration of the proteoglycan molecule) confined to the transitional zone. Moderately advanced lesions are characterized by a decrease in overall cartilage height, clefts which extend into the transitional and upper portions of the radial zone, and increased numbers of cells in the form of cell clusters or "clones" in the transitional and radial zones. Many clones in the superficial region of the carti-

lage are devoid of a proteoglycan halo, while those in the basilar portion of the transitional zone are surrounded by intense proteoglycan halos. The loss of proteoglycans extends through the transitional and into the radial zone.

In early lesions ultrastructural observations of the matrix show minute surface irregularities, loss of lamina splendens, and a decrease in interfibrillar matrix most evident in the transitional zone. With progression to moderately advanced lesions, clefts take the form of progressively deepening infoldings (Fig. 4-13) of the articular surface.[183] Collagen fibers of small diameter are arranged perpendicular to the joint surface.[80,183] It is probable that the compressive forces of weight bearing and the shearing forces of movement in vivo result in a flattening of these clefts resulting in a functional realignment so that fibers are arranged parallel or tangential to the "true" articular surface.[183] Individual collagen fibers in moderately advanced lesions appear smaller than those found in age-matched controls.[183] This may indicate that either collagen fibers break down secondary to enzymatic degradation[2,3,29,48,75,186] or that there is synthesis of new fibers.[183] In view of recent metabolic studies the latter explanation seems most plausible.[104,105]

Electron microscopic studies of early to

FIG. 4-14. Cells in the tangential zone of moderately advanced osteoarthritic cartilage. The cells are more rounded than those of normal articular cartilage, a dense groundplasm and well developed rough endoplasmic reticulum (*R*), large Golgi apparatus (*G*) and many vacuoles (*V*) filled with electron-dense material. (6,500X)

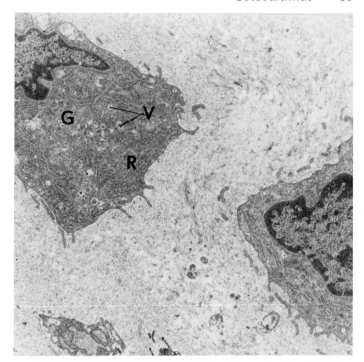

moderately advanced osteoarthritic cartilage show striking cellular changes.[183] An increase in the number of degenerating cells is found in the superficial and deep zones. These cells are characterized by increased intracellular filaments and a corresponding decrease in other intracellular organelles as well as dead cells devoid of a nuclear or cell membrane and consisting of aggregates of phospholipid membrane remnants.[117,147,183] In the superficial zone viable cells undergo hypertrophy, are surrounded by collagen fibers of small diameter, and appear similar to fibroblasts (Fig. 4-14).[147,183] Clones of cells in the deeper zones consist of viable hypertrophied cells that contain well de-

FIG. 4-15. Chondrocyte clone in moderately advanced osteoarthritic lesion. Collagen fibers run perpendicular to the articular surface and have a low interfiber density compared to the pericellular halo (*). Degenerating cells are present within this clone (*D*). Chondrocytes have well developed rough endoplasmic reticulum (*R*), extensive Golgi apparatus (*G*), numerous vacuoles (*V*) and mitochondria (*M*). Large lipid droplets (*L*) and lysosome-like structures are (*LY*) also present. (6,500X)

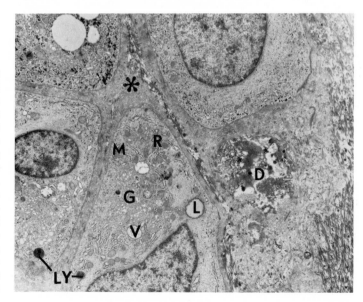

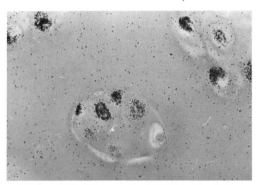

FIG. 4-16. Autoradiograph of chondrocyte clones in middle (transitional) zone of moderately advanced osteoarthritic lesion on human femoral condyle. Cartilage was incubated for 1 hour in H³ glycine. Activity is present in the cells as well as in the extracellular matrix, at a considerabe distance from the cells. This indicates that the cells have picked up the amino acid, synthesized a protein containing glycine, and secreted it into the extracellular matrix. Some cells, do not appear active and upon ultrastructural examination degenerating cells are frequently found within chondrocyte clones. (H≃E; 750X)

veloped rough endoplasmic reticulum, Golgi apparatus, mitochondria and numerous secretory vacuoles.[183] These clones are surrounded by halos of fibrillar matrix, probably proteoglycans (Fig. 4-15). Centrioles possibly indicative of cell division are present.[183] Cells in various stages of degeneration are commonly found within or adjacent to these clusters[183] (Figs. 4-15, 4-16).

Metabolic and biochemical studies have confirmed these histologic, histochemical, and ultrastructural impressions. Despite increased numbers of dead cells in early and moderately advanced osteoarthritic lesions,[183] there is an increase in the number of cells per unit volume of tissue.[93,104,105] These lesions are characterized by a progressive increase in thymidine-H³ incorporation, an indicator of mitotic activity.[104,105] Metabolic activity of the tissue is also increased.[36,37,118,119] While there is a progressive decrease in hexosamine with increased severity of the disease, there is a considerable increase in hexosamine synthesis on a per-cell basis indicating that although the individual cells are producing increased amounts of matrix, it is insufficient to compensate for the progressive degradation of matrix components that occurs with advancing disease.[104] The matrix synthesized by the "blastic"-appearing cells in the osteoarthritic lesion differs from that of normal adult cartilage by having a high content of chondroitin-4 sulfate.[105] Chondroitin-4 sulfate is normally found in large quantities only in immature cartilage. The fact that these cells are again able to divide and to synthesize a more "immature" matrix may indicate that in the early and moderately advanced stages of this disease chondrocytes are stimulated to dedifferentiate in an attempt to reconstitute the altered cartilage.

In the advanced osteoarthritic lesion cartilage height is markedly decreased, clefts extend to subchondral bone, there is a marked depletion of proteoglycans, the tissue is hypocellular, and the tide mark is disrupted (Fig. 4-12). Ultrastructural studies show a marked decrease in interfibrillar matrix, an increased number of microscars, and extracellular lipids.[183] The cells are often in advanced stages of degeneration.[183] Metabolic studies show a progressive decrease in DNA and hexosamine synthesis and a pronounced decrease in total hexosamine content.[16,17,30,104,105,160] There is a progressive increase in acid hydrolase activity in the advanced stages of the disease.[48,75] In summary, the early to moderately advanced osteoarthritic lesion represents an abortive attempt at tissue repair. This attempt takes the form of progressive cellular dedifferentiation, hypertrophy, cell replication, and increased synthesis of a more immature matrix. However, a simultaneous increase in matrix degradation secondary to the release of increased amounts of lysosomal (catheptic) enzymes and a decreased ability to withstand mechanical stress exceeds this attempt at repair, and the tissue proceeds unalterably to destruction. The ability of chondrocytes to multiply, and to synthesize increased amounts of matrix suggests that biochemical augmentation of these processes and/or inhibition of the degradative enzymes may eventually provide a solution to some of the problems of the osteoarthritic lesion.

REFERENCES

1. Adamson, L., Gleason, S., and Anast, C.: Sulfate incorporation by embryonic chick bone. Biochem. Biophys. Acta, *83*:262, 1964.
2. Ali, S. Y.: The presence of cathepsin-B in cartilage. Biochem. J., *102*:10c, 1967.
3. Ali, S. Y., Evans, L., Stainthorpe, E., and Lack, D. H.: Characterization of cathepsins in cartilage. Biochem. J., *105*:549, 1967.
4. Ali, S. Y.: Personal communication.
5. Anderson, A. J.: Some studies on the occurrence of sialic acid in human cartilage. Biochem. J., *78*:399, 1961.
6. Anderson, B., Hoffman, P., and Meyer, K.: The O-serine linkage in peptides of chondroitin-4 or -6 sulfate. J. Biol. Chem., *240*:156, 1965.
7. Anderson, C. E., Ludowieg, J., Harper, H., and Engleman, E. P.: The composition of the organic component of human articular cartilage. J. Bone Joint Surg., *46A*: 1176, 1964.
8. Balazs, E. A., Bloom, G. D., and Swann, D. A.: Fine structure and Glycosaminoglycan content of the surface layer of articular cartilage. Fed. Proc., *25*:1813, 1966.
9. Barland, P., Janis, R., and Sandson, J.: Immunofluorescent studies of human articular cartilage. Ann. Rheum. Dis., *25*: 156, 1966.
10. Barnett, C. H., and Cobbold, A. F.: Lubrication within living joints. J. Bone Joint Surg., *44B*:662, 1962.
11. Barnett, C. H., Cochrane, W., and Palfrey, A. J.: Age changes in articular cartilage of rabbits. Ann. Rheum. Dis., *22*:389, 1963.
12. Barnett, C. H., Davies, D. V., and MacConnaill, M. A.: Synovial Joints, Their Structure and Mechanics. Springfield, Charles C Thomas, 1961.
13. Benmaman, J. D., Ludowieg, J., and Anderson, C. E.: Glucosamine and galactosamine in human articular cartilage: Relationship to age and degenerative joint disease. Clin. Biochem., *2*:461, 1969.
14. Bennett, G. A., Waine, H., and Bauer, W.: Changes in the Knee Joint at Various Ages. With Particular Reference to the Nature and Development of Degenerative Joint Disease. New York, The Commonwealth Fund, 1942.
15. Benninghoff, A.: Form und Bau der Gelenk-Knorpel in ihren Beziehungen zur Funktion. S. Anat. Entwicklungsgesch., *76*:43, 1925.
16. Bollet, A. J.: Connective tissue polysaccharide metabolism and the pathogenesis of arthritis. Advances Intern. Med., *13*: 33, 1967.
17. Bollet, A. J., Handy, J. R., and Sturgill, B. C.: Chondroitin sulfate concentration and protein polysaccharide composition of articular cartilage in osteoarthritis. J. Clin. Invest., *42*:853, 1963.
18. Bollet, A. J., and Nance, J. L.: Biochemical findings in normal and osteoarthritic articular cartilage. II. Chondroitin sulfate concentration and chain length, water and ash content. J. Clin. Invest., *45*:1170, 1966.
19. Brandt, K. D., and Muir, H.: Characterization of protein-polysaccharides of articular cartilage from mature and immature pigs. Biochem. J., *114*:871, 1969.
20. Brower, T. D.: The localization of chloride in hyaline cartilage by histochemical techniques. J. Bone Joint Surg., *38A*:655, 1956.
21. Brower, T. D., Akohoshi, Y., and Orlic, P.: The diffusion of dyes through articular cartilage in vivo. J. Bone Joint Surg., *44A*:456, 1962.
22. Butler, W. T., and Cunningham, L. W.: Evidence for the linkage of a disaccharide to hydroxylysine in tropocollagen. J. Biol. Chem., *241*:3382, 1966.
23. Cameron, D. A., and Robinson, R. A.: Electromicroscopy of epiphyseal and articular cartilage matrix in the femur of the newborn infant. J. Bone Joint Surg., *40A*: 163, 1958.
24. Campo, R. D., and Dziewiatkowski, D. D.: Intracellular synthesis of protein polysaccharides by slices of bovine costal cartilage. J. Biol. Chem., *237*:2729, 1962.

25. Campo, R. D., and Tourtelotte, C. D.: The composition of bovine cartilage and bone. Biochem. Biophys. Acta, *141*:614, 1967.
26. Campo, R. D., Tourtelotte, C. D., and Brelin, R. J.: The protein-polysaccharides of articulars, epiphyseal plate and costal cartilages. Biochem. Biophys. Acta, *177*:501, 1969.
27. Charnley, J.: The lubrication of animal joints in relation to surgical reconstruction by arthroplasty. Ann. Rheum. Dis., *19*:10, 1960.
28. Chrisman, O. D.: The ground substance of connective tissue. Clin. Orthop., *36*:184, 1964.
29. Chrisman, O. D., Semonsky, C., and Bensch, K. G.: Cathepsins in articular cartilage. *In* Workshop on the Healing of Osseous Tissue, Washington; N.A.S. - N.R.C., 1967.
30. Chrisman, O. D.: Biochemical aspects of degenerative joint disease. Clin. Orthop., *64*:77, 1969.
31. Clark, I. C.: Surface characteristics of human articular cartilage – A scanning electron microscope study. J. Anat. (London), *108*:23, 1971.
32. Clark, I. C.: Human articular cartilage surface contours and related surface depression frequency studies. Ann. Rheum. Dis., *30*:15, 1971.
33. Clark, I. C.: Articular cartilage: A review and scanning electron microscope study. J. Bone Joint Surg., *58*:732, 1971.
34. Collins, D. H.: The Pathology of Articular and Spinal Disease. London, E. Arnold and Co., 1949.
35. Collins, D. H., Chadially, F. N., and Meachim, G.: Intracellular lipids of cartilage. Ann. Rheum. Dis., *24*:123, 1965.
36. Collins, D. H., and McElligott, T. F.: Sulphate ($^{35}SO_4$) uptake by chondrocytes in relation to histological changes in osteoarthritic human articular cartilage. Ann. Rheum. Dis., *19*:318, 1960.
37. Collins, D. H., and Meachim, G.: Sulphate ($^{35}SO_4$) fixation by human articular cartilage compared in the knee and shoulder joints. Ann. Rheum. Dis., *20*:117, 1961.
38. Cooper, G. W., and Prockop, D. J.: Intracellular accumulation of protocollagen and extrusion of collagen by embryonic cartilage cells. J. Cell Biol., *38*:523, 1968.
39. Crelin, E. S., and Southwick, W. O.: Mitosis of chondrocytes induced in the knee joint articular cartilage of adult rabbits. Yale J. Biol. Med., *33*:243, 1960.
40. Crelin, E. S., and Southwick, W. O.: Changes induced by sustained pressure in the knee joint articular cartilage of adult rabbits. Anat. Rec., *149*:113, 1964.
41. D'Abramo, F., and Lipmann, F.: The formation of adenosine 3' phosphate-5' phosphosulfate in extracts of chick embryo cartilage and its conversion into chondroitin sulfate. Biochem. Biophys. Acta, *25*:211, 1957.
42. Davies, D. V., Barnett, C. H., Cochran, W., and Palfrey, A. J.: Electron microscopy of articular cartilage in the young adult rabbit. Ann. Rheum. Dis., *21*:11, 1962.
43. Dawson, D., Wright, V., and Lozfield, M. D.: Human joint lubrication. Biomed. Eng., *160*, 1969.
44. Dickens, F., and Weil-Malherbe, H.: Metabolism of cartilage. Nature, *138*:30, 1936.
45. Dingle, J. T.: Studies on the mode of action of excess vitamin A 3. Release of a bound protease by the action of vitamin A. Biochem. J., *79*:509, 1961.
46. Dintenfass, L.: Lubrication in synovial joints: A theoretical analysis. J. Bone Joint Surg., *45A*:1241, 1963.
47. Dorfman, A.: Metabolism of Acid Mucopolysaccharides. *In* Connective Tissue: Intercellular Macromolecules. Boston, Little Brown & Co., 1964.
48. Ehrlich, M. G., Mankin, H. J., and Treadwell, B. V.: Acid Hydrolases in Osteoarthritic and Normal Cartilage. J. Bone Joint Surg., *55A*:1068, 1973.
49. Eichelberger, L., Akeson, W. H., and Roma, M.: Biochemical studies of articular cartilage. I. Normal values. J. Bone Joint Surg., *40A*:142, 1958.
50. Ekholm, R.: Articular cartilage nutrition. Acta Anat., *11*:1, 1951.
51. Elmore, S. M., Sokoloff, L., Norris, G., and Carmeci, P.: The nature of "imperfect" elasticity of articular cartilage. J. Appl. Physiol., *18*:393, 1963.

52. Fell, H. B., and Dingle, J. T.: Studies on the mode and action of excess of vitamin A: G. lysosomal proteases and the degradation of cartilage matrix. Arthritis Rheum., 7:398, 1964.

53. Fell, H. B., and Thomas, L.: Comparison of the effects of papain and vitamin A on cartilage. J. Exp. Med., 111:719, 1960.

54. Fessel, J. M., and Chrisman, D. D.: Enzymatic degradation of chondromucoprotein by cell free extracts of human cartilage. Arthritis Rheum., 7:398, 1964.

55. Gardner, D. L., and McGillivray, D. C.: Living cartilage is not smooth. Ann. Rheum. Dis., 30:3, 1971.

56. Gardner, D. L., and McGillivray, D. C.: Surface structure of articular cartilage: Historical review. Ann. Rheum. Dis., 30:10, 1971.

57. Gardner, D. L., and Woodward, D.: Scanning electron microscopy and replica studies of articular surfaces of guinea pig synovial joints. Ann. Rheum. Dis., 28:379, 1969.

58. Gardner, D. L.: The influence of microscopic technology on knowledge of cartilage surface structure. Ann. Rheum. Dis., 31:235, 1972.

59. Ghadially, F. N., Meachim, G., and Collins, D. H.: Extracellular lipid in the matrix of human articular cartilage. Ann. Rheum. Dis., 24:136, 1965.

60. Glimcher, M. J., and Krane, S. M.: The organization and structure of bone, and the mechanism of calcification. In Gould, B. S. (ed.): Treatise on Collagen, vol. II. New York, Academic Press, 1968.

61. Godman, G. C., and Lane, N.: On the site of sulfation in the chondrocyte. J. Cell Biol., 21:353, 1964.

62. Gregory, J. D., Laurent, T. C., and Roden, L.: Enzymatic degradation of chondromucoprotein. J. Biol. Chem., 239:3312, 1964.

63. Hamerman, D., Rosenberg, L. C., and Schubert, M.: Diarthrodial joints revisited. J. Bone Joint Surg., 52A:725, 1970.

64. Harrison, M. H. M., Schajowicz, F., and Trueta, J.: Osteoarthritis of the hip: A study of the nature and evolution of the disease. J. Bone Joint Surg., 35B:598, 1953.

65. Hascall, V. C., and Sajdera, S. W.: Protein-polysaccharide from bovine nasal cartilage: The function of glycoprotein in the formation of aggregates. J. Biol. Chem., 244:2384, 1969.

66. Herring, G. M.: The chemical structure of tendon, cartilage, dentin and bone matrix. Clin. Orthop., 60:261, 1968.

67. Honner, R., and Thompson, R. C.: The nutritional pathways of articular cartilage. J. Bone Joint Surg., 53A:742, 1971.

68. Hunter, W.: On the structure and diseases of articulating cartilage. Phil. Trans., 42:514, 1743.

69. Ingelmark, B. E., and Saaf, J.: Ueber die Ernahrung des Gelenkknorpels und die Bildung der Gelenkflussigkeit unter verschiedenen funktionellen Verhaltnissen. Acta Orthop. Scan., 17:303, 1948.

70. Jeanloz, R.: The nomenclature of mucopolysaccharides. Arthritis Rheum., 3:233, 1960.

71. Kantor, T. G., and Schubert, M.: The difference in permeability of cartilage to cationic and anionic dyes. J. Histochem. Cytochem., 5:28, 1957.

72. Kiuirikko, K. I., and Prockop, D. J.: Purification and partial characterization of the enzyme for the hydroxylation of proline in protocollagen. Arch. Biochem. Biophys., 118:611, 1967.

73. Krane, S., Parson, V., and Kunin, A. S.: Studies of the metabolism of epiphyseal cartilage. In Bassett, C. A. L. (ed.): Cartilage Degradation and Repair. Washington, N.A.S. - N.R.C., 1967.

74. Kuhn, R., and Leppelmann, H. J.: Galaktosamin und Glucosamin im Knorpel in Abhangigkeit vom Lebensalter. Liebig Ann. Chem., 611:254, 1958.

75. Lack, C. H., and Ali, S. Y.: The degradation of cartilage by enzymes. In Bassett, C. A. L. (ed.): Cartilage Degradation and Repair. Washington, N.A.S. - N.R.C., 1967.

76. Leidy, J.: On the intimate structure and history of articular cartilage. Am. J. Med. Sci., 17:277, 1849.

77. Levene, C.: The patterns of cartilage canals. J. Anat., 98:515, 1964.

78. Lindahl, O.: Ueber den Wassergehalt des Knorpels. Acta Orthop. Scand., 17:134, 1958.

79. Linn, F. C., and Sokoloff, L.: Movement and composition of intrastitial fluid of cartilage. Arthritis. Rheum., *8*:481, 1965.

80. Little, K., Pimm, L. H., and Trueta, J.: Osteoarthritis of the hip: An electron micrographic study. J. Bone Joint Surg., *40B*:123, 1958.

81. Loewe, G.: Localization of chondromucoproteins in cartilage. Ann. Rheum. Dis., *24*:528, 1965.

82. Loewe, G.: Changes in the ground substance of aging cartilage. J. Pathol. Bacteriol., *65*:381, 1963.

83. Lucy, J. A., Dingle, J. T., and Fell, H. B.: Studies on the mode of action of excess vitamin A. II. A possible role of intracellular proteases in the degradation of cartilage matrix. Biochem. J., *79*:500, 1961.

84. Lutfi, A. M.: Mode of growth, fate and functions of cartilage canals. J. Anat., *106*:135, 1970.

85. Lutwak-Mann, C.: Enzyme systems in articular cartilage. Biochem. J., *34*:517, 1940.

86. McConnaill, M. A.: The movements of bone and joints. 4. The mechanical structure of articulating cartilage. J. Bone Joint Surg., *33B*:251, 1951.

87. McCutchen, C. W.: Sponge, hydrostatic and weeping bearings. Nature., *184*:1284, 1959.

88. McCutchen, C. W.: The frictional properties of animal joints. Wear, *5*:1, 1962.

89. McCutchen, C. W.: Why did nature make synovial fluid slimy? Clin. Orthop., *64*:18, 1969.

90. McElligott, T. F., and Collins, D. H.: Chondrocyte function of human articular and costal cartilage compared by measuring the in vitro uptake of labelled (^{35}S) sulphate. Ann. Rheum. Dis., *19*:31, 1960.

91. McKibben, B., and Holdsworth, F. S.: The nutrition of immature joint cartilage in the lamb. J. Bone Joint Surg., *48B*:793, 1966.

92. Mankin, H. J.: Unpublished data.

93. Mankin, H. J.: Biochemical and metabolic aspects of osteoarthritis. Ortho. Clin. N. Am., *2*:19, 1971.

94. Mankin, H. J.: Localization of tritiated thymidine in articular cartilage of rabbits. II. Repair in immature cartilage. J. Bone Joint Surg., *44A*:688, 1962.

95. Mankin, H. J.: Localization of tritiated thymidine in articular cartilage of rabbits. I. Growth and immature cartilage. J. Bone Joint Surg., *44A*:682, 1962.

96. Mankin, H. J.: Localization of tritiated cytidine in articular cartilage of immature and adult rabbits after intraarticular injection. Lab. Invest., *12*:543, 1963.

97. Mankin, H. J.: The calcified zone (basal layer) of articular cartilage of rabbits. Anat. Rec., *145*:73, 1963.

98. Mankin, H. J.: Localization of tritiated thymidine in articular cartilage of rabbits. III. Mature articular cartilage. J. Bone Joint Surg., *45A*: 529, 1963.

99. Mankin, H. J.: The articular cartilages: A review. AAOS Instructional Course Lectures, *XIX*:204, 1970.

100. Mankin, H. J., and Baron, P. A.: The effect of aging on protein synthesis in articular cartilage of rabbits. Lab. Invest., *14*:658, 1965.

101. Mankin, H. J., and Boyle, C. J.: The acute effects of lacerative injury on DNA and protein synthesis in articular cartilage. *In* Bassett, C. A. L. (ed.): Cartilage Degradation and Repair. Washington, N.A.S.-N.R.C., 1967.

102. Mankin, H. J., and Conger, K. A.: The effect of cortisol on articular cartilage of rabbits. Lab. Invest., *15*:794, 1966.

103. Mankin, H. J., and Conger, K. A.: The acute effects of intraarticular hydrocortisone on articular cartilage in rabbits. J. Bone Joint Surg., *48A*:1383, 1966.

104. Mankin, H. J., Dorfman, H., Lippiello, L., and Zarins, A.: Biochemical and metabolic abnormalities in articular cartilage from osteoarthritic human hips. II. Correlation of morphology with biochemical and metabolic data. J. Bone Joint Surg., *53A*: 523, 1971.

105. Mankin, H. J., and Lippiello, L.: Biochemical and metabolic abnormalities in articular cartilage from osteoarthritic human hips. J. Bone Joint Surg., *52A*: 424, 1970.

106. Mankin, H. J., and Lippiello, L.: The turnover of the matrix of articular cartilage. J. Bone Joint Surg., *51A*:1591, 1969.

107. Mankin, H. J., and Orlic, P. A.: A method of estimating the "health" of rabbit articular cartilage by assays of ribonucleic acid and protein synthesis. Lab. Invest., *13*: 465, 1964.

108. Maroudas, A.: Physiochemical properties of cartilage in the light of ion exchange theory. Biophys. J. *8*:575, 1968.

109. Maroudas, A.: Distribution and diffusion of solutes in articular cartilage. Biophys. J., *10*:365, 1970.

110. Maroudas, A., and Bullough, P.: Permeability of articular cartilage. Nature., *219*: 1260, 1968.

111. Maroudas, A., Bullough, P., Swanson, S. A. V., and Freeman, M. A. R.: The permeability of articular cartilage. J. Bone Joint Surg., *50B*:166, 1968.

112. Maroudas, A., Muir, H., and Wingham, J.: The correlation of fixed negative charge with glycosaminoglycan content of human articular cartilage. Biochem. Biophys. Acta, *177*:492, 1969.

113. Martin, G. R., Gross, J., Piez, K. A., and Lewis, M. S.: On the intramolecular cross linking of collagen in lathyretic rats. Biochem. Biophys. Acta, *53*:599, 1961.

114. Mathews, M. B.: The interaction of collagen and acid mucopolysaccharides: A model for connective tissue. Biochem. J., *96*:710, 1965.

115. Mathews, M. B., and Glagov, S.: Acid mucopolysaccharide patterns in aging human cartilage. J. Clin. Invest., *45*:1103, 1966.

116. Meachim, G.: The histology and ultrastructure of cartilage. In Bassett, C. A. L. (ed.): Cartilage Degradation and repair. Washington, N.A.S. - N.R.C., 1967.

117. Meachim, G.: Age changes in articular cartilage. Clin. Orthop., *64*:33, 1969.

118. Meachim, G.: The effect of scarification on articular cartilage in the rabbit. J. Bone Joint Surg., *45B*:150, 1963.

119. Meachim, G., and Collins, D. H.: Cell counts of normal and osteoarthritic articular cartilage in relation to the uptake of sulfate ($^{35}SO_4$) in vitro. Am. Rheum. Dis., *21*:45, 1962.

120. Meachim, G., Ghadially, F. N., and Collins, D. H.: Regressive changes in the superficial layer of human articular cartilage. Ann. Rheum. Dis., *24*:23, 1965.

121. Meachim, G., and Roy, S.: Intracytoplasmic filaments in the cells of adult human articular cartilage. Ann. Rheum. Dis., *26*:50, 1967.

122. Meachim, G., and Roy, S.: Surface ultrastructure of mature adult human articular cartilage. J. Bone Joint Surg., *51B*:529, 1969.

123. Miles, J. S., and Eichelberger, L.: Biochemical studies of human cartilage during the aging process. J. Am. Geriat. Soc., *12*:1, 1964.

124. Miller, E. J., and Matukas, V. J.: Chick cartilage collagen: A new type of $\alpha 1$ chain not present in bone or skin of the species. Proc. Nat. Acad. Sci. (US), *64*:1264, 1969.

125. Miller, E. J., Vanderkorst, J. K., and Sokoloff, L.: Collagen of human articular and costal cartilage. Arthritis Rheum., *12*:21, 1969.

126. Miller, E. J.: Isolation and characterization of collagen from chick cartilage containing three identical α chains. Biochem., *10*:1652, 1972.

127. Muir, H.: Chemistry and metabolism of connective tissue glycosaminoglycans (mucopolysaccharides). In Hall, D. A. (ed.): International Review of Connective Tissue Research, vol. 2. New York, Academic Press.

128. Pal, S., Doganges, P. T., and Schubert, M.: The separation of new forms of the protein polysaccharides of bovine nasal cartilage. J. Biol. Chem., *241*:4261, 1966.

129. Palfrey, A. J., and Davies, D. V.: The fine structure of chondrocytes. J. Anat., *100*:213, 1966.

130. Partridge, S. M., Davis, H. F., and Adair, G. S.: The chemistry of connective tissues. 6. The constitution of the chondroitin sulfate-protein complex in cartilage. Biochem. J., *79*:15, 1961.

131. Pasternak, C. A.: The synthesis of 3′ phosphoadenosine 5′ phospho-sulfate by mouse tissue: Sulfate activation in vitro and in vivo. J. Biol. Chem., *235*:438, 1960.

132. Piez, K. A.: Characterization of a collagen from codfish skin containing three chromatographically different α chains. Biochem., *4*:2590, 1965.

133. Prockop, D. J.: The intracellular biosynthesis of collagen. Arch. Internal. Med., *124*:563, 1969.

134. Quintarelli, G.: Methods for the histochemical identification of acid mucopolysaccharides: A critical evaluation. *In* Quintarelli, G. (ed): The Chemical Physiology of Mucopolysaccharides. Boston, Little, Brown & Co., 1968.

135. Raden, E. L., and Paul, I.: Joint function. Arthritis Rheum., *13*:276, 1970.

136. Raden, E. L., Swann, D., and Weisser, P. A.: Separation of a hyaluronate-free lubricating fraction from synovial fluid. Nature, *228*:337, 1970.

137. Redfern, P.: A Normal Nutrition in the Articular Cartilage. Edinburgh, Sutherland & Knox, 1850.

138. Redler, I., and Zimny, M. L.: Scanning electron microscopy of normal and abnormal articular cartilage and synovium. J. Bone Joint Surg., *52A*:1395, 1970.

139. Roden, L.: The protein carbohydrate linkages of acid mucopolysaccharides. *In* Quintarelli, G. (ed.): The Chemical Physiology of Mucopolysaccharides. Boston, Little, Brown & Co., 1968.

140. Rosenberg, L.: Chemical basis for the histological use of safranin-O in the study of articular cartilage. J. Bone Joint Surg., *53A*:69, 1971.

141. Rosenberg, L., Johnson, B., and Schubert, M.: Protein polysaccharides from human articular and costal cartilages. J. Clin. Invest., *44*:1647, 1965.

142. Rosenberg, L., Pal, S., Beale, R., and Schubert, M.: A comparison of protein polysaccharides of bovine nasal cartilage isolated and fractionated by different methods. J. Biol. Chem., *245*:4112, 1970.

143. Rosenthal, O., Bowie, M. A., and Wagoner, G.: Studies on the metabolism of articular cartilage. II. Respiration and glycolysis of cartilage in relation to its age. J. Cell Comp. Physiol., *17*:221, 1941.

144. Roy, S.: Ultrastructure of articular cartilage in experimental hemarthrosis. Arch. Pathol., *86*:69, 1968.

145. Roy, S.: Ultrastructure of articular cartilage in experimental immobilization. Ann. Rheum. Dis., *29*:634, 1970.

146. Roy, S., and Meachim, G.: Chondrocyte ultrastructure in adult human articular cartilage. Ann. Rheum. Dis., *27*:544, 1968.

147. Ruttner, J. R., and Spycher, M. A.: Electron microscopic investigations on aging and osteoarthritic human cartilage. Pathol. Microbiol., *31*:14, 1968.

148. Sajdera, S., and Hascall, V. C.: Protein polysaccharide complex from bovine nasal cartilage: A comparison of low and high stream extraction procedures. J. Biol. Chem. *244*:79, 1969.

149. Schubert, M.: Intercellular macromolecules containing polysaccharides. *In* Connective Tissue: Intracellular Macromolecules. Boston, Little, Brown & Co., 1964.

150. Schubert, M., and Hamerman, D.: A Primer on Connective Tissue Biochemistry. Philadelphia, Lea & Febiger, 1968.

151. Seno, N., Meyer, K., Anderson, B., and Hoffman, P.: Variations in keratosulfates. J. Biol. Chem., *240*:1005, 1965.

152. Silberberg, R.: Ultrastructure of articular cartilage in health and disease. Clin. Orthop., *57*:233, 1968.

153. Silberberg, R., Silberberg, M., and Feir, D.: Life cycle of articular cartilage cells: An electronmicroscopic study of the hip joint of the mouse. Am. J. Anat., *114*:17, 1964.

154. Silberberg, M., Silberberg, R., and Hasler, M.: Effects of fasting and refeeding on the ultrastructure of articular cartilage. Pathol. Microbiol., *30*:283, 1967.

155. Silberberg, R., Silberberg, M., Vogel, A., and Wettstein, W.: Ultrastructure of articular cartilage of mice of various ages. Am. J. Anat., *109*:251, 1961.

156. Silberberg, R., Stamp, W. G., Lesker, P. A., and Hasler, M.: Aging changes in ultrastructure and enzymatic activity of articular cartilage of guinea pigs. J. Gerontol., *25*:184, 1970.

157. Smith, J. W., Peters, T. J., and Serafini-Fracassini, A.: Observations in the distribution of the protein polysaccharide complex and collagen in bovine articular cartilage. J. Cell Comp. Physiol., *2*:129, 1967.

158. Sokoloff, L.: Elasticity of articular cartilage: Effect of ions and viscous solutions. Science, *141*:1055, 1963.

159. Sokoloff, L.: Elasticity of aging cartilage. Fed. Proc., *25*:1089, 1966.

160. Sokoloff, L.: The biology of degenerative joint disease. Chicago, University of Chicago Press, 1969.

161. Spicer, S., Horn, R. G., and Leppi, T. J.: Histochemistry of connective tissue mucopolysaccharides. *In* Wagner, B. M., and Smith, D. E. (eds.): The Connective Tissue. Baltimore, Williams & Wilkins, 1967.

162. Stevens, F. S.: Multiple stage depolymerization of collagen fibrils. Biochem. Biophys. Acta, *130*:202, 1966.

163. Stockwell, R. A.: The cell density of human articular and costal cartilage. J. Anat., *101*:753, 1967.

164. Stockwell, R. A.: Lipid content of human costal and articular cartilage. Ann. Rheum. Dis., *26*:481, 1967.

165. Stockwell, R. A.: Changes in the acid glycosaminoglycan content of the matrix of aging human articular cartilage. Ann. Rheum. Dis., *29*:509, 1970.

166. Stockwell, R. A.: The lipid and glycogen content of rabbit articular hyaline and nonarticular hyaline cartilage. J. Anat., *102*:1, 1967.

167. Stockwell, R. A., and Scott, J. E.: Distribution of acid glycosaminoglycans in human articular cartilage. Nature, *215*:1376, 1967.

168. Stone, A. L.: Optical rotary dispersion of mucopolysaccharides and mucopolysaccharide-dye complexes. Biopolymers, *3*:617, 1965.

169. Strangeways, T. S. P.: Observations on the nutrition of articular cartilage. Brit. Med. J., *1*:661, 1920.

170. Strominger, J. L.: Nucleotide intermediates in the biosynthesis of heteropolymeric polysaccharides. *In* Connective Tissue: Intercellular Macromolecules. Boston, Little, Brown & Co., 1964.

171. Thomas, L.: The effects of papain, vitamin A, and cortisone in cartilage matrix in vivo. *In* Connective Tissue: Intercellular Macromolecules. Boston, Little, Brown & Co., 1964.

172. Thomas, L., McCluskey, R. T., Potter, J. L., and Weissmann, G.: Comparison of the effects of papain and vitamin A on cartilage. I. The effects in rabbits. J. Exp. Med., *111*:705, 1960.

173. Toda, N., and Seno, N.: Sialic acid in the keratan sulfate fraction from whole cartilage. Biochem. Biophys. Acta, *208*:227, 1970.

174. Toynbee, J.: *In* Redfern, P.: Abnormal Nutrition in the Articular Cartilages. Edinburgh, Sutherland and Knox, 1850.

175. Underfriend, S.: Formation of hydroxyproline in collagen. Sci., *152*:1335, 1966.

176. Wagoner, G., Rosenthal, O., and Bowie, M. A.: Studies of the cells in normal and arthritic bovine cartilage. Am. J. Med. Sci., *201*:489, 1941.

177. Walker, P. S., Dowson, D., Longfield, M. D., and Wright, V.: Boosted Lubrication in synovial joints by fluid enlargement and enrichment. Ann. Rheum. Dis., *27*:512, 1968.

178. Walker, P. S., et al.: Behavior of synovial fluid on surfaces of articular cartilage. Ann. Rheum. Dis., *28*:1, 1969.

179. Walker, P. S., et al.: Mode of aggregation of hyaluronic acid protein complex in the surface of articular cartilage. Ann. Rheum. Dis., *29*:591, 1970.

180. Weiss, C., and Mankin, H. J.: Unpublished data.

181. Weiss, C., Mankin, H. J., and Treadwell, B. V.: Diffusion rates in articular cartilage: Evidence for an active transport system. (abstract) J. Bone Joint Surg., *55A*:657, 1973.

182. Weiss, C.: An ultrastructural study of aging human articular cartilage (abstract). J. Bone Joint Surg., *53A*:803, 1971.

183. Weiss, C., Mirow, S.: An ultrastructural study of osteoarthritic changes in the articular cartilage of human knees. J. Bone Joint Surg., *54A*:954, 1972.

184. Weiss, C., Rosenberg, L., and Helfet, A. J.: An ultrastructural study of normal young adult human articular cartilage. J. Bone Joint Surg., *50A*:663, 1968.

185. Weissman, G., and Spilberg, I. L.: Breakdown of cartilage protein polysaccharide by lysosomes. Arthritis Rheum., *11*:162, 1968.

186. Woessner, J. F., Jr.: Acid cathepsins of cartilage. *In* Bassett, C. A. L. (ed.): Cartilage Degradation and Repair. Washington, N.A.S. - N.R.C., 1967.

187. Woessner, J. F.: Personal communication.

5

The Physical Properties of Synovial Fluid and the Special Role of Hyaluronic Acid

Endre A. Balazs, M.D.

This chapter was written with two aims in mind. First, to give a brief review of the chemical composition and rheological properties of the synovial fluid in normal and pathological joints; and second, to present, with critical comments, various current hypotheses on the importance of this fluid in the function of the joint with special emphasis on the biological role of hyaluronic acid.

There is considerable data available in the literature on the chemical composition and rheological properties of synovial fluid of various species. This review does not intend to be all-inclusive, rather it presents primary data on human joint fluids only. A large number of speculations and hypotheses are recorded in the literature on the lubricating and nutritive functions of the synovial fluid in the joint. This review aims to be selective in this area as well and present only the most important recent findings and speculations on this subject.

SYNOVIAL FLUID AS AN INTERCELLULAR MATRIX

From a rheological point of view, the natural environment of cells in a tissue can be liquid or solid. The liquid or solid extracellular matter around and between cells is called matrix. In the solid matrix, certain macromolecular components (mostly colla-

gen or elastin, or both) and their aggregates form a continuous solid phase. The rheological qualities of the solid matrix, that is, the rigidity, elasticity, and viscosity, vary considerably as exemplified by the differences between cartilage and the vitreous of the eye.

The solid matrix consists of fixed and fluid components. The fixed components are made up of such microscopic elements as collagen and elastin fibrils, basal laminae, and the structural network of proteoglycans. The fluid component comprises water and those solutes (salts, small organic molecules, peptides, proteins, etc.) that, dissolved in water, are distributed between the fixed components of the solid matrix.

The liquid matrix, on the other hand, is water in which molecules of various sizes are dissolved or dispersed. The rheological qualities of liquid matrices also vary considerably, as exemplified by the differences between the aqueous humor of the eye and synovial fluid.

The joint contains both solid and liquid matrices. From the four tissue elements forming a joint: articular cartilage, synovial tissue, intraarticular ligaments, and synovial fluid, the first three have solid matrices and the last is a liquid matrix.

It is of primary importance to recognize that all three solid matrix compartments of

63

TABLE 5-1. Proteins and Hyaluronic Acid in the Synovial Fluid
of Knee Joints of Human Subjects of Various Ages

Age Group (yrs.)	Knees Investigated	Protein (mg./ml.)	Hyaluronic Acid mg./ml.	Limiting Viscosity Number (ml./g.)
18-20	36	20.5 ± 0.8	3.8 ± 0.1	5200 ± 100
21-23	24	21.0 ± 0.9	3.8 ± 0.2	5300 ± 100
24-27	20	19.4 ± 1.3	3.4 ± 0.1	5000 ± 150
28-35	18	18.5 ± 2.6	2.5 ± 0.04	5800 ± 300
52-78	34	18.5 ± 1.6	2.5 ± 0.2	5400 ± 200

(Data taken from unpublished work of E. A. Balazs, N. W. Rydell, P. O. Seppälä, I. F. Duff, E. W. Merrill and D. A. Gibbs)

the joint are directly adjacent to the liquid matrix compartment, the synovial fluid. Another important morphological fact is that the solid matrix compartments of the articular cartilage, ligaments, and synovial tissue are not separated from the fluid matrix compartment by a continuous cell layer or basal lamina. Therefore, no visible, morphological barrier separates these two types of matrix compartments.

Other adajacent liquid and solid matrices such as are present in the peritoneal, pericardial, and pleural spaces and in the anterior chamber of the eye, are separated by microscopically recognizable cellular (epithelium) and matrix (basement membrane) barriers. The joint, however, is not the only tissue in which the liquid and solid matrices are not separated by these barriers. Other tissues in the musculoskeletal systems are similarly structured, such as the tendons and their sheaths and the space between fasciae and the bursal space.

CHEMICAL COMPOSITION OF THE SYNOVIAL FLUID

Proteins

The protein content of normal synovial fluid in all species studied is much lower than in serum.[34] The general statement can be made that the very large protein molecules of the serum, such as γ-1 macroglobulin, β-lipoprotein, fibrinogen, and α-2 macroglobulin, are absent, and others, such as α-1 antitrypsin and plasminogen, are present in traces in the normal synovial fluid.

In addition, some smaller proteins, such as haptoglobulins and prothrombin present in the serum are also absent from normal synovial fluid.[3,14,18,33,39] Because of the absence of fibrinogen and prothrombin, the normal fluid does not clot.

The total protein content of synovial fluid aspirated from normal human knee joints does not change with age of the donor (Table 5-1). In all inflammatory joint diseases, however, the concentration of protein in synovial fluid increases, and the missing plasma proteins appear. Fibrinogen appears, and, after aspiration, the fibrin precipitates, or often, the fluid clots. From the point of view of protein content, inflammatory synovial fluid is more "plasmalike" than normal synovial fluid.

In most degenerative type joint diseases, the protein concentration also increases in the fluid, but it does not necessarily become "plasmalike." While there is no clear proof, there are indications that in these cases, proteins appear in the synovial fluid that originate from the cells and matrix of neighboring tissues.[38]

Proteins with enzymatic activity also appear in the inflammatory synovial fluid. Enzymes present in the lysosomes of leucocytes, such as acid phosphatases, β-glucuronidase, and β-N-acetylglucosaminidase, are released from the destroyed cells. Other enzymes, such as lactic dehydrogenases, collagenase, and muramidase (lysozyme) are also found in pathological synovial fluids.[1,16,21]

Most importantly, inflammatory synovial

fluid contains immune complexes and antibodies that are not present in the normal fluid. In rheumatoid arthritis, the appearance of the so-called rheumatoid factors (primarily antibodies to γG-globulin) and their complexes with immunologically active proteins, as well as activation of components of the complement system are typical examples of the drastic changes occurring in the protein composition and immunological characteristics of synovial fluid during inflammation.[29,37,43-45] The extremely complex alteration in the immunologically active proteins of the synovial fluid indicate that the neighboring tissues—first of all, the synovial tissue—are the sites of very intensive protein synthesis during inflammation.

Hyaluronic Acid

The viscoelastic nature of synovial fluid is due to its hyaluronic acid content. This polyanion is present in the synovial fluid of all species investigated. In equine, bovine, and human joints a considerable variation was found in the hyaluronic acid concentration of synovial fluid collected from various joints of the same subject.[40]

Hyaluronic acid concentration also varies with age.[36] In the synovial fluid of human knee joints the hyaluronic acid concentration is highest between 18 and 25 years, after which it decreases. Between the ages of 30 and 80, no change could be observed in normal joints.[6]

The size of the hyaluronic acid molecules in the synovial fluid of human knee joints was determined by various physicochemical methods. The results vary somewhat, depending on the method used for the purification of the hyaluronic acid and for the determination of the molecular weight.

This large molecule occupies an extremely large volume when dissolved in water that contains a physiological concentration of salts and hydrogen ions. A single molecule of Na-hyaluronate, with a weight of 5 million, occupies a spheroidal domain with a diameter of 0.5 μ. This means that one gram dissolved in physiological saline fills 3 liters of solvent. In other words, the individual molecules, in close contact with one another but without overlapping, occupy the whole volume of solution at a concentration of only 0.33 mg./ml. The concentration of hyaluronic acid in synovial fluid of the human knee joint is 2 to 3 mg./ml. This means that the molecules are "crowded"; they overlap, and, therefore, such a solution must be considered as a continuous network of interacting, entangled molecular chains. Any other molecules, large or small, dissolved in the solution, are within the domain of this hyaluronic acid network, and any molecule or particle that moves in it must pass through this feltlike molecular network. The chemical activity of the molecules that can penetrate this network may be changed, and other large molecules cannot find space to penetrate the network. In this sense, one speaks about the exclusion effect and the dynamic filtration effect of hyaluronic acid solutions.[26]

Experiments in vitro carried out by many investigators, have demonstrated that large protein molecules can be filtered from solution by passage through a filter layer of synovial fluid or hyaluronic acid. Furthermore, due to the exclusion effect, molecules dissolved in hyaluronic acid solutions are altered in their chemical activity (solubility, aggregation, osmotic effect, charge effect, etc.).[23]

Limiting viscosity number (intrinsic viscosity) is a widely-used index for characterizing polymers such as hyaluronic acid. The limiting viscosity number of hyaluronic acid in synovial fluid can be measured without separating the polysaccharide from proteins. This measurement gives a meaningful parameter of one hyaluronic acid molecule which expresses the size, volume, and shape of the molecule as well as its interaction with the solvent (water with ions dissolved in it[8,14,36]). The limiting viscosity number of the synovial fluid of normal human knee joint does not change with age (Table 5-1).[6] This indicates that the molecular size of the hyaluronic acid in the joint remains the same during a lifetime, but the concentration of this polymer drops suddenly around 28 to 35 years of age.

THE ELASTOVISCOUS NATURE OF SYNOVIAL FLUID

Normal Fluid

Synovial fluid exhibits viscous and elastic properties. Both depend on its size, conformation, interactions, and number of hyaluronic acid molecules present in the fluid.

In recent years, a considerable amount of work has been reported on the elastoviscous nature of human knee synovial fluid obtained from normal and pathological joints.[5,6,12,14] These studies clearly show that, from a rheological point of view, the synovial fluid and the protein-free (<1.0 per cent) hyaluronic acid prepared from other tissues (umbilical cord and rooster comb) are identical. Up to now, no evidence has been found that would indicate that the presence of proteins in the synovial fluid significantly alters the elastoviscous properties of the pure sodium salt of hyaluronic acid. Of course, this does not eliminate the possibility that some interaction may occur between proteins and Na-hyaluronate molecules, which could cause minor modifications in the viscoelastic properties of synovial fluid. The important fact is, however, that Na-hyaluronate without proteins exhibits the same molecular relaxation mechanism as synovial fluid when it is exposed to strain of various frequencies.[20]

To demonstrate the elastoviscous nature of synovial fluid, one has to measure the

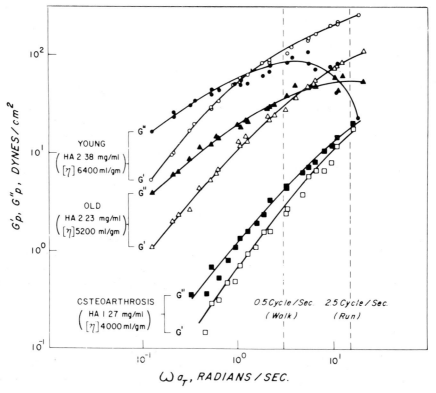

Fig. 5-1. Dynamic elastic modulus, G' (open symbols) and dynamic viscous modulus, G'' (filled symbols) of three human synovial fluid samples aspirated from the normal knee joint of one young (20 yrs.) and one old (67 yrs.) subject and from the osteoarthritic knee joint of an old subject (63 yrs.), plotted against strain frequency. The broken vertical lines indicate the frequencies that correspond approximately to the movement of the knee joint in walking and running. The concentration (HA) and limiting viscosity number ([η]) of hyaluronic acid in the aspirated fluid are given in parentheses. (From Balazs, E. A.: Univ. of Michigan Med. Ctr. July, [Special Arthritis issue]: 255, December, 1968)

TABLE 5-3. Concentration and Limiting Viscosity Number of Hyaluronic Acid and the Rheological Properties of Synovial Fluids Aspirated from Human Pathological Knees.*

Pathological Condition	Fluids Analysed	Volume Fluid Collected (ml.)	Hyaluronic Acid		Elastic Modules G' (dyn./ sec.⁻²)	Viscous Modules G" (dyn./ sec.⁻²)	Crossover Point of Two Modules (G', G") (cycles/sec.⁻¹)
			mg./ml.	[η] ml./g.			
Osteoarthritis	11		1.55 ± 0.14	3800 ± 350	85 ± 54	48 ± 28	4.7 ± 1.9
Traumatic Arthritis	3	7-20	0.69-1.76	2100-4200	2-41	2-29	1.3-2.9
Gout	4	3-5	1.28 ± 0.14	3500 ± 690	30 ± 10	15 ± 7	0.9 ± 0.3
Chondrocalcinosis	2	2.5	0.75	3700	5	5	1.7
			1.22	3900	22	13	0.9

* Data taken from unpublished work of E. A. Balazs, P. O. Seppälä, N. W. Rydell, I. F. Duff, E. W. Merrill and D. A. Gibbs.

later. Thus, the rheological properties of synovial fluids in all three age groups studied are significantly different. The fluid from young subjects is very highly elastic and rigid at relatively low frequencies. The fluid from middle-aged subjects is less rigid but still highly elastic at higher frequencies. The synovial fluid from older subjects is less rigid, less viscous, and less elastic at all frequencies.

The frequencies at which these measurements were carried out were in the same range as the frequencies at which the joints are loaded and flexed during natural movements of the body. Therefore, some conclusions can be drawn about the rheological behavior of the fluid in the joint submitted to various rates of strain. Between the ages of 18 and 39, the synovial fluid undergoes a substantial decrease in rigidity, but retains its generally elastic character. With further aging the elasticity decreases in such a way that under the frequency conditions of normal knee motion the synovial fluid changes from the highly elastic fluid in the young to a nonelastic viscous fluid in the old.

Since the concentration, size, shape, and limiting viscosity number of individual hyaluronic acid molecules does not change in the synovial fluid of normal human knee joint between the ages of 27 and 78 but the elastoviscous properties of the fluid radically decrease, one has to assume that the interaction between the chains of the neighbor-

ing molcules is altered. Recent studies on hyaluronic acid, carried out using X-ray diffraction and optical rotation measurements, indicate that a certain amount of the individual polysaccharide chains form double helical junction points or crosslinks that increase the elastoviscous properties of the polymer. It is possible that during aging the amount of these double helical crosslinks between the chains of neighboring molecules decreases. This in turn would make the molecular chain segments less stiff and the solution less elastic.

Pathological Fluids*

In the synovial fluids aspirated from joints with osteoarthritis, traumatic arthritis, gout, chondrocalcinosis, and rheumatoid arthritis, the concentration, limiting viscosity number, and molecular weight of hyaluronic acid is lower than in normal joints.[14,35,40] Consequently, all rheological properties of the fluid, such as the dynamic viscous and elastic moduli and the crossover point of the two moduli are also much below normal values (Table 5-3; Fig. 5-1). Thus, in the pathological joint, the synovial fluid does not have those rheological properties that protect the synovial tissue and cartilage against mechanical stress.

---

* Data reported here are from the work of Balazs, Seppälä, Rydell, Gibbs, Duff and Merrill. While the details of this work are not yet published, a brief review of it can be found in Balazs 1968.[5]

THE SURFACE OF
THE ARTICULAR CARTILAGE

There is some indication that hyaluronic acid is not evenly distributed in the entire joint space. On the surface of the articular cartilage and on the surface of the synovial tissue, a hyaluronic acid layer was observed which cannot be easily washed away from these tissue surfaces. The concentration of the hyaluronic acid in these layers is higher than in the fluid aspirated from the joint. It is not clear what kind of molecular interaction is responsible for the "accumulation" of hyaluronic acid on these tissue surfaces.

Electron microscopic studies showed that a 1- to 2-μ-thick layer of hyaluronic acid-protein complex covers the surface of the articular cartilage. This layer is anchored to the fibrillar collagen matrix of the cartilage and can be removed from it by treatment with proteolytic enzymes or hyaluronidase. With aging, and in osteoarthritic cases, this layer becomes thicker. It is now known, however, how the hyaluronic acid-and protein content of the layer change with aging and with various pathological conditions.[8]

Histochemical and chemical analyses carried out on the cartilage close to the articular surface indicate the presence of hyaluronic acid 50 to 100 μ deep into the cartilage where it shares the space between the collagen fibrils with sulfated proteoglycans.[8] The deep layers of the cartilage matrix contain only sulfated proteoglycans (proteoglycans of chondroitin 4-sulfate and keratan sulfate) but no hyaluronic acid.

Scanning electron microscopy also showed an accumulation of synovial fluid (hyaluronic acid and proteins) on the surface of articular cartilage[19,24,42] (1970). Under conditions of extreme load, experiments in vitro show, this fluid layer protects the cartilage surface.[42]

One can only speculate about the importance of this layer in the normal function and pathology of the joint. Since it represents the only morphologically visible barrier between the cartilage matrix and the joint space, it is tempting to assume that it is responsible for the protection of the cartilage surface. Since the synovial fluid of the normal joint does not contain appreciable amounts of sulfated proteoglycans, it is possible that the surface layer of the cartilage impregnated with hyaluronic acid forms an effective barrier against diffusion or flow (under pressure caused by compressing the cartilage when the joint is loaded) of the sulfated proteoglycans into the synovial fluid. In various pathological conditions sulfated glycosaminoglycans were found in the synovial fluid,[35] suggesting that the integrity of the surface layer of the articular cartilage impregnated with hyaluronic acid is responsible for the normal maintenance of the cartilage by preventing the leakage of proteoglycans into the synovial space and the subsequent loss of this important component of the cartilage matrix. The missing link in this argument, of course, is the complete lack of knowledge of the chemical composition of the cartilage surface layer in pathological conditions.

THE EFFECT OF HYALURONIC ACID
ON CELL ACTIVITIES

Recently, several effects of hyaluronic acid on cells in vitro and in vivo have been reported. None of these effects have been directly connected to the pathological processes in the joint. Nevertheless, the effect of hyaluronic acid on cell activities is so general that the assumption that it is operative in wound healing and inflammation of the joint is justified.[12]

Na-hyaluronate was found to be a cell-immobilizing agent. The movement of cells of the lymphomyeloid system (lymphocytes, granulocytes, macrophages) is inhibited by this biopolymer and by the tissue fluids that contain this molecule (synovial fluid, liquid vitreous). The fast-moving cells of the lymphomyeloid system exhibit different sensitivities to hyaluronic acid. This cell-immobilizing effect is specific for these types of cells because cells that move slowly in vitro (fibroblasts) are not affected. The effect of hyaluronic acid on the motility of cells is not directly related to the bulk viscosity of the solution in which the cells are moving. The effect is dependent on the limiting viscosity number of the hyaluronic acid used. Hyaluronic acid preparations with low limiting viscosity numbers are less effective cell movement inhibitors than preparations with high limiting viscosity numbers. Pathological synovial fluids, with low limiting viscosity numbers, are less effective than normal fluids.[13]

Hyaluronic acid also inhibits the modulation of lymphocytes to lymphoblasts. When blood lymphocytes, stimulated by mitogens (phytohemagglutinin, pokeweed mitogen, streptolysin O or purified protein derivative of tuberculin) are placed in viscous hyaluronic acid solution, the transformation of lymphocytes to lymphoblasts and the subsequent mitosis is prevented as long as the cells are surrounded and separated from each other by viscous Na-hyaluronic solutions.[17]

Na-hyaluronate can also prevent the targets cells from killing sensitized lymphocytes. The cytotoxic effect of lymphocytes is inhibited when the Na-hyaluronate concentration in the medium separating the target cells from the lymphocytes reaches a certain concentration.[11]

The graft-versus-host reaction could be inhibited with Na-hyaluronate when the donor cells are injected into the peritoneal cavity. Apparently, the spleen cells injected with Na-hyaluronate do not find their target organ (spleen, liver); or, if they do, their proliferation is inhibited.[13]

Na-hyaluronate seems also to influence the wound healing of articular cartilage, tendons, and fasciae. Relatively few experiments have been reported in this area and therefore, one has to regard these results as preliminary. When the dorsal fasciae of rabbits and guinea pigs and the long extensor tendons of the legs of rabbits were traumatized by mechanical damage and, after the trauma, viscous Na-hyaluronate solution (sterile and pyrogen-free) was applied to the damaged area, the subsequent formation of granulation tissue and fibrous adhesions was considerably suppressed. Na-hyaluronate also suppressed formation of granulation tissue around foreign bodies (polyethylene).[17,30,32] All these investigations suggest that hyaluronic acid has a cell regulatory function which specifically affects the lymphomyeloid system during the inflammatory process.

Effect on Frictional Resistance

It has been generally accepted for a long time that the frictional resistance of those parts of the joint that move adjacent to each other (articular cartilage, synovial tissue, ligaments, tendons within their sheaths, walls of bursae) is decreased by the viscous synovial fluid. The viscosity of the fluid has been regarded as the key to this lubricating effect, and the high-molecular-weight hyaluronic acid as the essential component of the lubricating fluid.[25,27,42]

Recently, this joint lubrication was further defined by separating it into two problem areas: the lubrication of the "soft tissues" (ligaments and synovial tissue) and the lubrication of the cartilage surfaces.[27] The role of hyaluronic acid in diminishing the frictional resistance of "soft tissues" sliding across each other was confirmed. On the other hand, the same action of hyaluronic acid on cartilage sliding over cartilage was questioned. A glycoprotein fraction was found in the synovial fluid that decreased the coefficient of friction between moving cartilage surfaces.[41] The importance of hyaluronic acid as an agent that reduces the frictional resistance between the moving surfaces inside the joint, and between tendons and their sheaths, is still not fully understood.

Role of the Cartilage Surface

As described above, the surface layer of articular cartilage is impregnated with hyaluronic acid. One can visualize the two opposing cartilage surfaces and the thin layer of synovial fluid between as a continuous hyaluronic acid network. The hyaluronic acid network is anchored onto the collagen fibrillar matrix of the surface layer of cartilage of both sides. The space beween the two collagen matrices is filled with the same hyaluronic acid molecular network that impregnates the collagen matrix. Therefore, dislocations between the two moving cartilage surfaces occur not between two rheologically different systems (solid cartilage and synovial fluid), but within the hyaluronic acid network. This concept has two important biological implications. One, there are no asperities or ripples on the sliding surfaces. That is, the beautiful scanning electron micrographs showing the unhydrated cartilage-synovial fluid surface with its many crevices do not picture the real sliding surface. The real sliding surface is not that which one exposes by breaking the continuity of the hyaluronic acid network and its dehydrated picture in the electron microscope does not give the proper impression of a highly hydrated hyaluronic acid molecular network. Two, the hyaluronic acid impregnated cartilage surface that serves as a barrier against the movements of macromolecules in and out of the cartilage is not distributed by the movements in the joint. Therefore, the integrity of this layer and the composition of the cartilage matrix is maintained. According to this hypothesis, the major role of hyaluronic acid on the cartilage surface is to provide the real sliding surfaces and to maintain the integrity of the cartilage matrix.

Control of Cell Invasion

There is no epithelial barrier on the surface of the synovial tissues that would prevent cell migration from these tissues into the synovial space and on the surface of the soft tissues and the cartilage of the joint. It was proposed that hyaluronic acid prevents the invasion of cells into joint space.[7,9] This concept is especially important in view of the fact that in all acute or chronic inflammatory processes of the joint, both the concentration and size of the hyaluronic acid

molecules decrease and, at the same time, the cell population in the joint space increases. It is important to note that the pathological fluid is less effective in preventing the migration of the lymphomyeloid cells in vitro than the normal fluid. These findings, while suggestive, do not present direct proof of the role of hyaluronic acid as a cell movement controlling factor in the joint.

HYALURONIC ACID AS A THERAPEUTIC AGENT

In acute and chronic inflammation and in most degenerative processes of the joint, the concentration and molecular size of hyaluronic acid decreases in the synovial fluid. Consequently, the viscosity and elasticity of the fluid also decreases. We suggested that intraarticular application of highly purified (protein content <0.3%) concentrated (10 to 20 mg./ml.) Na-hyaluronate that contains fairly large molecules (molecular weight 1 to 3 million) of this biopolymer can influence the healing and regeneration of the cartilage and soft tissues of the joint. The rationale for this suggestion is that the injected hyaluronic acid will accumulate on the articular and synovial tissue surfaces, thereby "reinforcing" the natural barriers which are most probably deteriorated in the course of the pathological process. Thus, the injection of hyaluronic acid into a diseased connective tissue compartment in which it is normally present can properly be called a macromolecular implantation. The main objective of the implantation is to increase the hyaluronic acid concentration in the joint well above the pathological and even the normal level. Since this biopolymer is a natural component of the joint, it metabolizes by diffusion and probably by phagocytic activity of macrophages. Consequently, the elevated concentration in the joint caused by the injection decreases to normal level within days. Nevertheless, one expects that the invasion of the lymphomyeloid cells into the joint space is halted by the temporary increase of hyaluronic acid concentration by the same mechanism as the movement of these cells is inhibited by this biopolymer in vitro. Furthermore, the hyaluronic acid accumulated on the surface of the cartilage and soft tissues may block inflow of proteins (immune complexes) and proteoglycans into the joint space, thereby triggering a healing process in the cartilage and decreasing inflammation in the synovial tissue.

Experiments carried out in dog and rabbit joints indicate that intraarticular cartilage heals better when the Na-hyaluronate concentration of the synovial space is increased after wounding by implantation of this biopolymer.[32] It was also found that the granulation reaction in subcutaneous tissue after surgical wounds[30] and in adhesion formation between tendon and tendon sheaths after mechanical damage is decreased when Na-hyaluronate is applied to the wounded surfaces.[32]

Treated with intraarticular administration of Na-hyaluronate traumatic arthritis in horses, rapidly improved and, in most cases, the normal function of the joint was restored after one or two treatments.[31]*

Na-hyaluronate was administered intraarticularly for human osteoarthritis by several investigators. (Rydell, Helfet, Peyron). Results of these investigations are reported elsewhere in this book (see p. 142)

Na-hyaluronate was also implanted into human vitreous during surgical procedures for retinal detachment. Since hyaluronic acid is present in the vitreous in its highest concentration adjacent to the retina, it was thought that in chronic inflammation caused by retinal wounds, the healing would be promoted by implantation of this biopolymer. Furthermore, it was stipulated that viscoelastic Na-hyaluronate solution would facilitate the reattachment of the retina in cases where other surgical techniques failed.[4] Several investigators found that Na-hyaluronate implanted into human vitreous in complicated cases of retinal detachment facilitated the reattachment of retina to choroid, thus improving the healing of the vitreoretinal wound.[2,15,22,28]

One has to point out that the Na-hyaluronate used for implantation into the joint, vitreous, or other connective tissue compartments must be free from impurities that can cause immunological reaction or tissue irritation. Furthermore, the preparation must exhibit specific biological activity on lymphomyeloid cells. Such Na-hyaluronate fractions have been prepared from both human (umbilical cord) and avian (comb) tissues;† it was used in most of the experimental and clinical work cited above.

---

* J. L. Butler and A. Asheim, personal communications.

† Available from Biotrics, Inc., Arlington, Mass., USA.

REFERENCES

1. Alexandersson, R., Nettelbladt, E., and Sundblad, L.: Lactic dehydrogenase isoenzymes in arthritic synovial fluid: Effect of cortisol. Acta Rheumatol. Scand., *14*:243, 1968.
2. Algvere, P.: Intravitreal injection of high-molecular-weight hyaluronic acid in retinal detachment surgery. Acta Ophthalmol., *49*:975, 1971.
3. Andersen, R. B., and Gormsen, J.: Fibrin dissolution in synovial fluid. Acta Rheumatol. Scand., *16*:319, 1970.
4. Balazs, E. A.: Physical chemistry of hyaluronic acid. Fed. Proc., *17*:1086, 1958.
5. ———: Viscoelastic Properties of Hyaluronic Acid and Biological Lubrication. Univ. Michigan Med. Ctr. J., [Special Issue]: 255-259, December, 1968.
6. ———: Some aspects of the aging and radiation sensitivity of the intercellular matrix with special regard to hyaluronic acid in synovial fluid and vitreous. *In* Engel, A., and Larsson, T. (eds.): Thule International Symposium: Aging of Connective and Skeletal Tissue. Stockholm, Nordiska Bokhandelns Forlag, 1969.
7. ———: Structure and metabolism of connective tissue under physiological and pathological conditions. *In* Rüttner, J., *et al.* (eds.): Arthritis and Osteoarthrosis. Bern, Stuttgart, Verlag Hans Huber, Wien, 1971.

8. Balazs, E. A., Bloom, G., and Swann, D. A.: Fine structure and glycosaminoglycan content of the surface layer of articular cartilage. Fed. Proc., *25*:1817, 1966.

9. Balazs, E. A., and Darzynkiewicz, Z.: The effect of hyaluronic acid on fibroblasts, mononuclear phagocytes and lymphocytes. *In* Kulonen, E., and Pikkarainen, J. (eds.): Biology of the Fibroblasts. London, Academic Press, 1973.

10. Balazs, E. A., Friberg, S., and Freeman, M. I. (unpublished data).

11. Balazs, E. A., Friberg, S., and Darzynkiewicz, Z. (unpublished data).

12. Balazs, E. A., and Gibbs, D. A.: The rheological properties and biological function of hyaluronic acid. *In* Balazs, E. A. (ed.): Chemistry and Molecular Biology of the Intercellular Matrix III. New York, Academic Press, 1970.

13. Balazs, E. A., Skopinska, E., and Darzynkiewicz, Z. (unpublished data).

14. Balazs, E. A., Watson, D., Duff, I. F., and Roseman, S.: Hyaluronic acid in synovial fluid. I. Molecular parameters of hyaluronic acid in normal and arthritic human fluids. Arthritis Rheum., *10*:357, 1967.

15. Balazs, E. A., *et al.*: Hyaluronic acid and the replacement of the vitreous and aqueous humor. *In* Modern Problems in Ophthalmology, *10*:1, 1972.

16. Bartholomew, B. A., and Perry, A. L.: Alpha-mannosidase activity in synovial fluid. Acta Rheumatol. Scand., *16*:304, 1970.

17. Darzynkiewicz, Z., and Balazs, E. A.: Effect of connective tissue intercellular matrix on lymphocyte stimulation. I. Suppression of lymphocyte stimulation by hyaluronic acid. Exp. Cell Res., *66*:113, 1971.

18. Decker, B., McKenzie, B. F., and McGuckin, W. F.: Zone electrophoretic studies of proteins and glycoproteins of bovine serum and synovial fluid. Proc. Soc. Exp. Biol. Med., *102*:616, 1959.

19. Gardner, D. L., and Woodward, D.: Scanning electron microscopy and replica studies of articular surfaces of guinea pig synovial joints. Ann. Rheum. Dis., *28*:379, 1969.

20. Gibbs, D, A., Merrill, E. W., Smith, K. A., and Balazs, E. A.: Rheology of hyaluronic acid. Biopolymers, *6*:777, 1968.

21. Jasani, M. K., Katori, M., and Lewis, G. P.: Intracellular enzymes in synovial fluid joint diseases. Origin and relation to disease category. Ann. Rheum. Dis., *28*: 497, 1969.

22. Klöti, R.: Hyaluronsäure als Glasköpersubstituent. Ophthalmologica, *165*:351, 1971.

23. Laurent, T.: Structure of hyaluronic acid. *In* Balazs, E. A. (ed.): Chemistry and Molecular Biology of the Intercellular Matrix II. New York, Academic Press, 1970.

24. McCall, J. G.: Scanning Electron Microscopy of Articular Surfaces. *The Lancet,* 1194, 1968.

25. McCutchen, C. W.: Boundary lubrication by synovial fluid: Demonstration and possible osmotic explanation. Fed. Proc., *25*: 1061, 1966.

26. Ogston, A. G.: The Biological Functions of the Glycosaminoglycans. *In* Balazs, E. A. (ed.): Chemistry and Molecular Biology of the Intercellular Matrix *III*. New York, Academic Press, 1970.

27. Radin, E. L., and Paul, I. L.: A Consolidated View of Joint Lubrication. J. Bone Joint Surg., *54A*:607, 1972.

28. Regnault, F.: Acide hyaluronique intravitreen et cryocoagulation dans le traitment des formes graves de decollement de la retine. Bull. Mem. Soc. F. Ophthalmol., *84*:106, 1971.

29. Ruddy, S., and Austen, K. F.: The complement system in rheumatoid synovitis. I. An analysis of complement component activities in rheumatoid synovial fluids. Arthritis Rheum., *13*:713, 1970.

30. Rydell, N. W.: Decreased granulation tissue formation after installment of hyaluronic acid. Acta Orthop. Scand., *41*:307, 1970.

31. Rydell, N. W., Butler, J., and Balazs, E. A.: Hyaluronic acid in synovial fluid. VI. Effect of intra-articular injection of hyaluronic acid on clinical symptoms of arthritis in track horses. Acta Vet. Scand., *11*:139, 1970.

32. Rydell, N. W., and Balazs, E. A.: Effect of intra-articular injection of hyaluronic acid on clinical symptoms of osteoarthritis and on granulation tissue formation. Clin. Orthoped., *80*:25, 1971.

33. Schmidt, K., and MacNair, M. B.: Characterization of the proteins of certain post mortem human synovial fluids. J. Clin. Invest., *37*:708, 1958.

34. Schubert, M., and Hamerman, D. A.: A Primer on Connective Tissue Biochemistry. Philadelphia, Lea and Febiger, 1968.

35. Seppälä, P. O.: Synovial Fluid in Rheumatoid Arthritis. Scan. J. Clin. Lab. Invest., *16*[Suppl.]:79, 1964.

36. Seppälä, P. O., and Balazs, E. A.: Hyaluronic acid in synovial fluid III. Effect of maturation and aging on chemical properties of bovine synovial fluid of different joints. J. Gerontol., *24*:309, 1969.

37. Sliwinksi, A. J., and Zvaifler, N. J.: The removal of aggregated and nonaggregated autologous gamma globulin from rheumatoid joints. Arthritis Rheum., *12*:504, 1969.

38. ———: In vivo synthesis of IgG by Rheumatoid synovium. J. Lab. Clin. Med., *76*: 304, 1971.

39. Sundblad, L., Jonsson, E., and Nettelbladt, E.: Permeability of the synovial membrane to glycoprotein. Nature, *192*:1192, 1961.

40. ———: Glycosaminoglycans and glycoproteins in synovial fluid. *In* Balazs, E. A., and Jeanloz, R. W. (eds.): The Amino Sugars *IIA*, New York, Academic Press, 1965.

41. Swann, D. A., Radin, E. L., and Weisser, P. A.: Separation of a hyaluronate-free lubricating fraction from synovial fluid. Nature, *228*:377, 1970.

32. Walker, P. S., *et al.*: Mode of aggregation of hyaluronic acid protein complex on the surface of articular cartilage. Ann. Rheum. Dis., *29*:591, 1970.

43. Ward, P. A., and Zvaifler, N. J.: Complement-derived leucatactic factors in inflammatory synovial fluids of humans. J. Clin. Invest., *50*:606, 1971.

44. Winchester, R. J., Agnello, V., and Kunkel, H. G.: Gamma globulin complexes in synovial fluids of patients with rheumatoid arthritis. Partial characterization and relationship to covered complement levels. Clin. Exp. Immunol., *6*:689, 1970.

45. Zvaifler, N. J.: Breakdown products of C3 in human synovial fluids. J. Clin. Invest., *48*:1532, 1969.

6

Common Derangements of the Knee Joint and the Manner of Their Production

Arthur J. Helfet, M.D.

SEMILUNAR CARTILAGES

When bearing weight, the tibia rotates laterally as the knee joint straightens. It rotates medially when the knee bends. If this synchrony is prevented forcibly, as by the weight of the falling body, the rotator mechanism of the knee is injured. Certain cartilage tears are caused by nothing more than this disruption of the rotator mechanism of the knee. As far as I can determine, only the transverse fracture of the fibrotic medial meniscus of the elderly, which takes place at the junction of the anterior two thirds and the posterior one third, may be due to pressure or grinding between the femur and the tibia. All others can be explained by the violent stretching which must occur if medial rotation of the tibia in flexing the knee, or lateral rotation in extending it, is prevented. Similar forces are brought into play if while weight is taken when squatting or kneeling, a sudden twist occurs without extension or further flexion, or the tibia twists outwardly while the body lurches backward and increases flexion of the knee.

These are the common causes of injury described by patients. The footballer catches his toe, trips and falls, while the foot and the leg are rotated outward—flexion occurs without medial rotation (Fig. 6-1). The miner squats with knees fully flexed. An uncontrolled twist—rotation without synchronous extension—is followed by a searing pain, the signal of a tear in the cartilage (Fig. 6-2). One patient, a carpenter, was working in front of a chest of drawers in this attitude. A drawer had jammed. He wrenched vigorously to open it, and the drawer gave suddenly. He twisted on his right knee, and immediately he felt a searing pain over the medial cartilage. To relieve the agony he threw himself onto his left knee with identical consequences to that joint. At operation bucket-handle tears of both medial cartilages were found (Fig. 6-3).

In another instance a housewife knelt on her kitchen sink to open the cupboard above it (Fig. 6-4). The door opened suddenly. She lurched backward, increasing the flexion of the knee, but the thigh twisted inwardly instead of outwardly on the leg. A stab of pain signaled detachment of the anterior end of her medial cartilage. While synchronous rotation is prevented, the knee will flex completely only if the rotator mechanism is stretched the full distance that the tibia normally rotates—in the adult, approximately ½ inch.

At first, presumably, the meniscus straightens out. To allow it to do so, a transverse or oblique split forms in the shorter or free edge (Fig. 6-5). This minor split is the most frequent finding and, as expected and observed also by Smillie,[6] is usually deeper in

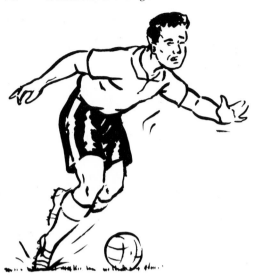

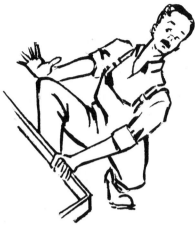

Fig. 6-1. The soccer player catches his toe, trips, and falls. The foot and the tibia are rotated outwardly while the knee flexes. Flexion occurs without medial rotation.

Fig. 6-3. A carpenter twisted violently on his flexed right knee when the drawer gave suddenly. He felt a searing pain over the medial cartilage. To relieve the agony he threw himself on to his left knee, with identical consequences to that joint.

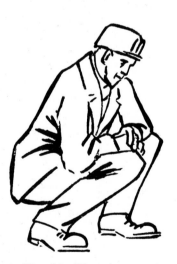

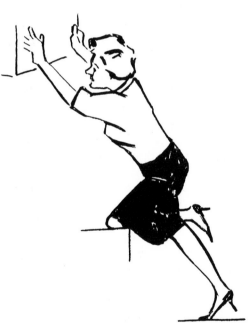

Fig. 6-2. The miner squats with knees fully flexed; an uncontrolled twist causes rotation without synchronous extension.

Fig. 6-4. A housewife knelt on her kitchen sink to open the cupboard above. The door opened suddenly. She lurched backward, increasing flexion of knee, but the thigh twisted inwardly instead of outwardly on the leg.

the lateral than in the medial meniscus because of the longer curve in the latter (Fig. 6-6). If no more than this occurs, the knee might well be symptomless after recovery from the acute injury, although the split itself would not heal. Occasionally, however, the split extends obliquely to form a mobile tag, which causes an irritating and recurring painful catch in the knee (Fig. 6-7).

It is interesting to note that the split usually occurs at the apex of the curve or in the anterior portion of the meniscus. This is to be expected, for the straightening out under tension would take place first in the more mobile portion. The posterior segments are more firmly fixed to the capsule.

A newspaper photographer, who often squatted and knelt in awkward positions to photograph dramatic moments in football matches, suffered this lesion. During clinical examination a twist would occasion a minor click which would "lock" the knee. The signs due to blocking of outward rotation of the tibia, which will be described later, were all present. Another twist and a further click unlocked the knee, which then moved freely and painlessly. He could perform these maneuvers himself with facility. At operation, no more than a pedicled tag on the free border of the medial meniscus was found. The cartilage was removed, and he has had no symptoms since.

Should the range of unaccommodated movement be greater, it is achieved either by pulling the cartilage away from its attachments to the anterior cruciate (Figs. 6-8 and 6-9) or from its capsular moorings at the back (Fig. 6-10) or by splitting the cartilage longitudinally to allow the free border to bowstring across the joint (Figs. 6-11 and 6-12). Occasionally, instead of a longitudinal

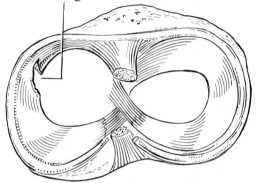

FIG. 6-6. This minor split is the most frequent finding.

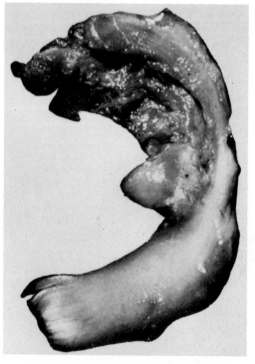

FIG. 6-7. Split posterior horn and a mobile tag, which causes an irritating and recurring painful catch in the knee.

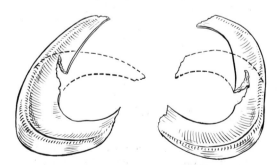

FIG. 6-5. The meniscus straightens out. To allow it to do so, a transverse or oblique split forms in the shorter or free edge.

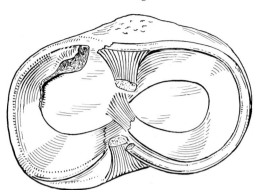

FIG. 6-8. After detachment from the cruciate ligament and tibial spine the anterior horn retracts. Note the ruffled inner edge of the retracted meniscus.

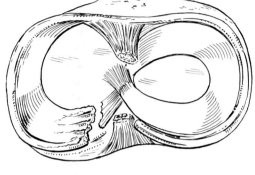

FIG. 6-10. Rupture of its firm attachments to the cruciate ligament and posterior capsule produces the ragged refracted posterior horn.

split nearly the whole cartilage or the anterior half is wrenched from its peripheral attachments and bowstrings across the intercondylar space (Fig. 6-13).

As the complete range of rotation is in the order of ½ inch or a little more than 1 cm., the displacement need not be great. Allowing for the elasticity of the cartilage, it is always within this measurement.

Whatever the case, the figure-of-eight rotator mechanism is interrupted. As the

anterior end of the cartilage is detached, the whole cartilage retracts, and a gap forms between the attachment of the cruciate ligament and the torn edge. At operation the gap may be recognized; in a young patient, the free edge of the cartilage will present a ruffle which raises it from the surface of the tibia (Fig. 6-8). The front half of the cartilage is slack and looks too long, and the inexperienced may consider it a "lax cartilage." Sometimes the torn tip of cartilage is coiled up on itself, as Sir Robert Jones[5] aptly described, "had undergone changes in the loose anterior extremity of the semilunar of the nodular type, some being as lumpy

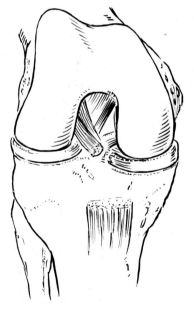

FIG. 6-9. Retracted anterior horn of the medial meniscus.

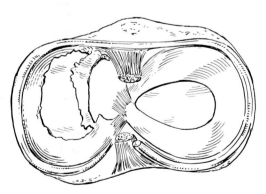

FIG. 6-11. The "bowstring" or buckethandle results from splitting of the cartilage longitudinally to allow the free border to bowstring across the joint. The separation is roughly equivalent to the distance the tibia normally rotates.

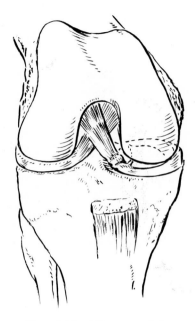

FIG. 6-12. Diagram of bow-string (or bucket-handle) tear from the front.

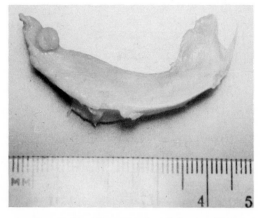

FIG. 6-14. The torn tip of the cartilage is coiled up on itself and "had undergone changes in the loose anterior extremity of the semilunar of the nodular type, some being as lumpy and large as a pea."

and large as a pea" (Fig. 6-14). In an older patient with fibrotic and less resilient carti-lages, retraction causes a thickening of the anterior half of the cartilage, which is yel-lowish, hard, and triangular in section, and a heaped-up mass is formed in the anterior compartment of the joint (Fig. 6-15). The lump so formed produces a pattern of ero-sion over the corresponding area of articular cartilage on the anteromedial part of the weight-bearing surface of the medial femoral condyle. After the joint is opened at opera-tion the observation of this mark or depres-sion or erosion immediately confirms the diagnosis (Fig. 6-16). As this type of carti-lage tear presents its own clinical features and sequelae, it should be known as the "retracted" cartilage to distinguish it from the "bucket-handle" cartilage, which itself should be more aptly named the "bowstring" cartilage. In the latter type of injury the whole or part of the cartilage is bowstrung across the joint, and the symptoms are more severe than in the case of the retracted carti-lage. But if in the first attack, or subse-

Complete peripheral detachment of meniscus

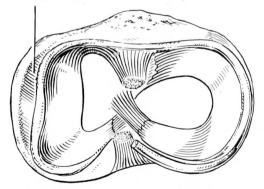

FIG. 6-13. Nearly the whole cartilage is wrenched from its peripheral attach-ments and bowstrings across the joint.

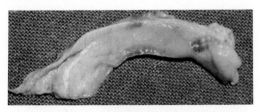

FIG. 6-15. In an older patient retrac-tion causes a thickening of the anterior half of the cartilage, and a heaped-up mass is formed in the anterior compartment of the joint.

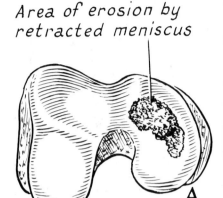

Area of erosion by
retracted meniscus

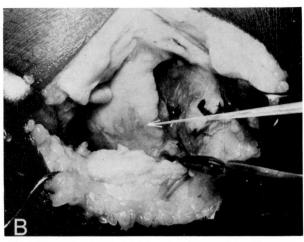

FIG. 6-16. (A) The arrow points to the pattern of erosion created by heaped-up
retracted anterior horn of medial meniscus. (B) Erosion by detached anterior horn.

quently, the bowstring snaps and coils up at the fixed end in the anterior compartment, the clinical picture resembles that of the retracted variety (Fig. 6-17). The first reaction to the snapping of the bowstring is a

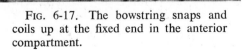

Coiled-up
bowstring

FIG. 6-17. The bowstring snaps and coils up at the fixed end in the anterior compartment.

measure of relief, for the retracted cartilage is so much more comfortable to the patient than is the bowstring. Only later do the sequelae cause symptoms. Manipulation for reduction of the displaced bowstring frequently results in snapping of the bowstring again with relief although temporary. Eventually meniscectomy is necessary. The "bowstring" injury produces a pattern of erosion on the articular cartilage covering the intercondylar border of the condyle of the femur (Fig. 6-18).

Less frequently, the posterior end of the cartilage is torn or detached (Fig. 6-19). Only twice have I found the whole back end of the cartilage wrenched from its attachments and the entire cartilage coiled in the anterior compartment. The first of these injuries was sustained during an amateur wrestling match and the second during a football scrimmage. We were unable to reconstruct the exact mechanism, except to establish that the injury in each case took place while the knee was well flexed. It is significant that these were the only cartilage injuries in which limitation of extension of the knee was more than 20 degrees and the block had the elastic consistency mentioned by Sir Robert Jones.

Occasionally violent distraction of the cartilage causes a horizontal split, but rarely

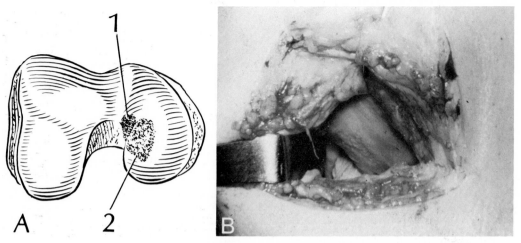

FIG. 6-18. (*A*) The drawing shows the pattern of erosion from the cruciate ligament in the bowstring meniscus (*arrow 1*) and the approximate pattern from the bowstring meniscus itself (*arrow 2*). (*B*) An operative photograph of the same area is included for comparison.

FIG. 6-19. (*A*)Tears of the posterior end of the meniscus. (*B*) Squashed pedunculated tags in triangular fibrotic cartilage of older patient the "fish-tail meniscus.

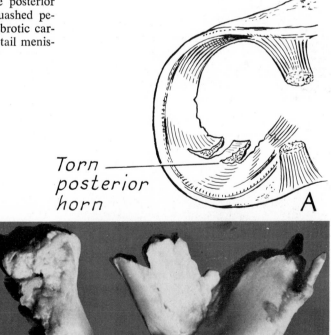

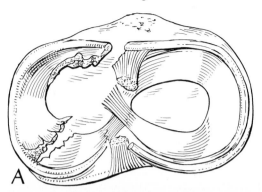

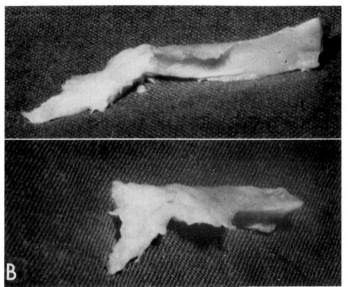

Fig. 6-20. In older people the anterior half or two thirds of the retracted cartilage thickens. Later, another traumatic incident causes a transverse tear in the posterior half of the cartilage. The torn back end of the front part has a splayed, squashed and scalloped edge (*A, B*). (*C*) Two fragments which have obviously been separated by a complete transverse tear for some time.

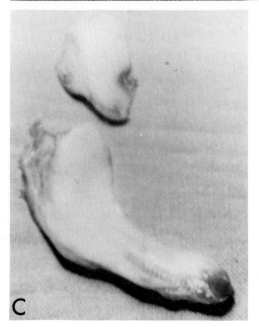

over the whole length of the meniscus. A tear of the inferior layer may pedicle towards the center of the joint and in two instances was found insinuated peripherally between the meniscus and capsule, locking the joint in a particularly painful manner (see Plate 6-1).

When distracted, the hard, fibrotic meniscus in an elderly person tends to pull off from its anterior attachments to the cruciate ligaments and retracts backwards. The anterior half or two thirds of the cartilage, as described earlier, thickens and forms a heaped-up mass which causes grumbling and increasingly severe symptoms.

Often another and minor traumatic incident causes an acute exacerbation of symptoms that necessitates surgery. At operation a complete transverse tear in the posterior half of the cartilage is found (Fig. 6-20). The torn back end of the front part has a splayed, squashed, and scalloped edge, the fish-tail meniscus. The remaining fragment of the meniscus is relatively normal for the age of the patient. The condition of the fractured end does suggest that it has been nipped off by pressure between the femur and the tibia. It seems that the heaping up or thickening caused by the anterior retraction is all taken up in the front portion and that the weight-bearing surfaces eventually grind through the junction between the thickened and the normal portions of the cartilage.

Alternatively, the second traumatic incident distracts the cartilage, but, as the anterior portion is too thick to glide between the weight-bearing surfaces, the posterior end is wrenched off at the line of the obstruction. Detachment of the anterior horn with retraction occurs frequently, while detachment of the posterior horn is uncommon. On the other hand, multiple longitudinal splits of the posterior horn with or without anterior extensions to form a bowstring, are comparatively frequent, but these splits are rare in the anterior horn. This is understandable. The more mobile and loosely bound anterior horn tears more easily from its attachments.

The more firmly held posterior horn tears in its substance. In the young where the meniscus is stretchable, the splits are longitudinal. In the old fibrotic cartilage, the split is transverse.

PATTERNS OF ARTICULAR EROSION

Lesions of the semilunar cartilages result in specific patterns of articular erosion. Each has its own clinical features, though they do tend to merge. Some indication has been given already of the effects of undue tension on the cruciates and the patella by the displaced bowstring tear and by the heaped-up retracted cartilage. They are repeated here for completeness.[3,4]

When rotation of the tibia is prevented during extension of the knee, the cruciate is tensed. It impinges on the lateral side of the medial femoral condyle and in time erodes the surface of the articular cartilage in this area. In turn, the cruciate ligament suffers from the continuous or recurring tension and is slowly stretched, with consequent laxity of the joint; at operation it may show a raw area of granulation on its otherwise shining surface.

The string of the bowstring cartilage etches its pattern medially and posteromedially to that of the cruciate ligaments (Fig. 6-18).

The effect of the retracted cartilage differs with age. The youthful soft semilunar cartilage is heaped up or ruffled. The anteromedial part of the weight-bearing surface of the medial femoral condyle comes into contact with the thickened anterior part of the retracted cartilage when the knee is extended and thus is slowly worn away (Fig. 6-16). But, because of the protrusion of the femoral condyle, the area of erosion never reaches the edge (see Fig. 7-4). Consequently, after the torn cartilage is removed and full extension and rotational alignment of the femur and the tibia are regained, normal articular cartilage is brought back to the weight-bearing area; this is one reason why, however long its history and whatever

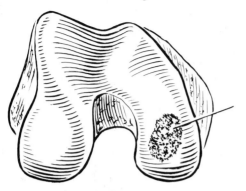

FIG. 6-21. The posterior horn tear etches its pattern (*arrow*) farther back.

the age of the patient, it is worthwhile removing the retracted cartilage.

At operation on older patients the semilunar cartilage may be seen to be yellowish and hard. It forms a shorter triangle on section because the free edge has contracted. The narrow hard cartilage tends to erode a more linear groove on the femoral condyle, and the area of erosion seems to extend further backward (Fig. 6-21). At this age, too, transverse tears in the middle third of the cartilage are more common (Fig. 6-20). The torn end of the front part has a splayed, squashed and scalloped edge. It seems that the heaping up or thickening caused by the anterior retraction is all taken up in this front portion and that eventually the weight-bearing surfaces nip it off at this junction between the thickened and the normal portions of the cartilage. Therefore, the anterior erosion extends and broadens out further back (Fig. 6-22). Tears of the posterior horn of the cartilage produce a broadish pattern, but these have not been observed as often as the anterior patterns—probably because this series includes very few patients, such as miners, who normally work in a squatting position.

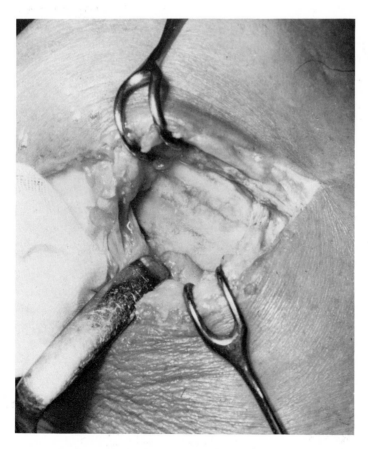

FIG. 6-22. The posterior horn tear extends and widens the area of erosion further back. The harder meniscus of the older patient scores the surface more deeply.

FIG. 6-23. In this cadaveric specimen note the tear in the cruciate ligament with retraction of the anterior horn of the lateral meniscus and the corresponding patterns of erosion. The medial condyle is unaffected. (Courtesy Royal College of Surgeons, England)

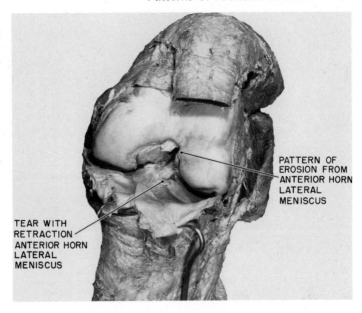

PATTERN OF
EROSION FROM
ANTERIOR HORN
LATERAL
MENISCUS

TEAR WITH
RETRACTION
ANTERIOR HORN
LATERAL
MENISCUS

In time the posterior horn tear etches its pattern of erosion, as is to be expected, further back on the medial condyle (Figs. 6-21 and 6-22).

The lateral condyle has a smaller, rounder articular surface (Figs. 6-23 - 6-25).

The third pattern of erosion concerns the medial border of the patella and the surface of the femur with which it is in contact (Fig. 6-26). Attention has been drawn to the effect produced by inadequate excursion of the tibial tubercle on the relationships of the patella and the femur. Normally, in full extension, the line of action of the quadri-

FIG. 6-24. Cadaveric specimen of displaced anterior half of lateral meniscus. The ligament uniting the anterior horn of the lateral meniscus and the cruciate ligament is partly torn. The infrapatellar pad of fat has been removed to demonstrate the imprint of the scar of the fat pad and the anterior horn of the meniscus on the upper surface of the tibia and the opposing articular surface of the lateral femoral condyle. (Courtesy Royal College of Surgeons, London)

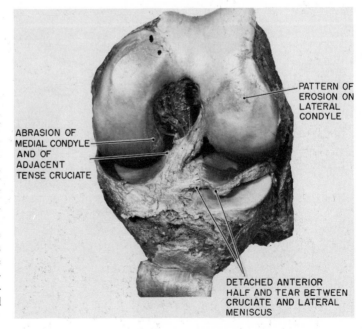

PATTERN OF
EROSION ON
LATERAL
CONDYLE

ABRASION OF
MEDIAL CONDYLE
AND OF
ADJACENT
TENSE CRUCIATE

DETACHED ANTERIOR
HALF AND TEAR BETWEEN
CRUCIATE AND LATERAL
MENISCUS

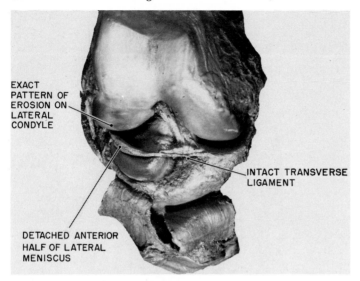

EXACT
PATTERN OF
EROSION ON
LATERAL
CONDYLE

INTACT TRANSVERSE
LIGAMENT

DETACHED ANTERIOR
HALF OF LATERAL
MENISCUS

FIG. 6-25. Cadaveric specimen of bowstring lateral meniscus. Nearly the whole lateral meniscus has been wrenched from its peripheral attachments. Note the pattern of erosion on the lateral condyle. (Courtesy Royal College of Surgeons, London)

ceps on the patellar ligament settles the patella comfortably on the trochlear surface of the femur. When the tibial tubercle halts short of this line, the patella will deviate medially as the knee extends, particularly when the quadriceps contracts against in-

creased resistance, as in climbing and descending stairs.

It is tensed against the medial slope of the trochlear surface of the femur, and the tension is greatest over the area A and B in Figure 1-17 of the patella and area T (see

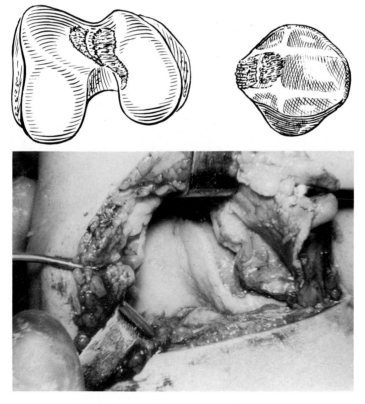

FIG. 6-26. The drawings show areas of erosion due to local compression on the medial trochlear slope of the femur. The operative photo shows erosions on the medial slope of the trochlear groove.

FIG. 6-27. (*Left*) Axial view of right patella showing erosion of articular cartilage in area B and of corresponding area of trochlear surface of femur. (*Right*) Degenerative changes on medial articular surface of patella.

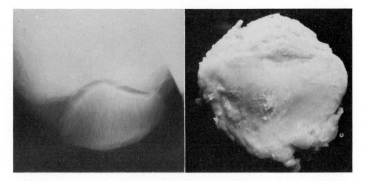

Fig. 1-19) of the femur. These are the sites of articular cartilage erosion (see also Fig. 6-27).

During flexion from complete extension, the increased medial pull on the whole mechanism produces increased pressure by the patella as it slips downward and backward on the extension of the trochlear surface on the medial condyle of the femur, and gradually the complete pattern of traumatic arthritis of the knee is etched (Fig. 6-28).

Normally, in the flexed position the patella tilts onto its medial articular surface. This tilt is accentuated in the blocked knee and will be present even in the position of fullest extension (Figs. 6-29 and 6-30).

A review of two personal series of operations for cartilage injuries reveals that retracted and bowstring cartilages are the most frequent consequences of injury (80.6% — see Table 6-2). In the series, the bowstring tears exceeded the retracted cartilages by 11 per cent, and in the medial cartilages by

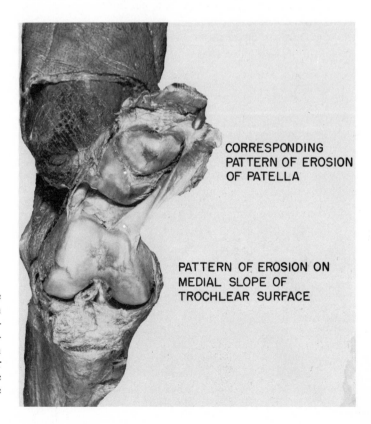

CORRESPONDING
PATTERN OF EROSION
OF PATELLA

PATTERN OF EROSION ON
MEDIAL SLOPE OF
TROCHLEAR SURFACE

FIG. 6-28. This perspective of the retracted anterior horn of medial meniscus demonstrates the comparable scarring of articular cartilage on the patella and the trochlear surface of the femur. Note the preponderance of damage on the medial surfaces.

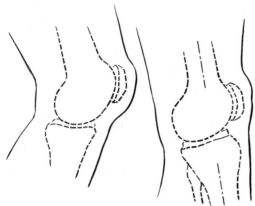

FIG. 6-29. (*Left*) Extension and lateral rotation are limited in traumatic arthritis of the knee. In the fullest extension possible the patella remains perched on the trochlear extension on the medial femoral condyle. (*Right*) In normal full extension the patella rests comfortably in the trochlear groove.

6.8 per cent (Table 6-3), but with increasing age the relative incidence of anterior tears increased (Tables 6-5 and 6-6). This must mean that as the cartilage becomes less resilient and more fibrotic, it is more liable to tear from its ligamentous moorings than to split in its substance.

TABLE 6-1. Incidence of Tears of the Semilunar Cartilage— Percentage of 627 Cases by Age Group

Age Group	Percentage
Under 16	3
10 to 20	12
20 to 44	53
45 and over	32

TABLE 6-2. Types of Cartilage Injury (Series 1—232 Cases)

	Number	Per Cent
Retracted cartilages	81	34.9
Bowstring or bucket-handle cartilage	106	45.7
Posterior tears	26	11.2
Other tears	19	8.2

TABLE 6-3. Types of Medial Cartilage Injury (Series 2—627 Cases)

	Number	Per Cent
Retracted cartilages	191	44.7
Bowstring cartilages	220	51.5
Isolated posterior tears	16	3.8

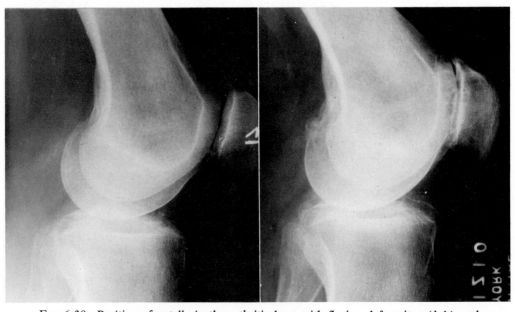

FIG. 6-30. Position of patella in the arthritic knee with flexion deformity: (*left*) early osteoarthritis, (*right*) late osteoarthritis.

TABLE 6-4. Types of Lateral Cartilage Injury
(Series 2—627 Cases)

	Number	Per Cent
Anterior tears	28	71.8
Posterior tears	11	28.2

TABLE 6-5. Types of Injury
Related to Age of Patient
(Series 1—232 Cases)

Age	Number and Percentage of Cases	
	Retracted Cartilage	Bowstring Cartilage
10 to 19	14 (35%)	26 (65%)
20 to 44	53 (43%)	70 (57%)
45 and over	14 (58%)	10 (42%)

TABLE 6-6. Types of Injury
Related to Age of Patient
(Series 2—627 Cases)

Age	Number and Percentage of Cases	
	Retracted Cartilage	Bowstring Cartilage
10 to 19	28 (28%)	72 (72%)
20 to 44	60 (39%)	93 (61%)
45 and over	103 (65.5%)	54 (34.5%)

CYSTS OF THE SEMILUNAR CARTILAGES

Cysts of the cartilages should be mentioned, for most if not all are probably traumatic in origin and degenerative in character. I have never seen a cystic cartilage at operation in which there was no evidence of injury. An interesting feature is that the cyst forms in the vascular edges of the cartilages. A cyst in a bowstring cartilage is invariably found in the part attached to the capsule. Although they are sometimes found in the medial meniscus, the majority of cysts form in the middle third of the lateral meniscus, where the meniscus is separated from the capsule by the popliteus tendon and two folds of synovium. Smillie[6] reports an incidence of 2.5 per cent of cystic change in medial and of 22.5 per cent in lateral meniscus tears (Fig. 6-31).

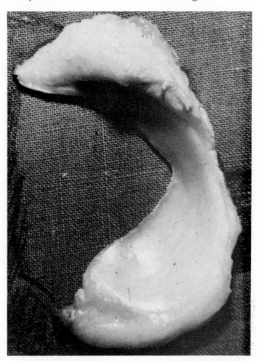

FIG. 6-31. Cyst of anterior horn of medial meniscus.

Synovial Cysts. Synovial cysts or ganglia arising completely intra-articularly in the intercondylar space are rare. Only four have been found in my experience of over 2500 knee operations. Two developed in the torn attachments between the anterior horn of the medial meniscus and the cruciate ligament (Fig. 6-32) and two from the synovium enveloping the cruciate ligaments. One patient in his early fifties suffered for four months from unceasing and finally almost constant pain in the knee. At first swelling and limitation of movement were not remarkable. When, after this time, he sought orthopedic opinion, an indefinite but tender swelling could be felt presenting in the posterolateral joint line. Clinically, the posterior horn of the lateral cartilage was tender. Flexion and internal rotation were limited by pain and on maneuver a click was elicited. At operation for excision of the lateral meniscus, the posterior horn was found to be torn, and during the approach and its detachment an enormous cyst con-

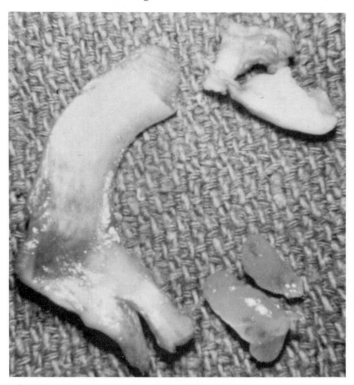

FIG. 6-32. Two synovial cysts developed in the attachments between the anterior horn of the medial meniscus and the cruciate ligament. Note the fractured posterior horn.

taining thick yellowish fluid was opened. It stemmed from the attachment and synovial sheath of the cruciates and was tense in the intercondylar and posterolateral space. Removal of the meniscus and most of the wall relieved his pain and other symptoms. Unlike true cartilage cysts, these do not arise from the substance of the meniscus.

DISCOID LATERAL CARTILAGES

Discoid cartilages of all degrees are more liable to injury than the normal cartilage. The free edge is shorter and more curved than that of the normal lateral meniscus, and transverse and oblique splits are common. Also, the cartilage is thicker in its substance and therefore vulnerable to lesser strains.

THE CRUCIATE AND THE CAPSULAR LIGAMENTS

Isolated ruptures of the cruciate ligaments are rare and of little clinical significance. Occasionally, when operating for a torn medial cartilage, one finds that the anterior cruciate ligament has been torn from its insertions in the tibia. The injury was violent enough to disrupt the cartilage and the cruciate from their moorings at the same time. But this knee does not demonstrate anteroposterior instability preoperatively or postoperatively, and removal of the cartilage cures all symptoms. Moreover, it is not possible to diagnose the coincidental rupture of the cruciate ligament before operation. Loss of rotation is present because of the injury to the rotator mechanism. No abnormal movement is possible.

By orthopedic custom, anteroposterior instability of the tibia on the femur is considered pathognomonic of tears of the cruciate ligaments. However, this sign is present only if the capsule is weak and has been injured on one side or the other as well (see Fig. 16-4).

On no occasion has an isolated rupture of the cruciates been detected preoperatively, and it is difficult to imagine a knee in which anteroposterior laxity is possible without

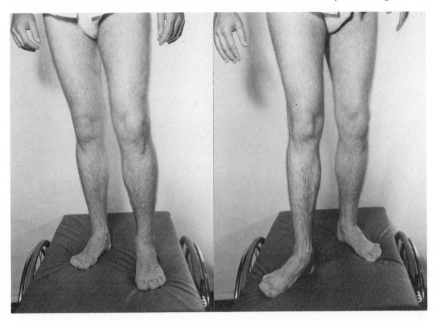

FIG. 6-33. (*Left*) To stabilize the weak knee, the foot is placed on the ground in lateral rotation. As weight is taken, the knee is straightened as the femur is rotated internally on the tibia. Compare this gait with the normal stride (*right*).

weakness in the capsule on one side. So that, whereas a displaced meniscus blocks the rotator mechanism, rupture of the cruciates with its concomitant capsular weakness results in loss of control of helical movement. Normally, the figure-of-eight mechanism keeps the tibia on a well-defined track on the medial condyle of the femur until it has wound itself to stability in full extension. Loss of control by rupture of the cruciates and the medial capsule results in a type of instability whereby the tibia leaves the curved track and slides straight forward from the medial condyle of the femur. This weakness, or anteroposterior glide, has become the standard test for cruciate ligament injury. However, in any such knee, if the tibia is first rotated outward to its full extent on the femur, i.e., if it is screwed home, anteroposterior glide can no longer be elicited.

Stabilization by external rotation of the leg may be demonstrated by the patient. Before weight-bearing, the foot is placed on the ground in lateral rotation. This means that the whole limb from the hip downward is turned outward. While the leg is straight-ened as weight is taken, the knee may be stabilized by turning the femur medially on the tibia (Fig. 6-33). Mitchell (quoted in Helfet[2]) reported one patient who, after 5 months of stumbling and falling, was ready for operation but refused further treatment when he discovered this trick movement. Stabilization by this method may be confirmed clinically on most patients.

Another observation is of clinical interest. When rupture of the cruciates is accompanied by displacement of a semilunar cartilage, anteroposterior glide may be elicited, but complete passive external rotation of the tibia is not possible. In this instance, treatment demands removal of the cartilage as well as the extra-articular tendon transposition.

Mechanism of Injury

When the helical element in movement of the knee joint is forcibly prevented, the rotator mechanism is disturbed. When the force is no more than the weight of the body, as in household and most athletic injuries, the semilunar cartilages seem to be

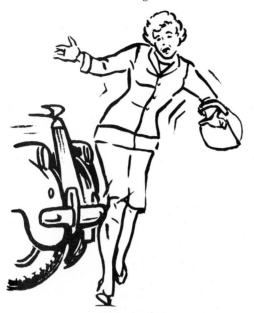

FIG. 6-34. When the foot is caught and the rest of the body is thrown violently! This accident caused rupture of the medial and the cruciate ligaments.

able to take the brunt. More violence is needed to disrupt the cruciate ligaments, for the capsule must be torn and the tibia must actually be wrenched away from the femur, i.e., the disruption is part of a subluxation or dislocation of the knee joint. This has happened to patients in heavy tackles at football, in a motor accident when the foot is caught and the rest of the body is thrown violently (Fig. 6-34), in a fall from a ladder when one foot was impeded or temporarily caught and in an awkward fall from a height when the patient landed with one leg twisted under the body.

Over a period of time the locked knee may stretch, but cannot rupture, the anterior cruciate ligament. The cruciates, as is proper for guide ropes, are at even tension at all phases of normal *active* movement of the knee. However, when the synchrony of outward rotation with extension is obstructed by a displaced meniscus, the cruciate ligament is tensed over the intercondylar edge of the medial femoral condyle (see Fig. 1-21). In the course of time extension is recovered at the expense of stretching

the cruciates and the capsule. Mild antero-posterior and general laxity develop. At operation the anterior cruciate shows the localized area of irritation with a corresponding area of erosion of articular cartilage on the affected edge of the femoral condyle (Fig. 6-18). The suggestion sometimes made that this is related to osteochondritis dissecans is unfounded. It is due to superficial traumatic erosion, and the pattern is etched in exactly the same way as other specific patterns of traumatic arthritis elsewhere in the knee and in other joints.

TEARS OF THE LATERAL LIGAMENTS

The capsular and the cruciate ligaments have been joined under the same heading in this chapter, for rupture of one or the other lateral ligament and adjacent parts of the capsule are components of the same traumatic incident that may cause weakness and profound instability of the knee joint. On the other hand, the lateral ligaments may be injured independently of rupture of the cruciates (Fig. 6-35). Sprains of the medial or

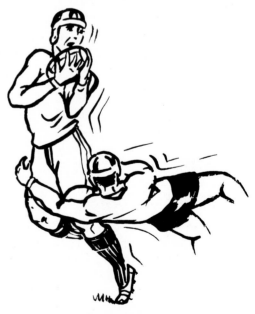

FIG. 6-35. Violent abduction or adduction injuries with the leg straight produce ruptures of the medial or the lateral ligaments.

the lateral capsule may follow twists of the knee, but ruptures of the ligaments are the result, in most instances, of violent abduction or adduction forces on the extended leg. Usually the nature of the injury is detachment of the ligament from its insertion to the tibia, the fibula, or the femur, sometimes with a flake of bone. Not infrequently rupture of the lateral ligament is accompanied by injury to the lateral popliteal nerve.

SPRAINS OF THE CAPSULAR LIGAMENTS

Abnormal strain on the knee joint from any direction may injure the capsular ligaments. As with all tissues that embody elastic elements, damage occurs at the attachments, i.e., where the elastic fibers join a less yielding structure. In the knee joint this implies the attachments of the capsule to bone and of the medial meniscus to the medial ligament. The term sprain includes many gradations of partial rupture of ligaments, but the exact distinction between rupture and sprain has not been clearly defined. For the purposes of this monograph the distinction will be clinical, viz., if passive stretching produces pain before or at the normal limit of any angled movement of the joint, the diagnosis will be that of sprain. If the extreme range or more is reached before discomfort is felt, the ligament has ruptured. Difficulties arise when both conditions are present, e.g., the medial ligament may be avulsed from the tibia while the adjacent capsular attachments are strained. Passive movement produces pain before instability is detected. When there is doubt, it becomes necessary to test the stability of the knee joint under local or general anesthetic. Arthrography by x-rays after the injection of contrast media is helpful in diagnosis. See Chapter 16.

Abduction, adduction and *hyperextension* sprains occur frequently. Pain, tenderness and swelling are maximal at, and usually localized to, the affected attachment to bone. Sprains of the fibular attachment of the

lateral ligament usually are associated with injury of similar severity to the insertion of the biceps.

Rotation Sprains

A rotational element complicates most strains, but the most obvious is probably the strain between the deep portion of the medial ligament and the medial meniscus. Differentiation clinically from the torn meniscus may be difficult unless the semilunar is displaced. Maximal swelling and tenderness is located *over* the midpoint of the meniscus (see Figs. 7-5 and 7-6).

Rotation Sprains of the Medial Semilunar Cartilage

W. Rowley Bristow in the 1930's described certain skiing injuries as "rotation sprain of the medial semilunar cartilage."[1,6] The clinical features are indistinguishable from those of a classic meniscus rupture. Injury is followed by locking and swelling of the knee joint. At operation the only

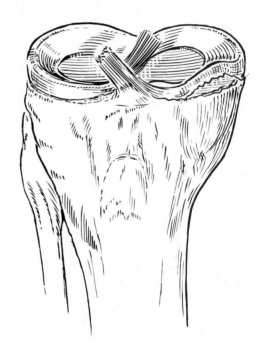

Fig. 6-36. Rupture of the coronary ligaments of the anterior half of the meniscus—a rotation sprain of the medial semilunar cartilage (see text).

lesion found is hemorrhagic suffusion of the coronary attachments of the medial meniscus to the tibia. It is probable that this is the repair stage after rupture of these vascular structures. The cartilage has been momentarily displaced but, because of the vascularity of the site of rupture, is able to heal (Fig. 6-36).

ACUTE DISLOCATION OF THE PATELLA

It is difficult to visualize the mechanism of traumatic dislocation of the patella in the normally-formed and -powered knee when it occurs without disruption of the medial ligament. Personal experience and the histories of patients suggest that it results from severe abduction-flexion force on the fully extended knee while the foot is fixed and the quadriceps are fully contracted, e.g., a tackle obliquely from behind on the rigid knee, while in the act of kicking a football

with the other leg (Fig. 6-37). In another instance, a forward was fully extended in the scrimmage when another player dived into his knee from the side and slightly behind. In both cases the quadriceps were powerfully contracted and the knee held straight when struck by a violent force into abduction and flexion.

George Dommisse, of the Pretoria General Hospital, and the author operated on the knee of a footballer who had suffered traumatic dislocation 2 days previously. Under the anesthetic, with the muscles relaxed, the patella was lax enough to be semiluxated to the outer side. The lesions in the fibrous capsule comprised a long vertical split immediately anterior to the medial ligament and a shorter split near the patella (Fig. 6-38). The synovium reproduced these lesions by a longitudinal parapatellar split the same length as the patella

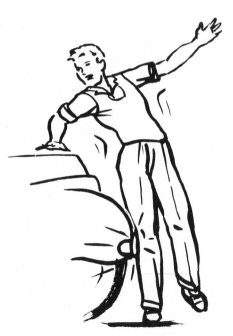

FIG. 6-37. This man's full weight is on the right leg with quadriceps braced. A pure abduction force would rupture the medial ligament. If he rotates his body and right thigh away from the car, he may dislocate the patella.

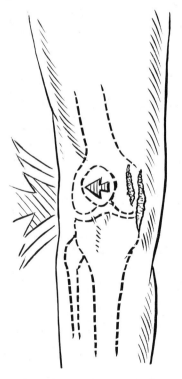

FIG. 6-38. The patella dislocates by virtue of vertical splits in the synovium and the medial capsule (see plate 6-2).

Plate 6-1. Lesions of semilunar cartilage.

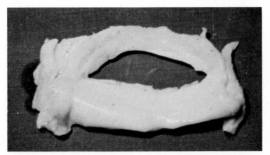

(A) A bow-string meniscus.

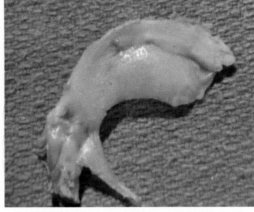

(B) Tear of the posterior horn

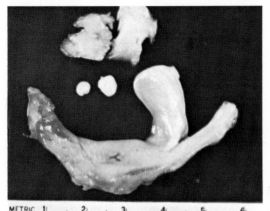

(C) Pedicled tear of posterior horn with loose bodies, fragments of abraded articular cartilage.

(D) A Peripheral tear of a discoid meniscus.

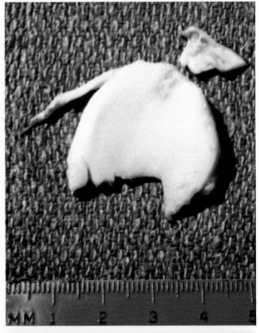

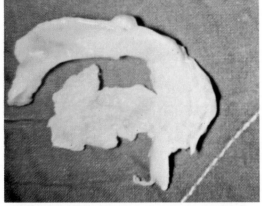

(E) Bow string tear of a discoid meniscus.

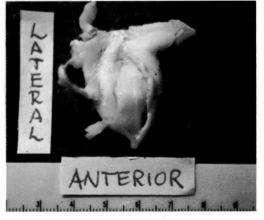

(F) Multiple ruptures in a discoid meniscus.

Plate 6-1. Lesions of semilunar cartilage.
(Continued)

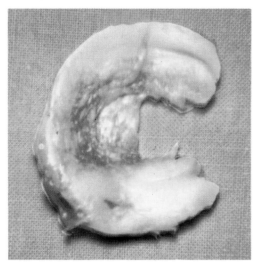

(G) Deplaced horizontal tear in a lateral meniscus.

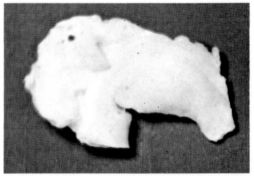

(H) Cyst of a medial meniscus.

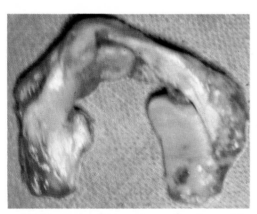

(J) Long standing rupture of a bow string meniscus with retraction.

(I) Cyst of a lateral meniscus.

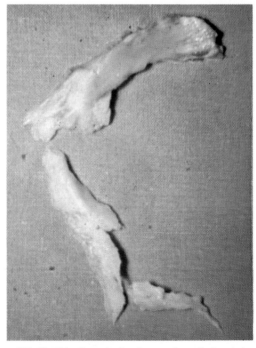

(L) Residual posterior horn of medial meniscus and regenerated anterior horn.

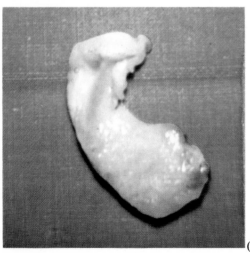

(K) Separated retracted meniscus.

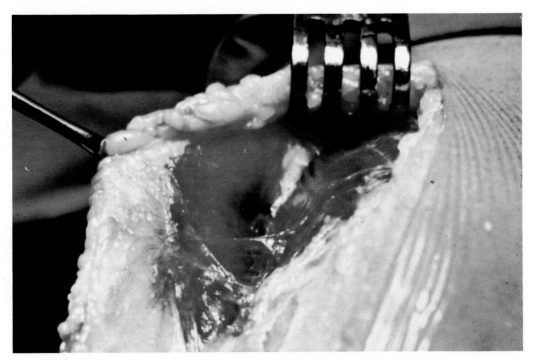

Plate 6-2. Vertical tear of the medial capsule in acute dislocation of the patella.

and a much longer vertical tear just anterior to the synovial reflexion, half way back in the joint. As soon as the synovium was sutured, the patella was harnessed and could no longer be moved out of the trochlear groove. Suture of the capsule reinforced the stability. In another case a 16-year-old girl suffered an abduction and rotation strain on the weight-bearing *fully extended* leg. The foot was fixed by weight-bearing, and the femur rotated fiercely medially on the tibia. Again at operation a vertical split in both synovium and capsule was found—in this case only one. Before suture the patella was easily displaceable, but repair brought complete stability.

When the quadriceps are contracted, the patella is at the limit of its upward excursion and at the level where the trochlear surface of the femur is shallowest. The vertical splits in the capsule permit the lateral shift.

RECURRENT DISLOCATION OF THE PATELLA

For many years the etiology of recurrent dislocation has stimulated considerable speculation, some of it confused. Because of the confusion a multitude of reconstructive operations have been devised and nearly as many discarded.

Since the realization that acute dislocation is accompanied by vertical splitting of the medial capsule, the role played by trauma has emerged more clearly. Any cause of transverse as opposed to longitudinal weakness of the medial capsule predisposes to further dislocations or subluxations of the patella. And a traumatic basis should be sought in any case in which the primary incident takes place in teenagers or adults. Careful questioning of patients in these age groups usually elicits a history that significant injury caused the first derangement and that minor but still abnormal strains were responsible for subsequent dislocations. This differs from the history of a knee with a congenital weakness in which the first incident occurs in childhood and recurrences are

associated habitually with specific and otherwise normal movements. For example, habitual dislocation may and often does occur on flexion of the knee, whereas post-traumatic recurring dislocation would occur when the knee is extending and is near or at full extension.

On closer examination we find that the same torsion injury that results in a derangement of the meniscus when the knee is *flexing* leads to dislocation of the patella when the knee is *extending*. For example, the footballer who through catching his toe causes external rotation of the tibia while the knee is falling into flexion, ruptures the meniscus—flexion without synchronous internal rotation of the tibia. On the other hand, in one authenticated instance a footballer caught his toe, causing increased external rotation of the tibia while his leg was straightening to kick. He suffered his second dislocation of the patella. On the first occasion his leg was powerfully and fully extended while pushing in the scrimmage. Another player hurtled into the scrimmage, striking his knee from the side and slightly behind. The patella dislocated. He was treated conservatively and presumably remained with a weakened medial capsule.

In the second incident the contracting quadriceps had elevated the patella into the shallowest part of the trochlear groove where the asynchronous and advanced lateral rotation of the tibial tubercle flicked the patella into malalignment over the lateral edge.

This introduces another consideration. Congenital foreshortening of the trochlear groove of the femur would be as conducive to dislocation of the patella as a shallow lateral slope (see Chap. 16 and Fig. 16-17).

In any event, treatment will be more certain and assessment of results of treatment more realistic if congenital or habitual dislocation were clearly distinguished from recurrent dislocation of traumatic origin, with which we are primarily concerned. In the former, the congenital abnormality must be treated, whereas the latter requires repair or reinforcement of the medial capsule. Failure is usually not the fault of the operation; it occurs because the particular operation is inappropriate.

SUPERIOR TIBIOFIBULAR JOINT

As instability and even osteoarthritis of the superior tibiofibular joint do not always incapacitate the patient, it has suffered clinical and literary neglect. Although material disability is rare, three patients suffered much distress, and their symptoms presented problems of diagnosis.

A staff nurse was running on wet sand when someone from behind flicked a towel around her left ankle. She stumbled and fell. Her recollection of the incident was uncertain, but she thought that her ankle had twisted before she fell forward onto her knee, which was almost fully flexed. Later that day she was able to walk and run, but during the evening the anterolateral part of the knee, the calf and the lower thigh became painful and swollen. She was forced to stay in bed for 3 days, by which time bruising from the superior tibiofibular joint downward had developed in the leg.

She suffered persistent disability. A year later, when examined for the first time, the superior tibiofibular joint was unstable. Although the maneuver was painful, the joint could be subluxated passively.

The violently twisting foot requires increased accommodation for equinovarus movement of the talus in the ankle mortise. When the knee bears weight, and/or is falling, this is provided by movement of the fibula on the tibia at their two articulations. If torque is excessive, diastasis of the lower tibiofibular or, less frequently, displacement of the superior tibiofibular joint takes place. Operative exploration revealed disruption of the anterior fibers of the capsule.

The second patient was a farmer who had injured his knee falling off a horse 5 years previously. Mistaken diagnosis had led to removal of the meniscus a year later, without relief. After 5 years the subluxating head of the fibula had eroded the joint sur-faces, and cystic degeneration from the torn capsular tissues was present.

In both patients tenderness from strain was present in the tendinous insertion of the biceps, and among other symptoms both complained of discomfort in the ankle on walking.

The third patient was a 23-year-old medical student who fractured the lower ends of the right tibia and fibula in 1959. The fractures healed in perfect position, but subsequently she suffered swelling of the ankle after standing. In December, 1961, she assisted at four operations, and increased swelling and discomfort eventuated. Next morning as she climbed out of bed she felt sharp pain in the right calf. She had to walk on her toes. Later pain was referred also up the right thigh. Although no veins were palpable, thrombosis of the deep veins was diagnosed. Anticoagulants and an elastic stocking gave no relief, and any period of standing resulted in intolerable discomfort. She despaired of continuing her interest in surgery.

On examination in April, 1962, the superior tibiofibular joint was tender. Rocking the head of the fibula firmly reproduced her pattern of pain. She could not take weight on the outer border of the right foot without pain, nor could she flex the knee and the ankle while taking full weight on the foot. Injection of procaine into the joint gave immediate though temporary relief. She has since been given three injections of procaine mixed with 25.0 mg. of prednisolone into the joint and gentle physiotherapy. Each injection has been followed by 3 or 4 weeks of comfort in spite of full activity before lesser symptoms on prolonged standing reappear. It may be necessary in due course to excise or arthrodese this joint.

Since publication of these observations in Management of Internal Derangements of the Knee in 1963 we have realized that *neither sprain nor frank derangement of the superior tibiofibular joint is uncommon.* Only in blatant dislocations, a rare disorder, is the diagnosis easily made. Often there has been associated major trauma to the foot or

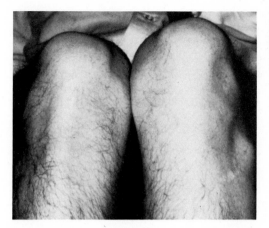

FIG. 6-39. Prominence of the head of the left fibula.

leg, and the injury to the small joint is overlooked. Physical impairment from injury is usually not dramatic, but symptoms are grumbling and persistent and are often mistaken for injury to the lateral meniscus or to thrombophlebitis. Some of our patients had undergone previous lateral meniscectomy or treatment for thrombophlebitis without benefit.

Clinical Picture

The presenting symptom is pain in the lateral aspect of the knee, the posterior aspect of the calf, or both. The patient is comfortable at rest. Pain develops with such activities as walking at a brisk pace, running, weight bearing on a semi-flexed knee or in actions which require full dorsiflexion of the ankle.

On examination tenderness is felt over the superior tibiofibular joint and at the insertion of the biceps femoris to the head of the fibula. Rocking the head of the fibula with the knee flexed, full dorsiflexion of the ankle, and walking with toe-in gait are all painful. Taking weight on the partially flexed knee or forceful contraction of the biceps femoris against resistance produces the characteristic symptoms. There may be prominence of the head of the fibula (Fig. 6-39). Knee movement itself is full and painless. Involvement of the peroneal nerve may be present when the joint has been dislocated. The lesion may be a simple sprain

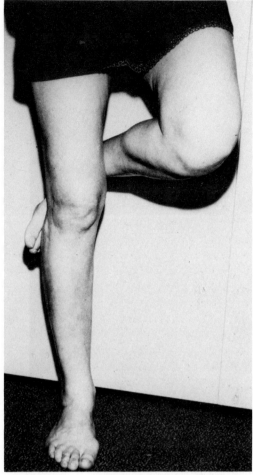

FIG. 6-40. Test for derangement or instability of the superior tibiofibular joint. (Helfet, A. J.: AAOS Instructional Course Lectures. vol. 19. St. Louis, C. V. Mosby, 1970)

or complete luxation. X-ray examination may show no change or occasionally evidence of joint irregularity or deformity of the head of the fibula. Taking an oblique view of the knee is most helpful in displaying the joint.

The importance of the superior tibiofibular joint in bearing body weight while the knee is flexed (see p. 3) provides a new diagnostic clinical test.[3]

If the patient with unstable joint is asked to flex the knee while bearing weight solely on the affected leg it will give way if he or she does not stabilize the leg with the opposite foot (Fig. 6-40). On the other hand

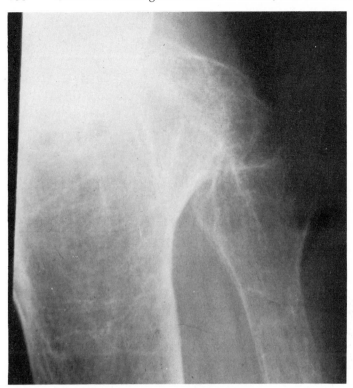

Fɪɢ. 6-41. Rheumatoid arthritis of the superior tibiofibular joint.

if the joint is arthritic or sprained he will find the test too painful to continue. Injection of 1 per cent solution of local anesthetic and 25 mgms. of hydrocortisone preparation into the joint provides instant relief of the painful symptoms and as this may last for a time gives an excellent therapeutic test in all but the unstable joint.

The most frequent cause of derangement is indirect trauma, the ankle being primarily involved. In our series, traumatic arthritis, rheumatoid arthritis and exostosis of the head of the fibula (Figs. 6-41 and 6-42) have also been a cause of the syndrome. Luxation of the joint has been reported among parachute injuries.

SUMMARY

1. Simple abduction or adduction force on the extended knee results in rupture of the medial or the lateral ligament, respectively (Fig. 6-35).

2. Forcible prevention of synchrony of medial rotation of the tibia when flexing and of lateral rotation when extending the knee produces rupture of a semilunar cartilage (Fig. 6-1).

3. The combination of (1) and (2) or either alone, with sufficient additional force to wrench the tibia away from the femur, results in disruption of the cruciate ligaments and capsule with or without concomitant rupture of a semilunar cartilage. It is interesting to note that when the cartilage is damaged the damage is usually of the "retracted" and not the "bowstring" variety, i.e., it has been wrenched away from its mooring to the cruciate ligaments and not split in its substance (Fig. 6-34).

4. Violent abduction and medial rotation of the thigh on the fixed tibia while the quadriceps are fully tensed may cause dislocation of the patella.

5. A twist of the ankle which cannot be accommodated by the falling knee may subluxate or strain the superior tibiofibular joint.

Fig. 6-42. Anteroposterior and lateral views of exostosis of the head of the fibula distracting the joint.

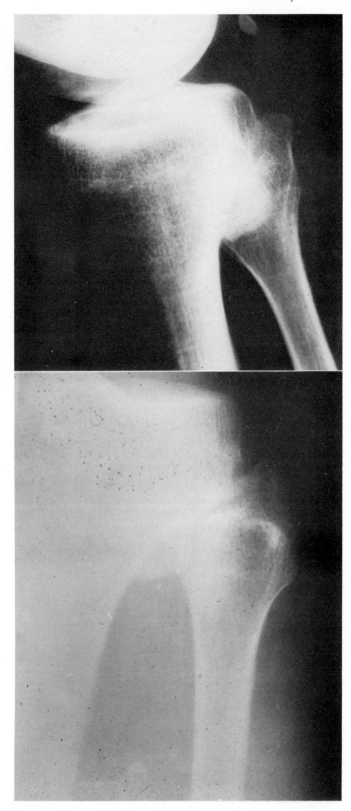

REFERENCES

1. Bristow, W. R.: Internal derangements of the knee joint. J. Bone Joint Surg., *17*:605, 1935.
2. Helfet, A. J.: Function of the cruciate ligaments of knee joint. Lancet, *1*:665, 1948.
3. ———: Diagnosis of internal derangements of the knee. AAOS Instructional Course Lectures. Vol. XIX. St. Louis, C. V. Mosby, 1970.
4. ———: Osteoarthritis of the knee and its early arrest. AAOS Instructional Course Lectures. Vol. XX. St. Louis, C. V. Mosby, 1971.
5. Jones, Sir Robert: Notes on derangements of the knee. Ann. Surg., *50*:969, 1909.
6. Platt, Sir Harry: Report 3rd Congress, Société Internationale de Chirurgie Orthopédique. 1936.
7. Smillie, I. S.: Injuries of the Knee Joint. Baltimore, Williams & Wilkins, 1970.

7

Clinical Features of Injuries to the Semilunar Cartilages

Arthur J. Helfet, M.D.

ONSET

An injury severe enough to damage the rotator mechanism of the knee joint must cause pain and swelling, but the quality and the severity of both vary considerably. The footballer who displaces a meniscus suffers immediate agony. He cannot straighten the knee and adamantly refuses to place weight on the limb. Once the knee is supported and at rest the pain eases. Should the cartilage not displace or not remain displaced, or be split at the back end only, the acute distress passes in minutes. The player limps but can walk and may even continue in the game. A posterior tear may signify its nature when the knee gives way, not necessarily very painfully, later in the game. This is one explanation of the situation in which a player whose knee is hurt continues after attention, only to leave the field following a second incident. Another explanation is that the cartilage is hurt in the first but displaced only in the second misadventure. In general, the injured players who remain on the field either have not displaced the meniscus or have torn only its posterior end.

The "retracted" cartilage provides a contrast to this acute onset, especially in middle-aged and older people in whom the trauma need be only minor in character. A twist while on bended knees, or a stumble, causes a stab of pain. When the knee is straightened, vague temporary discomfort remains. The whole incident is so brief that 3 weeks or more later the original mild accident is remembered with difficulty or dismissed as "I had a slight sprain only." In these cases the anterior end of the meniscus, usually the medial, is pulled off its mooring to the anterior cruciate. The cartilage retracts and, perhaps because the distraction is gentle, causes little pain. A similar reaction may follow complete rupture of ligaments or tendons. Sprains and partial tears cause much more pain than complete division, which is often relatively painless.

Mention must be made, though, of the acute reaction of the middle-aged knee to a transverse tear at the junction of the anterior two thirds and the posterior third of the medial meniscus. Often the patient has suffered for some time from recurring effusions, grumbling pain and limp, which have been diagnosed as osteoarthritis but usually have been due to a retracted anterior horn. Suddenly, after another, often minor injury, a transverse fracture has occurred, and the knee is acutely painful, swollen, partly flexed, and unable to bear weight. The severe and distressing disablement of the knee is due to displacement of part of the torn meniscus which "locks" the joint.

Synovial effusion, not unduly hemorrhagic if the split is in the avascular substance of the cartilage, will increase slowly and reach its maximum during the night—"when the joint became cold." Then, declares the patient, the knee, even at rest, is stiffer and more painful.

If the vascular structures of the joint are torn, frank hemarthrosis develops rapidly.

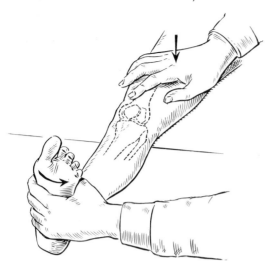

Fig. 7-1. Forced passive extension produces fingerpoint pain over the site of injury in the anteromedial or the anterolateral compartment of the joint.

The knee swells urgently and is much more painful than it is when a slow, simple effusion is present. The usual tests for fluid elicit signs of a tensely distended, very tender joint that is "rubbery" to the touch, in contrast to the softer, much less tender impression given by the simple effusion.

RESTRICTION OF MOVEMENT

Tears and displacements of the semilunar cartilages affect the smooth action of the rotator mechanism of the knee, and the presence of injury is signified in every instance by inability to rotate the tibia to its full extent and, therefore, to extend or flex the knee completely.

Lesions of the anterior half or more of either meniscus block lateral rotation and extension. To call it "locking" of the joint is inaccurate because only these movements are prevented. Flexion and medial rotation are unaffected and give comfort to the injured knee. The retracted cartilage causes the same limitations of movement but is not so painful. Since the anterior cruciate ligament exerts its guiding action on the tibia in part through the medial cartilage, it would seem reasonable to suppose that anterior

detachment of the cartilage would impair this function and leave the tibia unable to complete its normal excursion. But this cannot be so, for after excision of the torn cartilage the quadriceps regains full control of the range of rotation of the tibia and, incidentally, of extension as well. The cartilage is an accessory factor in the rotator mechanism. The abnormal cartilage disturbs function, but, when it has been excised, the knee can compensate for its absence.*

It appears that any increase in volume of the contents of the anteromedial compartment of- the knee prevents full lateral rotation of the tibia. This can be demonstrated experimentally at operation. Through the usual medial incision with the knee bent over the end of the table, the lateral rotation of the tibia during extension shows very well. If one puts a sterile rubber catheter across the medial joint space, the tibia cannot rotate fully. The reaction to the anterior tear is a blocking of movement by the "heaping-up" of the retracted cartilage.

Similarly, displacement of the posterior horn of the semilunar cartilage blocks full medial rotation of the tibia, and it is impossible to flex the knee completely. Attempts to force these movements cause pain, whereas full lateral rotation and extension of the knee is possible but painless.

The bowstring cartilage blocks extension and lateral rotation, and, if the split extends far enough back, flexion and medial rotation also are affected. It is usually the most painful type of cartilage tear, but, fortunately, is not always complicated by severe hemarthrosis.

---

* Sir Robert Jones commented on this point in the appendix to Timbrell Fisher's monograph[7]: "The question, What is the use of the semilunar cartilages? is a fundamental one. Whatever the conclusion to which we arrive, there is no doubt that men can perform the most arduous and expert acts with their joints after removal of the cartilages and without ill effects. I removed the semilunar cartilage in no less than six members of the same International football team. In one case, in which both cartilages were removed, he played through the season without a breakdown."

The extent of restriction of movement from a displaced or deformed meniscus is, within narrow limits, always the same for only rotation is blocked directly. Limitation of extension is usually some 5 degrees and at most, 10, and the same applies to flexion. This is understandable. If the knee was a hinge joint the block to movement would

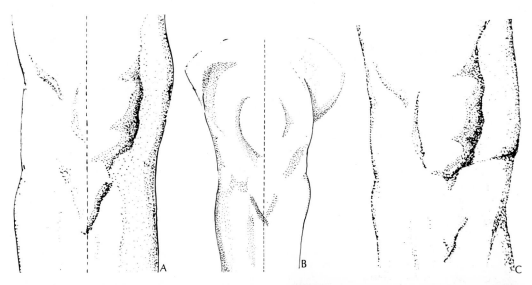

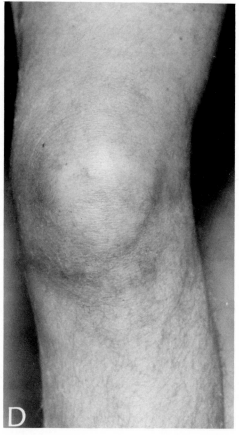

FIG. 7-2. (*A*) When the normal knee is straightened, the tibial tubercle rotates laterally into alignment with the outer half of the patella. (*B*) As the knee flexes the tubercle rotates medially toward the central axis. (*C*) When blocked by a deranged meniscus, the tibial tubercle of the extending knee cannot rotate beyond the central axis of the patella. The medial femoral condyle protrudes over the margin of the tibia. (*D*) the protrusion of the medial femoral condyle and the blocked rotation of the tibial tubercle are obvious in this knee with a retracted medial cartilage. (Helfet, A. J.: J. Bone Joint Surg., *41B*:319, 1959)

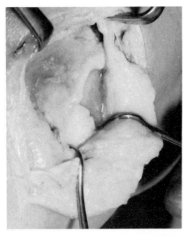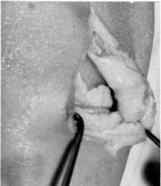

FIG. 7-3. (*Left*) The femoral condyle protrudes over the margin of the tibia when the knee is extended. The lower hook grips retracted meniscus. Note the heaping up of articular cartilage on the presenting surface of the femur. The area of erosion is in relation to the meniscus. (*Right*) After removal of the meniscus the margins of femoral condyle and tibia realign when the knee is extended.

be exactly proportional to the size and site of the obstruction, whereas any change in the volume between the articulating surfaces of a helix prevents rotation and converts the joint into a "condyloid joint," with its own range of movement in one plane. This is one of the reasons for limited movement obtained in the current fashion of knee replacements in which the helix is replaced by condyloid joint action.

Rotation Signs

The blocking of rotation gives us the following clinical signs, which are pathognomonic of injury to the cartilages:

1. When the anterior half of the meniscus is deranged, forced passive extension produces finger-point pain over the site of injury in the anteromedial or the anterolateral compartment of the joint. The patient can pinpoint the pain (Figs. 7-1; 7-4).

2. Any attempt to force the final degree of lateral rotation may cause pain localized to the same spot. Flexion and medial rotation of the knee are not affected and, indeed, give the patient comfort. This statement needs a word of qualification: if the effusion in the knee is tense, flexion is limited and painful because of the distention of the capsule as a whole, and if the split in the bowstring cartilage extends to the posterior compartment, the final degrees of flexion and medial rotation may be obstructed also.

3. Forced passive flexion and internal rotation produce finger-point pain in the posteromedial or the posterolateral compartments of the joint when the posterior horn of the meniscus is at fault. If only the posterior end of a cartilage has been injured, extension and lateral rotation are free and painless. The importance of the finger-point pain is readily understandable, as it indicates the site of injury of the cartilage.

4. Two additional signs are associated with anterior lesions. Compared with the normal knee, the outward excursion of the tibial tubercle is limited. When the normal knee is straightened, the tibial tubercle reaches the line of the lateral border of the patella. The tibial tubercle of the injured knee reaches approximately to the central axis of the patella (Fig. 7-2; see also Chap. 3).

5. The final screw-home of the knee in completing extension aligns the borders of the medial femoral condyle and the adjacent tibia exactly. When the screw-home is prevented by an injured cartilage, the femoral condyle is left protruding over the margin of the tibia. Unless the knee is very swollen, this is obvious to the eye (Figs. 7-2 and 7-3). In any case, it can be detected by palpation. If the examining finger follows the subcutaneous surface of the tibia upward, it will, when it reaches the knee, be obstructed by the protruding medial condyle of the femur, a feature that may be confirmed by com-

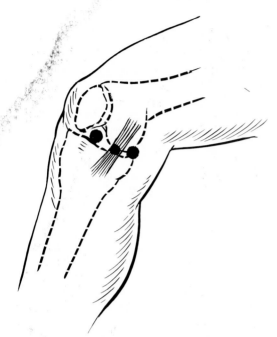
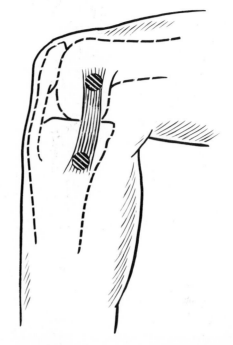

FIG. 7-4. Sites of fingerpoint tenderness associated with injuries to the medial meniscus are (*from left*) the anterior horn, attachment to the medial ligament, and the posterior horn.

parison with the normal knee. The protrusion is most obvious in the knee in which arthritic changes have become established.

At operation for a torn medial cartilage, these signs may be confirmed. After opening the joint through a medial incision, straighten the knee. The medial femoral condyle overlaps the tibial margin. Remove the cartilage and straighten the knee again. Complete extension is obtained, and the femur and the tibia are in perfect rotational alignment (Fig. 7-3).

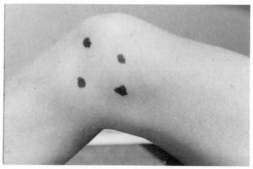

FIG. 7-5. (*Top*) Areas of tenderness from medial ligament sprains or tears are always at the attachment of the ligament to bone. The injured cartilage is tender fore and aft along the joint line. (*Bottom*) The knee in the photo is marked to show areas of tenderness from medial ligament or meniscal injuries.

TENDERNESS

Following injury the whole cartilage may be sensitive, but after a while the retracted cartilage will be tender in the anterior compartment, and the cartilage with a posterior tear, in the posterior compartment (Figs. 7-4 and 7-5). The complete bowstring cartilage may be tender at both ends. In the case of an untreated tear, tenderness subsequently develops in two other areas. The retracted cartilage, by virtue of its increase in bulk in the anterior compartment, gradually erodes an area of weight-bearing articular cartilage on the medial femoral condyle. The spot is adjacent to the area of condyle that protrudes over the tibia and is most easily located when the knee is flexed. The other site of tenderness is the medial border of the patella and the adjacent medial slope

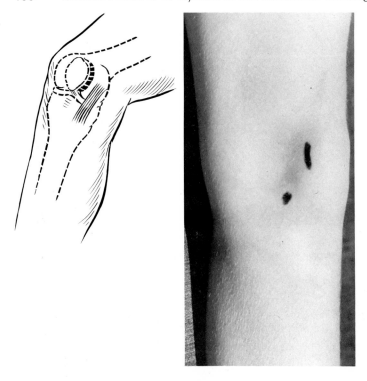

FIG. 7-6. (*Left*) The other site of tenderness is the medial border of the patella and the adjacent medial slope of the trochlear surface of the femur. (*Right*) The knee is marked to show areas of tenderness from the anterior horn of the medial meniscus and the medial border of the patella.

of the trochlear surface of the femur (Fig. 7-6); it is caused by injury to articular cartilage from undue tension between these surfaces of the patella and the femur.

Except in the case of the retracted cartilage, most injuries of the medial meniscus are accompanied by strain of the attachment of the deep fibers of the medial collateral ligament, and, therefore, there is tenderness over this point in the joint line (Fig. 7-5). Frank strains and rupture of the medial ligament itself occur at the upper or the lower insertion to bone with corresponding local tenderness (Fig. 7-5).

DIAGNOSTIC CLICKS

Maneuvers that elicit a click from an abnormal or displaced meniscus are useful aids in diagnosis. The well-established tests described by McMurray,[5] Fouche[2] and Apley[1] use the principle of rotation of the flexed knee with added compression or adduction or abduction to show up instability or displacement of a fragment of the *posterior half* of the cartilage. However, there are two other clicks that may be elicited and have diagnostic significance.

1. There is what may be called the *reducing* click, though sometimes the click signals displacement of the cartilage. The patient has an injured knee with positive rotation signs, limited lateral rotation of the tibial tubercle, prominence of the medial femoral condyle in extension and finger-point pain on forced extension. Flex the relaxed knee passively, and forcibly rotate it medially and laterally (Fig. 7-7). Suddenly, with a click, lateral rotation is freed. It is possible now to extend the knee fully, and the rotation signs are negative. The reduction often is felt by the patient as well as the surgeon. If rotation alone will not free the cartilage, extension with external rotation, or a kick by the patient into full extension, may do so (see Fig. 11-3). Sometimes it is possible to displace the cartilage by the opposite maneuver. Flex the knee passively while resisting medial rotation or extend it while resisting lateral rotation of the tibia. Again, there is a click, and the rotation signs reappear.

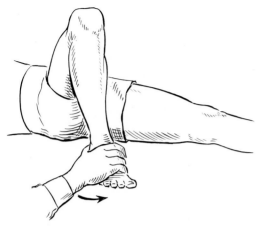

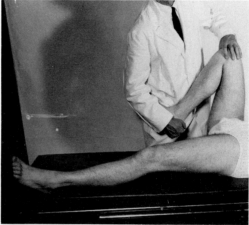

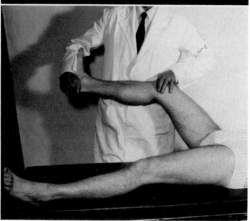

FIG. 7-7. Flex the relaxed knee passively and forcibly rotate it medially and laterally.

These reducing and displacing signs are present in *unstable* tears of four kinds—posterior horn, incomplete longitudinal, oblique pedicled tears of the inner margin and the retracted medial meniscus in youngish people in whom the structure is still reasonably resilient. It forms the basis of the manipulation for reduction of the displaced cartilage described on page 152.

2. This click is similar to the heavy thud felt over the congenital discoid cartilage. It is like the sensation of a wheel going over a bump. It is not felt often. A thickening in the meniscus is the cause, e.g., when a tag is folded back on the cartilage, or when the retracted cartilage shortens by becoming thicker fore and aft.

THE McMURRAY CLICKS

The late Professor McMurray described the maneuver to elicit his sign:

In making the examination the patient must be recumbent and relaxed, the surgeon standing at the side of the injured limb; he grasps the foot firmly and the knee is bent completely so that the heel approaches or touches the buttock. The foot is now rotated externally and the leg abducted at the knee whilst the joint is slowly extended [Fig. 7-8]. With the alteration of the angle of the joint any loose portion of the internal semilunar cartilage is caught between the femur and tibia, and the sliding of the femur

FIG. 7-8. The maneuvers to elicit the "McMurray click." (*Top*) The heel is gripped firmly in the surgeon's hand while the foot is held between the forearm and the side. After complete flexion of the knee, the foot is rotated externally and the leg rotated externally. (*Bottom*) Maintaining external rotation of the foot, the joint is extended slowly.

over the abnormal portion of cartilage is accompanied by a definite click and pain, which the patient states is similar to the feeling experienced each time the knee gives way. The angle at which this occurs gives the position of the cartilaginous lesion, and, if the maneuver is correctly followed out, the absence of such a click is a definite indication of the absence of any lesion in the posterior or middle portion of the cartilage.

It is difficult to maneuver the leg of a sturdy or heavy patient at the end of the forearm, but the task is facilitated by holding the foot against the examiner's side as shown in Figures 7-8 and 7-9. Movements

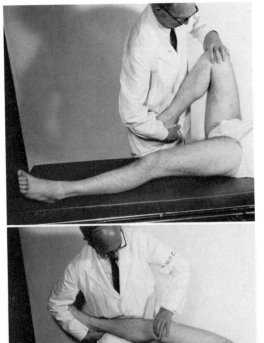

FIG. 7-9. Sometimes a positive click is obtained by the opposite maneuver. (*Top*) Rotating the foot internally and (*bottom*) adducting at the knee while slowly extending the joint.

then are controlled by the examiner's trunk.[3]

Sometimes a positive click is obtained by the opposite maneuver—rotating the foot internally and adducting at the knee while the joint is extended slowly (Fig. 7-9).

THE APLEY GRINDING AND DISTRACTION TESTS

With the patient lying on his face, the knee is flexed to 90 degrees and rotated while a compression force is applied; this, the grinding test, reproduces symptoms if a meniscus is torn. Rotation is repeated then while the leg is pulled upward with the surgeon's knee holding the thigh down; this,

the distraction test, produces increased pain only if there is ligament damage (Fig. 7-10).[1]

These *clicks* all are elicited by the examiner's fingers placed along the joint line and are usually palpable and only occasionally audible as well.

A click (especially if it produces in the patient the sensation of instability) is invaluable in placing the site of the lesion. On the other hand, failure to demonstrate a click does not always exclude a tear, for the sign may not be elicited unless the torn fragment is displaced. Nor will it be elicited in a complete bowstringing of the cartilage nor in the knee in which the displacement (such as the retracted anterior horn) has blocked lateral rotation of the tibia. In these instances the "rotation signs" are sufficient to diagnose the lesion and are pathognomonic.

"GIVING WAY" OR BUCKLING OF THE KNEE

The mechanics of this phenomenon are uncertain for we must rely on the patient's interpretation of symptoms. "Giving way" is a symptom of instability and may have one or more of six causes, namely:

1. Derangements of the posterior halves of the semilunar cartilages
2. Disruption of the capsular and/or cruciate ligaments
3. Vertical tears of the posteromedial capsule associated with a torn medial meniscus
4. Recurrent dislocation or subluxation of the patella
5. Instability of the superior tibiofibular joint
6. Weakness of the quadriceps

Any of these may actually cause the knee to give way and the patient to fall and should be distinguished from illusory "giving way," which occurs not infrequently as a symptom of *chronic strain of the medial lateral ligament* or of *adhesion of the fat pad to neighboring fixed structures as is described in Chapter 8.*

The infrapatellar pad of fat is a mobile structure that alters its shape to the changing accommodation in the anterior compartment of the knee joint during flexion and extension. Adhesions limit this movement. Sudden twists of the knee produce a twinge of pain and momentary weakness which the patient may mistake for "giving way," and these symptoms may also occur in chronic strains of the ligaments of the knee especially the medial. The diagnosis is determined by eliciting finger point tenderness and pain in the same place on reproducing the movement that causes the tension. Occasionally

"giving way" may also be simulated by slipping of a tendon such as the semitendinosis over the cancellous exostosis that forms between the hamstrings on the upper medial tibia.

Unstable tears of the posterior horn of the meniscus are a prime cause of giving way. Tears in or a detached anterior half of the medial meniscus are more liable to produce a painful "catch" than giving way. The following type of case illustrates the point: A torn cartilage that did not lead to giving

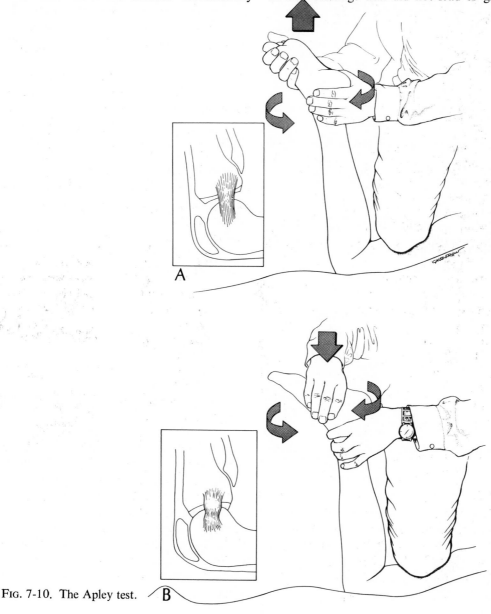

Fig. 7-10. The Apley test.

way before operation is inadequately re-moved. A loose posterior fragment remains. Subsequently, the only or the most trouble-some symptom is "giving way."

Giving way is not necessarily accom-panied by pain. Indeed more often than not, especially in the case of the lateral cartilage, it is painless. Patients describe a sensation similar to buckling when the unsuspecting straight weight-bearing leg is nudged gently from behind. The knee gives way, as far as we can be certain, during flexion. Presuma-bly, the medially rotating tibia loses control when it reaches the irregularity in its path and is precipitated into further flexion. It may be allied to the "reducing click" (p. 112) which, however, is elicited in the non-weight-bearing relaxed knee.

If the knee buckles after the cruciates and a medial or lateral ligament are torn it usually gives way during extension. Nor-mally, the intact rotator mechanism keeps the tibia on a well-defined track on the medial condyle of the femur until it has wound itself to stability in full extension. Loss of control by the cruciates and the medial capsule results in a type of instability in which the tibia leaves the curved track and slides straight forward from the medial condyle of the femur. Patients suffering from this injury find their main disability on slopes and ladders where quadriceps con-traction and control must be at their maxi-mum. This type of "giving way" tends to be painful and distressing.

In the experience of the author, buckling of the knee does not occur from isolated detachments or rupture of the anterior cru-ciate ligament, but only when accompanied by rupture or laxity of capsular ligaments. An isolated detachment of the anterior cru-ciate is detected when operation is necessary for associated disruption, with retraction of the anterior horn of the medial meniscus.

Both the anterior cruciate ligament and the anterior horn of the medial meniscus are pulled off the anterior tibial spine by the same twisting force, but the meniscus is responsible for the resulting symptoms. If the integrity of the capsular ligaments is intact, it is not necessary to replace the anterior cruciate. The stump of the liga-ment may be excised.

Vertical tears of the posteromedial capsule with accompanying rupture of the medial meniscus produces an unusual type of giving way. It seems to occur when the patient is standing and reaches near or full extension of the weight-bearing knee. Apparently, the medial condyle of the femur continues into uncontrolled abnormal internal rotation. The patient describes an odd sensation of weak-ness, often without pain. Excision of the torn meniscus does not cure, for the peculiar buckling continues until the tear is repaired.

Recurrent Dislocation of the Patella. Buckling of the knee due to a ruptured semi-lunar cartilage must also be differentiated from that recorded by the patient suffering from recurring dislocation or subluxation of the patella. The knee is said to give way, but the phenomenon seems to occur, and indeed can only occur, when the weight-bearing leg is straight or nearly straight and while the quadriceps are contracting or con-tracted. Abnormal internal rotation of the femur or external rotation with flexion of the tibia at this point forces the patella to be dislocated laterally out of the trochlear groove. In my experience medial dislocation has not been observed.

The leg gives way, or rather collapses, but the knee is locked in slight flexion. The dis-location is reduced by passively straightening the leg while relaxing the quadriceps. In cases of long standing, the quadriceps may be weak, and when the muscles are relaxed, there is gross laxity of the patella.

Instability of the Superior Tibiofibular Joint. As instability and even osteoarthritis of this joint do not always incapacitate the patient, it has suffered clinical and literary neglect. Although material disability is rare, patients may suffer much distress, and their symptoms present problems in diagnosis.

See Chapters 6 and 16.

Weakness of the Quadriceps. The knee gives way when walking especially down slopes and stairs as the knee flexes beyond a critical angle—this angle depending on the measure of weakness of the quadriceps. It is a common phenomenon in poliomyelitis. To maintain stability the patient has to lock the knee back in hyperextension. It occurs also after surgery on the knee if the patient walks before the power of the quadriceps has been adequately restored. As soon as the knee fatigues, buckling is experienced. This also troubles mountaineers with adequate quadriceps when they are overfatigued by a long and steep descent. Fixed flexion deformity with inability to extend the knee completely as in osteoarthritis, which is usually accompanied by weak quadriceps, aggravates this type of "giving way" and leads to the necessity of a knee brace.

DEVELOPMENT OF TRAUMATIC OSTEOARTHRITIS*

Traumatic osteoarthritis should be considered as a repair reaction after injury or wearing or abrasion of the articular surfaces.[4] As a reaction to the traumatic process, or possibly to the constituents of degenerating cartilage, adjacent bone becomes sclerotic, or patches of aseptic necrosis or small cysts develop. Heaped-up cartilage on the edges of the joint is ossified into osteophytes. The articular cartilage itself first loses its white glisten and tough compressibility or elasticity and becomes yellow, dull, and hard. In the young the cartilage is resilient, but with age it becomes more brittle and less durable, so that an irregularity that might need years to erode the cartilage of youth may do as much in weeks in the elderly.

Articular cartilage, generally considered to be aneural, after a period of abnormal pressure, whether constant or intermittent,

---

* See also Chapter 12.

becomes tender, but the patient does not apparently suffer "bone pain" until the underlying bone has been reached. "Bone pain" is of an aching, boring character, worse at night when the limb is warm. The patient often finds temporary relief by cooling the limb outside the bed clothes.

The clinical reaction to these changes is a knee progressively more susceptible to fatigue and strain. The knee tolerates less and less activity before it aches and swells. The discomfort and swelling is relieved by rest, but as time goes on the necessary rest periods are longer. Until the latest stages, complete rest in bed or by splinting is usually effective in bringing relief. Progress is aggravated by the tendency of the thigh muscles, which act on the joint, to waste and weaken. Fatigue and strain come on sooner. On the other hand, if the muscles are strengthened, the range of activity is improved, and, therefore, building up of muscle power is an important feature in treatment.

THE MECHANISM OF PAIN

It is interesting to establish a pathologic basis for the various sites and types of pain that follow injury to the medial cartilage. The bowstring tear causes immediate and severe pain. The patient cannot take weight on the leg. During the next 2 or 3 weeks the symptoms improve, though forcing the knee straight or turning suddenly are still painful. With time the cruciate ligaments stretch, the patient develops slight anteroposterior laxity, and the knee becomes more comfortable. Each recurrence of the derangement produces less severe symptoms until, finally, the articular cartilage is eroded and the symptoms of "arthritis" develop— namely pain and aching during activity referable mainly to the medial compartment of the knee, aching and swelling after effort, which subside with rest. Later when the patella is involved, increasing pain on descending or ascending stairs, from pressure between the medial border of the patella and the medial trochlear surface of the femur, is the disconcerting symptom.

The injury that causes the "retracted" cartilage produces less pain. The patient may experience a sharp, momentary stab, which is relieved when the twist is corrected. The joint swells, and there may be recurrent stabs of pain on sudden movements. Later, when the articular cartilage is eroded, the more distressing symptoms of arthritis become manifest—pain in the medial compartment of the knee on walking and aching after effort and, later, at night. The patient may feel that he is "walking with a stone in the knee." The ache is localized to the same area. The patellar symptoms, when they develop, are like those produced by the bowstring cartilage.

Occasionally, the bowstring snaps at an end, usually the anterior (see Fig. 6-17). It coils up in the front of the joint and then produces the clinical picture of a retracted cartilage. The first reaction to the snapping of the bowstring is a measure of relief, for the retracted cartilage is so much more comfortable to the patient than is the bowstring. Only later do the sequelae cause symptoms. Manipulation for reduction of the displaced bowstring frequently results in snapping of the bowstring, which is the reason for its apparent success.

Nonreferred Pain in the Knee with Osteoarthritis of the Hip

The patient suffering from osteoarthritis of the hip may feel referred pain in the knee. This referred pain is muscular in origin and is felt in front or on the sides of the knee depending on the muscle group that is contracted. A patient with flexion- and abduction- or adduction deformity may feel pain in front or on the sides of the knee. As extension contracture, if it ever occurs, is a rarity, pain is not felt behind the knee. It should be noted, too, that it is difficult to walk with a straight knee when there is fixed flexion of the hip. The trunk tends to

overbalance forward. The fixed deformities of osteoarthritis of the hip are *always* flexion, *either* adduction or abduction, and *usually* external rotation.

Surprisingly often, with long-established osteoarthritis of the hip, careful examination of the knee reveals fixed limitation of extension and external rotation of the tibia on the femur, prominence of the medial femoral condyle, and tenderness of the medial meniscus and medial border of the patella. Fixed adduction contracture of the hip may also lead to laxity of the medial ligaments of the knee. Referred pain therefore must be distinguished from that which is due to changes in the knee joint itself, secondary to fixed deformity of the hip.

Although pain in the knee need not necessarily be referred from the hip the question arises whether the changes in the knee are independent of the hip and part of a generalized osteoarthritis or whether they are secondary to and the consequence of fixed deformity of the hip. The latter is almost certainly the case, for the pattern of disorder in the knee depends on the particular deformity of the hip.

For example, fixed external rotation and flexion of the hip eventually leads to flexion and internal rotation contracture of the tibia on the femur with consequent internal derangement of the knee of the typical pattern. In normal walking, sinuous and synchronous adaptations of movement take place between hip and knee. During flexion, the hip rotates outwards while the tibia rotates inwards, and vice versa during extension. Walking with a fixed flexion-external rotation deformity of the hip demands compensation by flexion of the knee and—in order to point the foot forward—limiting external rotation of the tibia during extension. In time, these factors effect permanent fixed limitation of extension and external rotation of the tibia with retraction of the aging, hardening medial meniscus. This is shown in Figure 1-3 by the limitation of external rotation of the tibia and the prominent medial femoral condyle. These signs persist both while walking and at rest. When present, they represent or portend the typical patterns of erosion of the medial femoral condyle and medial border of the patella and are a frequent cause of pain— pain which may be relieved by simple meniscectomy and, when necessary, debridement of the medial border of the patella.

Adduction deformity adds a valgus strain to the knee and causes medial ligaments and sometimes cruciates to stretch, so producing instability of the knee. The medial meniscus may be and usually is retracted as seen in the patient depicted in Figure 1-3. For many years her left hip had been arthritic, flexed, adducted, and externally rotated. The roentgenographs of the knee with valgus stress showed the degree of medial capsule laxity, while the limited external rotation of the tibia and protrusion of the medial femoral condyle denote a retracted meniscus. These changes plus laxity of the cruciate ligaments were confirmed at operation. All were secondary to the fixed deformity of the hip and pain felt in the knee was local in origin and not referred.

To stabilize this knee, it was necessary to remove the meniscus and in addition to do an extra-articular tendon transplant of the semitendinosis into a groove in the medial femoral condyle, plus medial transfer of the tibial tubercle. An advanced example of change secondary to the arthritis of the hip joint, it stresses the importance of examination of the knee joint itself when pain is present with osteoarthritis of the hip.

MUSCLE WASTING

The quadriceps and, to a lesser extent, the hamstrings waste, often rapidly, after injury to the cartilages and the ligaments of the knee. This reaction is due to disturbance of the neurotrophic relationships between the joint and its controlling musculature and varies in degree. Muscle bulk, tone, and control are diminished rapidly and in some instances severely so. It is not due to muscle inactivity alone, though this factor does aggravate both wasting and weakness. In other words, conscientious muscle exercise cannot prevent but does minimize wasting. While effusion remains, wasting is generalized, but the tendency is for the medial vasti to show greater atrophy in sympathy with a medial meniscus injury, while lateral ruptures are associated with atrophy of the lateral vastus.

While muscle weakness is present, effusion tends to persist and is increased with any activity beyond the power and the endurance of the residual muscle bulk. In turn, the effusion affects the trophic reflexes, and further wasting occurs.

Watson-Jones[8] and Smillie[6] and later in this volume, Nicholas (Chap. 23), very properly stress the urgency in stimulation by controlled muscle exercises in all injuries of the knee, if the period of disability and impairment of function is to be kept to a minimum. The power of the thigh muscles, both quadriceps and hamstrings, must be developed sufficiently to cope with all strains to which the knee will be subjected, and, conversely, during convalescence the knee must not be subjected to any strain beyond the power and the endurance of the muscles. I stress "endurance," for the commonest form of strain to be countered is "fatigue."

While displacement of a meniscus remains, muscle bulk and tone cannot recover significantly, despite assiduous exercise. Recovery is impeded further as the patterns of osteoarthritic erosion develop. But should the cartilage be reduced, or removed by operation, so that the knee recovers full movement, both power and bulk of muscle will increase with exercise. And this happens even if roentgenograms show that preoperative changes in the joint outline persist.

REFERENCES

1. Apley, A. G.: A System of Orthopaedics and Fractures. London, Butterworth, 1959.
2. Du Toit, G. T., and Enslin, T. B.: Analysis of one hundred consecutive arthrotomies

for traumatic internal derangement of the knee joint. J. Bone Joint Surg., *27*:412, 1945.

3. Helfet, A. J.: Mechanism of derangements of the medial semilunar cartilage and their management. J. Bone Joint Surg., *41-B*: 319, 1959.

4. ———: The arrest of osteoarthritis of the hip and knee. In Apley, A. G. (Ed.): Recent Advances in Orthopaedics. London, J. & A. Churchill, 1969.

5. McMurray, T. P.: The Robert Jones Birthday Volume. London, Humphrey Milford, 1928.

6. Smillie, I. S.: Injuries of the Knee Joint. Baltimore, Williams & Wilkins, 1962.

7. Timbrell-Fischer, A. G.: Internal Derangements of the Knee Joint. Note 2, p. 189, New York, Macmillan, 1933.

8. Watson-Jones, Sir Reginald: Fractures and Joint Injuries. ed. 4. vol. 2. Baltimore, Williams & Wilkins, 1956.

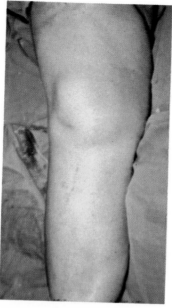

A

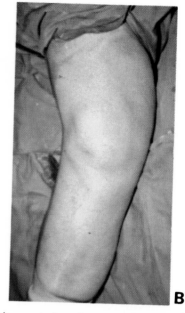

B

Plate 7-1. Knee of a patient who had a long-standing fixed flexion-adduction deformity of the hip. (*A*) The lack of rotation of the tibial tubercle and protrusion of the medial femoral condyle in extension are obvious, and denote an intraarticular block to rotation, probably by a meniscus. (*B*) Valgus stress demonstrates the laxity of the medial collateral ligament. A positive anterior drawer sign indicated cruciate instability. Roentgenogram in valgus stress showed the extent of medial laxity. (*C*) On opening the anteromedial joint space the loose medial meniscus with corresponding condylar abrasion are shown. The anterior cruciate ligament is lax. (*D*) The "anterior drawer sign" demonstrates that the anterior cruciate ligament is stretched and attenuated, not torn. (*E*) The loose medial cartilage is excised. After semitendinosus transfer (see Chap. 16). The patient walked with comfort and stability. The ligaments of this knee had been stretched and the meniscus deranged secondarily to the deformity of the hip.

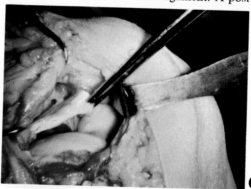

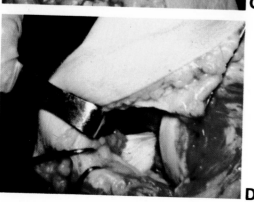

C

D

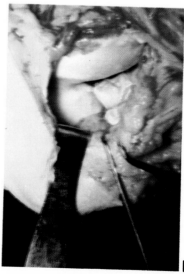

E

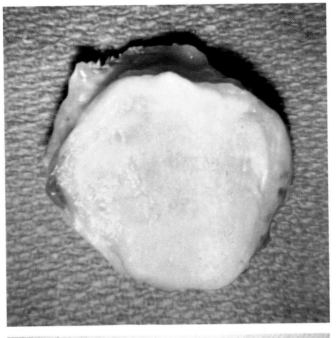

A

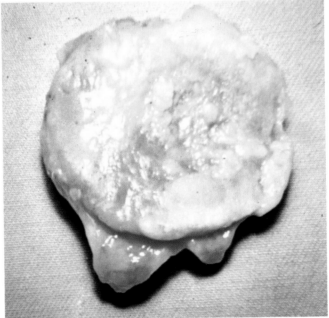

B

Plate 8-1. (*A*) Articular cartilage on both sides of the patella is eroded. (*B*) The cartilage is soft, fissured, and frayed with irregular patterns of disorganization.

8

Differential Diagnosis of Tears of the Semilunar Cartilages

Arthur J. Helfet, M.D.

Accurate diagnosis is essential for successful surgery of the knee. This finely adjusted joint brooks no unplanned or meddlesome surgery. There is little place for opening the joint "to have a look." Indeed, every endeavor should be made to diagnose not only a ruptured cartilage but also the site of rupture.

During the acute stage the knee is grossly swollen and limited in movement, but even then local tenderness and the rotation signs may be elicited. After 3 weeks, if displacement remains, swelling may have disappeared and local tenderness may be faint, but the typical pattern of restriction of movement remains. At a later stage new areas of tenderness of the articular cartilage, due to continuing tensions, develop on the medial condyle, the trochlear surface of the femur and on the patella.

MEDIAL OR LATERAL CARTILAGE?

The distinction is reasonably straightforward. After reflection most patients can indicate the site of injury and pain, or the side on which something "catches" or "slips." As the medial cartilage has a longer excursion during flexion and extension of the knee, symptoms on the medial side tend to be more severe. On occasion, a torn posterior end of the lateral cartilage may result in recurrent buckling of the knee, without remarkable "initial" injury, but forced extension and/or forced flexion usually result in pain that blocks further movement at the site of injury. This is confirmed by finger-point local tenderness and, when present, the palpable click. There is one exception. Very occasionally, pain is felt on one side, usually the medial, when the lesion exists in the opposite meniscus. This may also be due to the longer course that the medial meniscus has to travel. The rotary movement pivots on the posterior attachments of the lateral cartilage, while the medial side covers the curved tract on the longer medial condyle. If a tear of the lateral cartilage locks rotation, the tension of attempted movement may be felt more sensitively in the longer and more vulnerable medial cartilage and capsule. Although subjective pain may be felt on the opposite side, the site of tenderness and the diagnostic click usually coincide with the main lesion and are sufficient to localize it. If there is doubt, provocative exercise under a skilled physiotherapist accentuates the signs.

Tears of Both Semilunar Cartilages

Both cartilages are torn more often than one would expect. The presenting features of the injured medial meniscus may obscure those of the lateral side. A careful history may provide a clue in the severity of the accident or an atypical story. Pain may be reported on both sides, or, if the patient is uncertain in localizing the pain, one is led to even more elaborate examination. Again, provocative exercises may be helpful. Even

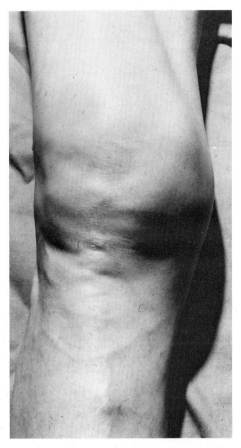

FIG. 8-1. The classical osteoarthritic knee with medially rotated tibial tubercle, prominent medial femoral condyle, prominent patella and wasted thigh.

so, the symptoms of the second rupture may be obvious only after the first cartilage has been removed. As will be discussed in the chapter on "the dashboard knee," severe contusions of the bent knee tend to injure both cartilages. So also does severe wrenching of the extended knee, as in the case of a rider who is dragged by a foot caught in the stirrup after being thrown from a horse.

ANTERIOR TEAR

The anterior tear also has its characteristics. The patient complains of locking or "catching" in the knee. The rotation signs—limitation of excursion of the tibial tubercle and protrusion of the medial femoral condyle—finger-point pain over the antero-

medial or the anterolateral compartment on forced extension and local tenderness in the same site all are present. A click can be elicited, but not consistently, if the anterior portion of the cartilage has been thickened and, more frequently, if a "pedicled" tag of the free margin can be manipulated in and out of position. In this latter event the rotation signs are switched on and off synchronously.

This picture includes the *retracted medial cartilage*. In the young, the onset and the course are less severe than they are with the tear with displacement, but the incidence of retracted medial cartilage is greatest in middle and old age when it is, in my opinion, *the most frequent cause of traumatic osteoarthritis of the knee.*

As with all injuries in older people, the onset may be very distressing, but more often it is mild and sometimes almost unnoticed. At intervals a typical sequence of attacks of discomfort and swelling follow any undue activity, and as the condition deteriorates it needs less strain to produce the same reaction. The joint swells on each occasion. Decrease in the patient's activity results in increased weight, which in turn adds to the strain on the knee. Eventually retropatellar pain is caused by going down and, later, going up stairs. The patient begins to feel that the bunched-up anterior horn is "like a stone in the knee." The final phase is bone pain at night.

At first, the physical signs are those of any anterior tear. The patient finds relief only by flexing the knee, and, as time goes on, the range decreases, and the fixed flexion is greater. Finally, the classical osteoarthritic knee with a medially rotated tibial tubercle, a prominent medial femoral condyle, a prominent patella and a wasted thigh (Fig. 8-1) is established. There are tender spots in the anteromedial compartment just in from the edge of the articular surface of the medial femoral condyle and on the medial border of the patella (Fig. 7-6, *right*). However, the lateral border of the patella and the lateral side of the joint are not as

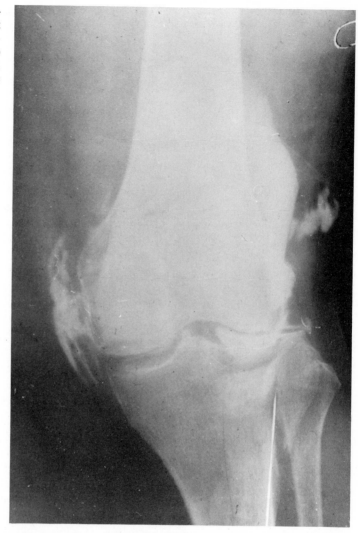

FIG. 8-2. Arthrogram showing ruptured medial ligament and fractured lateral tibial plateau, a combination difficult to diagnose clinically. (Helfet, A. J.: AAOS Instruction Course Lectures. Vol. 19. St. Louis, C. V. Mosby, 1970.)

tender or not tender at all. Painful retro-patellar grating may be elicited.

Sometimes, a fresh incident, usually fracture of the posterior third of the medial cartilage, results in grave aggravation of the condition of the knee as a whole. Should this be so, tenderness is felt also over the posterior horn, and a "click" may be elicited.

POSTERIOR TEAR

The characteristic symptoms of posterior tears of the meniscus are "giving-way" of the knee and pain on full flexion. Sometimes it is difficult for the patient to localize the pain to one side or the other, but tender-ness and a diagnostic click usually give a definite indication. The symptom of "giving-way" is often painless, especially on the lateral side. The torn posterior horn of the medial meniscus is the more frequently painful, while a residual tag after inadequate removal of a meniscus causes pain as well as buckling.

THE BOWSTRING CARTILAGE

The type of violence that produces the bowstring (bucket-handle) tear is usually followed by severe pain and swelling. The knee is limited in extension, and the rotation signs are present. If the split extends well aft, the later range of flexion and

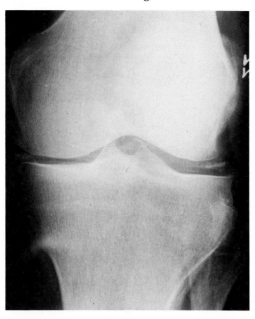

FIG. 8-3. The roentgenogram shows calcification of both the medial and the lateral meniscus.

medial rotations as well are limited and produce pain. While at rest the knee finds comfort anywhere in the intermediate range. Tenderness is felt over the front and the back of the joint line, and, as after all severe incidents, there is another tender spot half way back over the attachment of the deep fibers of the medial ligaments. Even if not reduced, swelling and pain subside after a week or ten days and the patient can take weight with a limp and with the knee slightly flexed. Eventually, the knee straightens, though at the expense of the capsule, for the rotation signs of limited movement of the tibial tubercle and protrusion of the femoral condyle remain. The stretch in the anterior cruciate ligament and the medial capsule is shown by slight laxity of the whole joint. A few degrees of anteroposterior glide and medial ligament laxity are demonstrable. Most often a diagnostic click is easily palpable.

ROENTGENOGRAPHY AS AN AID TO DIAGNOSIS

In the acute phase, and to some extent also in the later stages, roentgenograms have a negative rather than a positive value in diagnosis. Their main purpose is to differentiate internal derangements of the knee from fractures, loose bodies, and diseases that may produce comparable features. Arthrography and arthroscopy are of value in the hands of those who are practiced in their niceties. To the skilled and experienced clinician such aids are not always necessary, for the clinical patterns described are usually quite clear and are adequate for accurate diagnosis of ruptures of the semilunar cartilages. However, when there is any doubt, and especially in the presence of associated instability due to ligamentous and capsular weakness and tears and/or other disorders, these aids as demonstrated by distinguished exponents in Chapters 9 and 10 become invaluable (Fig. 8-2).

Of course, the semilunar cartilages themselves do not show up on x-ray, except in the rare instances when part of the meniscus is calcified. Even then the picture does not help in the diagnosis of rupture, for calcification is not continuous, and the meniscus does not tend to tear through the calcified portion (Fig. 8-3).

After recent injury the picture is usually negative. When traumatic erosion has occurred, irregularities of joint surface may be seen. Frank osteoarthritic changes, when these have supervened, are also visible. Of note are the tilted posture of the patella below the trochlear groove, and the changes in its outline, especially in the skyline view (Fig. 6-27, *left*). At this stage loose bodies and osteophytes also may be evident. Roentgenographic "loss of joint space" is a misleading description and is often due to an abnormal position of rotation of the femur on the tibia (Fig. 8-4). Hence the sometimes miraculous recovery of roentgenographic joint space after removal of the cartilage and restoration of normal movement and positioning. These features may be more accurately assessed in osteoarthritis by anteroposterior views taken when at rest and when bearing weight.

symptoms are aggravated by activity and relieved by rest, and the history suggests progressive deterioration as time passes.

On examination tender fullness on both sides of the patellar tendon can be observed. Squeezing the fat pad on both sides of the tendon between the thumb and the forefinger is painful. In an isolated injury of the anterior horn there is tenderness only on direct pressure over the lesion.

If adhesions form that anchor the mobile fat pad and/or the meniscus, the clinical picture may be complicated by painful limitation of rotation of the tibia and incidents that the patient wrongly interprets as "giving-way" due to acute stabs of pain. The progressive character of the condition and a careful local examination of the extent of swelling and tenderness are the keys to diagnosis. When the anterior horn is obviously damaged, the associated fat pad lesion may be detected only during the operation.

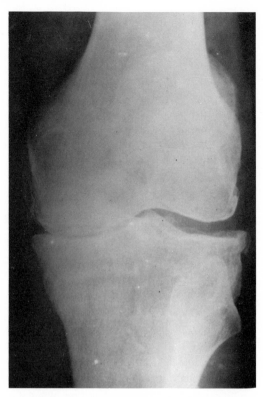

FIG. 8-4. Apparent loss of joint space largely due to rotation and flexion deformity.

INJURIES TO THE INFRAPATELLAR PAD OF FAT

Contusion, scarring, adhesions, and adherence of the fat pad to the tibia and the meniscus are difficult to distinguish from lesions of the anterior horns of the menisci, with which, of course, they may be associated (Fig. 8-5). The subject is considered in detail in Chapter 18 ("The Dashboard Knee"). The meniscus may be damaged coincidentally with the fat pad, with which it has intimate connections, or the alar flaps of the fat pad may be contused and become adherent to the meniscus. In either case the anterior horn and the fat pad acquire a point of fixation. This interferes with easy function, and disability ensues. The patient suffers vague aching in front of the knee joint with pain on forced extension and tension or pain in the same area at the extreme of flexion. The swelling and the

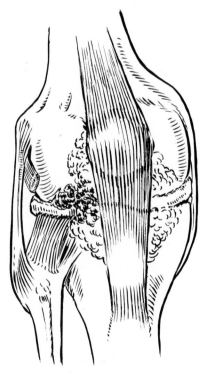

FIG. 8-5. Scar in the infrapatellar pad of fat involving the anterior horn of the lateral meniscus.

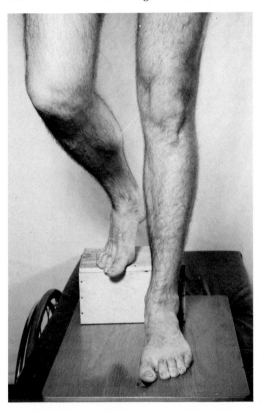

FIG. 8-6. On slopes and stairs, full contraction of the quadriceps pulls the tender patella tight against the trochlear surface of the femur.

CHONDROMALACIA OF THE PATELLA

In the absence of a meniscal injury chondromalacia of the patella presents a recognizable clinical picture, but when longstanding derangement has established the typical patterns of erosion on the medial surface of the patella and the trochlear slope of the femur, great difficulties in diagnosis may arise. It is possible that at least some of the early recorded cases of chondromalacia were these sequelae of semilunar cartilage displacement. The pathology and the clinical signs have been clarified by Hirsch[7] and Soto-Hall,[11] Cave et al.,[4] Wiles et al.,[14,15] and Devas.[5] The condition develops in young adults who complain of pain of aching character, worse after sitting, and transient swelling after exercise. Pain is in-

termittent, may be "catching" in character and is worse on slopes and stairs when the contracted quadriceps pulls the tender patella tight against the trochlear surface of the femur (Fig. 8-6). Slight stiffness, persistent swelling and wasting of the thigh muscles follow. Percussion of the patella against the underlying bone is painful. At a late stage momentary "catching" with a feeling of sudden insecurity may resemble locking or buckling of the knee joint. Retropatellar crepitation on active movement is characteristic. Soto-Hall[11] elicits this sign by having the patient lie on his back with knee and hip flexed. He is then asked to flex and extend the knee slowly without moving the hip.

Diagnosis is aided by finding that with the muscles relaxed full passive extension is possible without pain, for the patella then rests without tension in the trochlear groove of the femur. The articular surface of the patella is tender. This compares with the meniscal derangement of the knee when the medial border is the only tender part or is significantly more tender than the lateral border. Lateral roentgenograms of the extended knee show the normal patellar excursion, whereas, as shown in Chapter 13, when external rotation of the tibia is limited, the patella remains perched on the lower extension of the medial trochlear slope. Skyline views do not show the unilateral erosion or the osteophytic changes of the patella as in Figure 6-27, *left*. They may show thinning of the articular surface (Fig. 8-7).

When examined at operation, the distinction from the arthritic patella is usually obvious, for, instead of a specific pattern of erosion, the articular cartilage is soft, fissured, and frayed, with irregular patterns of disorganization in the late stages (Plate 8-1).

LOOSE BODIES IN THE KNEE

A loose body tends to reveal its presence without subterfuge. Frequently the patient is conscious of "a mouse in the joint" and

FIG. 8-7. Note thinning of the articular surface in these roentgenographic views of chondromalacia of the patella.

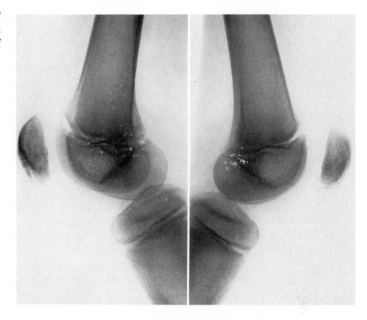

of the diagnosis. Recurrent attacks of momentary pain and locking, varying in site, followed by an effusion are characteristic. The loose body may be palpable. These incidents differ from those due to the recurrent derangement of a meniscus, in which pain and locking always occur at the same spot. A particularly unstable meniscal tear may also displace momentarily, and the attack then resembles that from the brief intrusion of the loose body between the articulating surfaces; usually derangement of the knee by a torn cartilage is a more protracted experience. When, as is common, the loose body is radiopaque, the roentgenogram is conclusive (Fig. 8-8).

The early stages of osteochondritis dissecans may be misleading clinically. This condition develops usually between adolescence and completion of growth and presents in three clinical phases. The first is that of a mildly irritable knee and is the reaction to the early products of degeneration of the affected area of articular cartilage. The knee swells and aches after exertion and may be uncomfortable at night. Roentgenograms usually, but not always, reveal the lesion at this stage (Fig. 8-9A). Both knees may be affected, but

clinical signs may be more marked or entirely absent on one side.

In 1967 Wilson[16] described the following sign:

The diagnosis of osteochondritis dissecans should be immediately considered in a child who presents a lateral rotation gait and complains of pain, and possibly swelling in the knee. The child may show the following sign which, I consider, is probably diagnostic of the condition. The child is examined in the supine position. The knee on the affected side is flexed through about 90 degrees, and the tibia is medially rotated. The

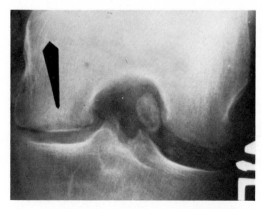

FIG. 8-8. Roentgenogram of third stage osteochondritis dissecans with separated fragment.

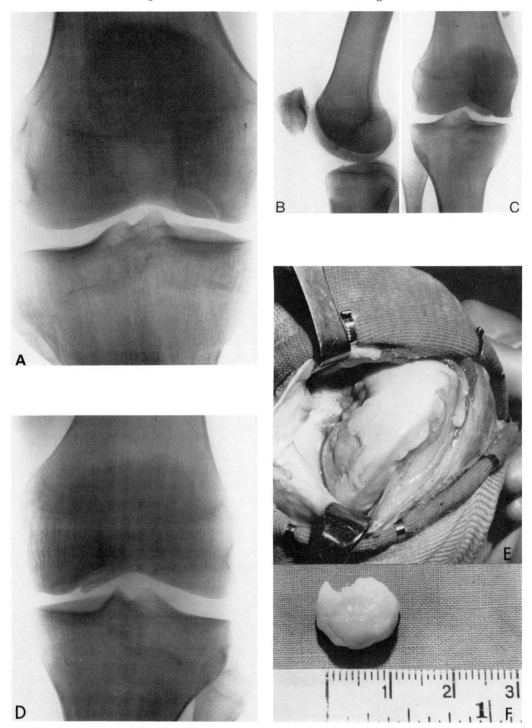

FIG. 8-9. (*A*) The first stage of osteochondritis dissecans in which detachment of the fragment has not commenced. (*B, C*) The second stage of osteochondritis dissecans; the fragment is separating and forming a mobile pedicle into the joint. (*D*) Another instance where the fragment has separated. (*E*) The site of separation of an osteochondritic fragment and (*F*) the loose body itself.

knee is then gradually extended, and at a point about 30 degrees short of full extension, the child will complain of pain over the anterior part of the medial femoral condyle. Lateral rotation of the tibia relieves this pain immediately.

The gradual separation of the fragment introduces the second clinical phase. When one edge is free, the fragment may be pedunculated into the joint and simulate the displacement of a semilunar cartilage (Fig. 8-9B, C, D). By this time the roentgenograms are diagnostic.

Once the fragment separates completely, the picture is that of a free loose body (Fig. 8-8, 8-9E, F) and see Chap. 21 on osteochondral fractures).

As a ruptured meniscus may coexist with the separating fragment—both lesions originating from the same injury—careful clinical examination is always essential. Positive rotation signs and finger-point tenderness suggest a second lesion.

The lesions in osteochondritis dissecans differ from the patterns of erosion of articular cartilage seen in osteoarthritis, the latter produced by recurrent pressure or friction of the displaced meniscus, the tensed cruciate ligament, or the friction between the medial facet of the patella and the trochlear groove in the "blocked" joint. In osteochondritis dissecans the surface of the articular cartilage of the separating or separated fragment is not eroded. The fragment of articular cartilage together with a wedge of underlying bone eventually separates from the joint surface.

Paul Aichroth in a scholarly survey of nearly 200 patients with osteochondritis dissecans of the knee joint at the Royal National Orthopaedic Hospital has tabulated the common sites of the osteochondritic lesion and implicates injury to the articular surface as the predominant etiological factor.[1] He adds that many patients had direct injuries and most had taken part in sports or athletics at a high level. In others, mechanical abnormality of the knee joint was found which subjected the joint surface to abnormal stress.

Seventy-five per cent of the lesions occurred in the classical site, on the lateral edge of the medial femoral condyle, 10 per cent on the inferocentral surface of the medial, and 13 per cent on the inferocentral surface of the lateral condyle. These are also common sites of erosive lesions. More than 60 per cent of the patients were classified as excellent or good athletes, and the higher the level of their participation the higher the incidence of osteochondritis dissecans. Sixteen of the patients had dislocated or subluxated the patella. Seventeen had a laterally rotated tibia, and in seven epiphyseal abnormalities were present. On the other hand 11 patients had osteoarthritic lesions of other joints, and similar lesions have been seen after steroid administration in rheumatic disease, and Gaucher's. Aichroth concludes: All features point to injury as the main etiological factor in osteochondritis dissecans of the knee.

In the early stages before separation of the fragment, when aching and swelling are the predominant symptoms, conservative treatment is indicated—an elastic knee guard reinforced with two whalebone struts, to limit the extremes of movement, and limited activity. The only exercise should be isometric muscle drill. The patience of both the young athlete and the surgeon may be tried, but the condition does tend to settle down. Once the fragment pedunculates into the joint or separates to become a loose body surgery is necessary. It has been my practice to excise the affected piece of cartilage with fragment of bone completely plus any loose bone debris. Often a crescent or disc of dull or yellowish cartilage larger than the attached bone fragment is raised from the underlying bone. This whole disc should be carefully excised. I have seen problems from leaving dead cartilage that subsequently separates and forms another loose body. This is obviated when the whole area is carefully removed. After the operation the joint should be protected from strain for 6 to 12 weeks until healing is

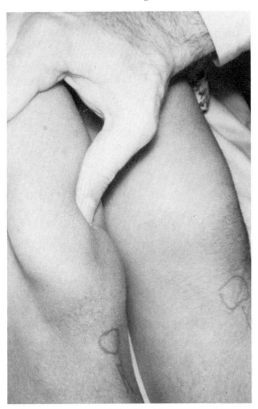

FIG. 8-10. The Apprehension Test. A patient resents and tries to prevent attempts to displace the patella laterally.

evidenced by comfortable functional recovery.

Replacement of the fragment with internal fixation has not been practiced. On the other hand, for patients referred after fixation but with continued or recurrent symptoms it has been necessary to remove pins and ununited or malunited bone fragments. In any event, it seems unnecessary to undertake an operation, which does not always result in perfection of surface or satisfactory union and which requires prolonged aftercare, to preserve a fragment without which the knee seems to be able to function perfectly well. The area concerned seldom takes part in weight bearing.

Every endeavor should be made to preserve the patella when it is involved. Prolonged protection by splinting and limited activity after adequate debridement, or after

semipatellectomy when indicated, is preferable to removal.[10] However good the initial results of patellectomy may be, in the long run a weak and painful knee eventuates, and this is a serious consideration for osteochrondritis dissecans, is most common in young people.

RECURRING SUBLUXATION AND DISLOCATION OF THE PATELLA

Dislocation of the patella presents little difficulty in diagnosis. Impaction of a meniscus causes acute pain and "giving way" of the knee, which cannot straighten completely but can flex, often by so doing bringing relief. Acute dislocation locks the knee which can neither straighten nor bend, and the patient falls forward as if tripped.

Recurring subluxation is more deceptive, and many a meniscus has been erroneously excised. The diagnosis should be suspected in the young and especially in young women, in whom it is more common than meniscal injuries. The patient has a feeling of "giving way," of momentary instability with or without a click, and pain on the medial side of the knee. Each incident is followed by an effusion. Tenderness is felt over the medial capsule in line with the border of the patella and chiefly above the joint line, whereas a meniscal tear is tender locally in the joint line. The lateral facet of the articular surface of the patella is tender.

An important sign is that the patient resents and tries to prevent attempts to displace the patella laterally—the apprehension test described by Fairbank[6] and Apley[2] (Fig. 8-10).

SUBLUXATION OF THE SUPERIOR TIBIOFIBULAR JOINT

Subluxation of the superior tibiofibular joint is a rare, or perhaps rarely diagnosed, lesion. A possible explanation of injury was suggested in Chapter 6. When present it must be differentiated from ruptures of the lateral meniscus.[3,8,9,12,13]

In retrospect, the symptoms and signs of

three patients are enlightening. During the first week after the accident the nurse suffered severe pain, swelling, and bruising of the anterolateral lower thigh, the knee and the tibial compartment of the leg. The case notes record a small effusion and stable ligaments, with full extension, but flexion of the knee limited to 110°. She felt cramp-like pain on walking, first on the inner and then on the outer side of the calf.

She returned to work after 3 weeks of physiotherapy and limited activity. A normally athletic girl, she gave up all games but still suffered increasing discomfort over the next year, after which she again reported for examination. She complained that although the knee was comfortable when she woke, halfway through the morning pain was felt over the lateral side of the knee and worsened as the day wore on. Examination revealed keen tenderness over the tendon of biceps and the superior tibiofibular joint, but not over the lateral joint line of the knee. The maneuver for the McMurray click resulted in a painful thud which might be confused with the click of a discoid cartilage but was, of course, the slip of the head of the fibula. It was produced by the forced rotation of the leg obtained through the grip on the foot and the ankle.

The diagnosis was confirmed by rocking the head of the fibula anteroposteriorly on the tibia, which produced the pain of which she complained. Comparable roentgeno-grams showed protrusion of the fibular head behind the posterior border of the tibia.

The second case also presented with pain over the outer side of the knee, cramps in the calf and aching in the ankle after walking. Rocking the head of the fibula resulted in the same knee pain. Roentgenograms showed displacement of the head of the fibula and signs of osteoarthritic change.

Pain induced by rocking the head of the fibula, tenderness of the joint and the distribution of pain also clinched the diagnosis in the third patient. In all patients, the new test (described on page 99, Fig. 6-40) confirms the diagnosis.

The first joint was repaired and reconstructed. The second was arthrodesed. In both cases the symptoms were completely relieved. Each patient returned to work in approximately 8 weeks. The third girl was kept comfortable for a long time by intra-articular injections of prednisolone. She finally required surgery.

Since 1963 six patients have required arthrodesis of the superior tibiofibular joint for instability and one for intractable osteo-arthritis. Eleven patients suffering from chronic sprain, osteo- or rheumatoid arth-ritis have been relieved by intraarticular in-jections of local anaesthetic and corticos-teroids. An elastic bandage or strap wound firmly round the upper calf has also given comfort.

TENOSYNOVITIS OF THE POPLITEUS TENDON

Another rare lesion! In this series only two cases were diagnosed and treated. Diagnosis was not difficult. The first patient, a radiologist, complained of pain but limited swelling on the outer side of the knee, ag-gravated by walking but chiefly on bending the knee. At its worst the pain was of a "burning, sharp, stabbing type" that oc-curred on kneeling when pressure was put on the joint, and, to a lesser extent, on passive hyperflexion. Flexion was limited and painful, and this is understandable, for then the tendon is actively engaged. The knee ached at night. Palpation revealed the tender swollen course of the popliteus tendon without effusion in the knee joint. Attempts to rotate the leg laterally against resistance were painful.

Injection of procaine and hydrocortisone acetate into the tendon sheath relieved the condition dramatically.

The second patient suffered from a dis-abling osteoarthritis of the right hip, which had been treated successfully by cup arthroplasty. Easy comfortable movement of the hip with good muscle control had been achieved.

He related that before the arthroplasty he had complained also of pain on the outer side of his knee which was worse postoperatively. A year later it was decided that the lateral meniscus was at fault, and it was removed. His symptoms were not relieved. He could not exercise the knee, and walking on crutches was accomplished only with discomfort. He could not take pressure on the outer side of the knee and so could not sleep on his right side. He suffered cramps in his calf from where pain radiated to the outer side of the knee.

On examination, tenderness was localized to the popliteus and the insertions of the lateral ligament and the biceps. With the muscles relaxed, movements of the knee, including rotation, were painless, but with the knee flexed, lateral rotation of the leg on the thigh against resistance caused pain. Taking weight standing was immediately painful, and bending the knee while bearing weight was impossible because of pain.

Injection of procaine into the lateral ligament had no effect, but injected into the tendon sheath of the popliteus it caused complete and immediate relief. He could move and walk a short while without pain.

ROTATION SPRAINS OF THE MEDIAL SEMILUNAR CARTILAGE

In the acute stage these lesions are often indistinguishable from derangements of the medial meniscus of the knee. The history of injury and locking followed by rapid swelling are typical, and properly so, for the lesion is probably a temporary displacement of the anterior half of the meniscus. The effusion is hemorrhagic and painful, for the vascular coronary attachments are strained or torn. The anteromedial compartment of the knee is tender, and forced extension is painful in the same place.

The "rotation sprains" differ from the ruptured semilunar in that after rest and physiotherapy the knee settles down without recurrence. Operation is not necessary, for the tear in the vascular coronary ligaments heals.

As we cannot diagnose peripheral detachments from ruptures in the substance of the meniscus, it is not customary to operate after the first accident (see Chap. 11). Therefore, the diagnosis is often negative and depends on whether the derangement recurs or not.

REFERENCES

1. Aichroth, P. M.: Osteochondritis dissecans of the knee. J. Bone Joint Surg., *53-B*:440, 1971.
2. Apley, A. G.: The diagnosis of meniscus injuries. J. Bone Joint Surg., *29*:78, 1947. Apley, A. G.: A system of orthopaedics and fractures. London, Butterworth, 1959.
3. Barnett, C. H., and Napier, J. R.: The axis of rotation at the ankle joint in man. Its influence upon the form of the talus and the mobility of the fibula. J. Anat., *86*:1, 1952.
4. Cave, E. F., Rowe, C. R., and Yee, L. B.: Chondromalacia of the patella. Surg., Gynec. Obstet., *81*:446, 1945.
5. Devas, M. B.: Chondromalacia of the patella. Clin. Orthop., *18*:54, 1960.
6. Fairbank, Sir, H. A. T.: Internal derangement of knee in children. Proc. R. Soc., *3*:11, 1937.
7. Hirsch, C.: A contribution to the pathogenesis of chondromalacia of the patella. Acta Chir. Scand., *90*[Suppl.]:83, 1944.
8. Lord, C. D., and Coutts, J. W.: A study of typical parachute injuries occurring in two hundred and fifty thousand jumps at the parachute school. J. Bone Joint Surg., *26*: 547, 1944.
9. Lyle, H. H. M: Traumatic luxation of the head of the fibula. Ann. Surg., *82*:635, 1925.
10. Sacks, S.: Semipatellectomy. S. Afr. Med. J., *36*:518, 1962.
11. Soto-Hall, R.: Traumatic degeneration of the articular cartilage of the patella. J. Bone Joint Surg., *27*:426, 1945.
12. Stratford, B. C.: Simple dislocation of the superior tibio-fibular joint. J. Bone Joint Surg., *41-B*:120, 1959.

13. Vitt, R. J.: Dislocation of the head of the fibula. J. Bone Joint Surg., *30-A*:1012, 1948.

14. Wiles, P., Andrews, P. S., and Bremmer, R. A.: Chondromalacia of the patella. J. Bone Joint Surg., *42-B*:65, 1960.

15. Wiles, P., Andrews, P. S., and Devas, M. B.: Chondromalacia of the patella. J. Bone Joint Surg., *38-B*:95, 1956.

16. Wilson, J. N.: A diagnostic sign in osteochondritis dissecans of the knee. J. Bone Joint Surg., *49-A*:477, 1967.

9

Arthrography of the Knee

R. H. Freiberger, M.D.

Arthrographic examination of the knee joint has been available for many years but has, in the past, been used only sporadically despite the fact that great accuracy of the procedure had been demonstrated.[1,3,4,5] The examination has become more widely used in recent years and is gaining acceptance as a routine diagnostic procedure because there is an increasing desire to obtain graphic confirmation of clinical diagnosis. The newer, water-soluble contrast media, particularly the meglumine salts, cause practically no irritation to synovial tissues and cause the patient little or no pain with inadvertent extraarticular injection. Fractional focal spot X-ray tubes are now generally available, and current flow and X-ray output are sufficient to produce high quality arthrograms. This is particularly important when fluoroscopic methods with spot filming are used, since the usual large focal spot used for spot filming does not provide the sharp radiographs necessary for adequate evaluation.

Arthrography is now used and taught in many medical centers and it is increasingly possible for the surgeon to request an arthrogram as he would any other radiographic examination.

The first arthrograms of the knee used air as contrast medium. The superiority of the water-soluble radiopaque contrast media now appears clearly established, and presently either positive contrast substance alone or a combination of air and positive contrast is used. The arthrograms illustrated were performed using double contrast, air and liquid positive contrast media, and a hori-zontal X-ray beam, a technique described by Andren and Wehlin. Equally good arthrograms can be obtained by fluoroscopic and spot film method using a fractional focal spot, although somewhat more gas distention of the knee joint is necessary than with the horizontal beam method. Arthrograms using radiopaque contrast substance only can be performed either by vertical X-ray beam or by the fluoroscopic method. Published data on large series of arthrograms by any of these three methods all show a high degree of accuracy of diagnosis of meniscus tear.

DOUBLE-CONTRAST HORIZONTAL BEAM METHOD

The knee is fluoroscoped briefly in lateral projection, and lines are drawn on the skin at the edge of the tibial plateau. These lines are later used to aim the central X-ray beam to obtain perfect tangential views of the meniscus. After antiseptic skin preparation, a 20-gauge needle is placed between the patella and femoral condyle, either medially or laterally. If fluid is present it is aspirated as completely as possible. Approximately 25 to 35 cc. of air is then injected followed by an injection of 5-10 cc. of meglumine diatrizoate 60 per cent. The needle is withdrawn; the patient walks a few steps to distribute the contrast substances and is then placed in the prone oblique projection for filming of the posterior portion of the medial meniscus (Fig. 9-1). A firm pillow is placed beneath the knee and a sandbag over the ankle to provide distraction of the medial

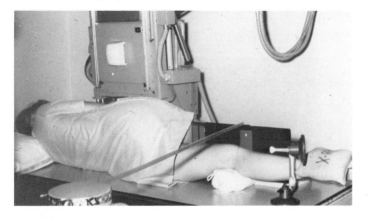

FIG. 9-1. The patient is positioned for the filming of the medial meniscus.

side of the knee. A film holder is used to provide six exposures on a 7 x 17 film, and the horizontal X-ray beam is aimed at the previously drawn line. A series of six exposures is made with the knee and the patient turned approximately 25 degrees between exposures, the last exposure providing a view of the most anterior portion of the medial meniscus. The patient is then placed in the opposite prone oblique projection with the leg to be examined on a low wooden table, and the same procedure is followed in filming the lateral meniscus (Fig. 9-2). Rapid film processing allows a review of the film of the medial meniscus before filming of the lateral meniscus has been completed, and if further exposures are deemed necessary they are taken immediately. The patient then stands up briefly and sits with his knee flexed at 90 degrees and a pillow behind the knee pushing the tibia forward. In this position the liquid

positive contrast agent falls to the bottom of the knee joint and covers the superior surface of the cruciate ligaments. Opacified popliteal cysts will be visible on this projection. Details of the roentgenographic technique have been published elsewhere.[1,4,5] The injection of the knee is performed by a radiologist, the filming, by a technician.

Meticulous attention to detail is necessary in performing the arthrogram to obtain practically perfect tangential views of the tibial plateau in order to evaluate the menisci that appear in cross section (Figs. 9-3 to 9-12).

ANATOMY PERTINENT TO ARTHROGRAPHY

The medial meniscus is firmly attached to the capsule along its periphery. Because of its complete peripheral attachment no contrast agent can normally be seen on the peripheral aspect of the medial meniscus nor

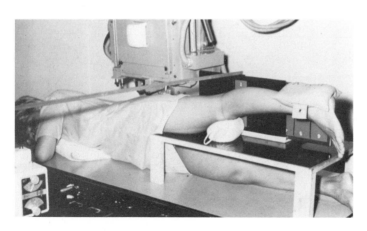

FIG. 9-2. The lateral meniscus is filmed with the patient in this position.

FIG. 9-3. The contrast agent enhances the free edges of this normal medial meniscus. No contrast agent is seen at the periphery marked by an arrow.

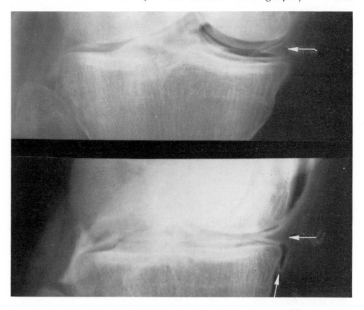

can contrast agent get within the meniscus except through a tear (Fig. 9-3). The arthrogram shows the tightness or laxity of the tibial attachment of the medial meniscus. Occasionally, the recess formed between the capsular attachment and the margin of the tibia is so irregular and deep that one can assume that the patient has had a coronary ligament tear. Most of the time the clinical significance of the loosely attached medial meniscus remains undetermined. The lateral meniscus is somewhat more circular than the medial meniscus, and therefore its most anterior and posterior portions at their attachment to the tibial plateau are not depicted on the tangential views of the arthrogram. In general, the lateral meniscus has a much looser tibial attachment nor-

mally allowing a greater degree of mobility, and we have not developed criteria as to when the laxity of the attachment of the lateral meniscus is of clinical significance. In addition, the lateral meniscus is separated from its capsular attachment posterolaterally by the sleeve of the popliteus tendon which communicates with the knee joint. The popliteus tendon sleeve is therefore always filled with contrast substance, and this normally gives the posterior portion of the lateral meniscus a peripherally detached appearance (Fig. 9-4). It is apparent that the combination of a more circular configuration, greater mobility, and the presence of the contrast-filled popliteus tendon sleeve make arthrographic evaluation of the lateral meniscus more difficult than that of the

FIG. 9-4. In the roentgenogram of the posterior portion of a normal lateral meniscus, the arrows point to the sleeve of the popliteous tendon which is filled with air. Its margins are enhanced by positive contrast, which gives the meniscus a peripherally detached appearance.

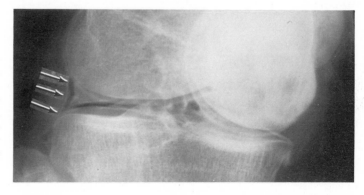

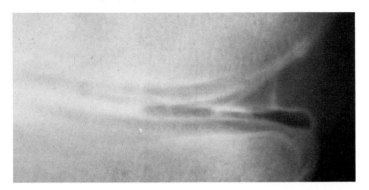

FIG. 9-5. Vertical tear with fragments in close apposition.

medial meniscus. Indeed, the accuracy of diagnosis of lesions of the lateral meniscus is somewhat less than of those of the medial meniscus.

The cruciate ligaments are extra-articular structures with broad, fan-shaped insertions into the tibial plateau and the intercondylar areas of the femur. They are covered by synovia which is reflected over both the anterior and posterior cruciate ligaments at their crossing in the center of the knee joint. Contrast agent, therefore, does not envelop each cruciate ligament completely, and their arthrographic examination has been difficult and not particularly accurate. Since tears of the cruciate ligaments can take place without a complete or persistent tear of their synovial surface, these ruptures are frequently undiagnosed by the arthrogram. We have managed to improve our diagnostic accuracy of cruciate ligament tears somewhat by taking a lateral view with the knee flexed 90 degrees over a firm pillow and the patient sitting. A further improvement has been made by tomography in this position, but this is a time consuming procedure and is only performed in selected cases.

DIAGNOSTIC FEATURES OF MENISCUS TEARS

The meniscus tears occur in two major types: vertical and horizontal. The vertical tear splits the meniscus from its superior to inferior surface, the bucket handle (bowstring) type tear falls in to this category. On the arthrogram the two fragments are seen either in close apposition (Fig. 9-5), slightly separated (Fig. 9-6), or with the inner fragment completely displaced and often visible with only the amputated outer fragment remaining (Fig. 9-7). The horizontal tear represents a splitting of the meniscus into superior and inferior portions.

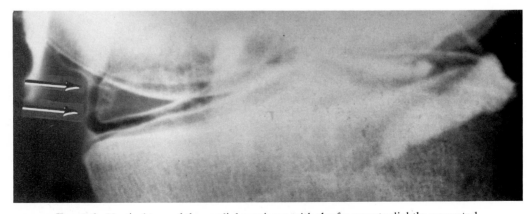

FIG. 9-6. Vertical tear of the medial meniscus with the fragments slightly separated.

FIG. 9-7. Tear of the medial meniscus with the inner fragment displaced into the intercondylar notch.

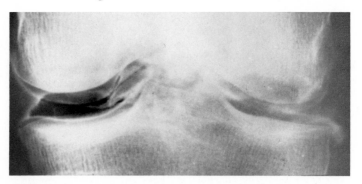

No major displacement of fragments is usually present (Fig. 9-8). Combinations of these types of tears are frequently present, and we do not usually describe the type of tear in great detail but try to describe its extent and whether it is located predominately in the anterior middle or posterior portion of the meniscus. Diagnosis of the discoid or partially discoid lateral meniscus recognized by its abnormal width is usually not difficult (Figs. 9-9, 9-10). We have encountered occasional difficulties in making a diagnosis of torn discoid lateral meniscus. An oblique tear in a discoid meniscus with the displacement of the inner fragment may leave the peripheral portion of normal width, and the tear may thus not be recognized.

Cysts of the lateral meniscus are frequently associated with degenerative horizontal tears, and the contrast agent in such a tear extending irregularly beyond the margin of the tibial plateau is indicative of

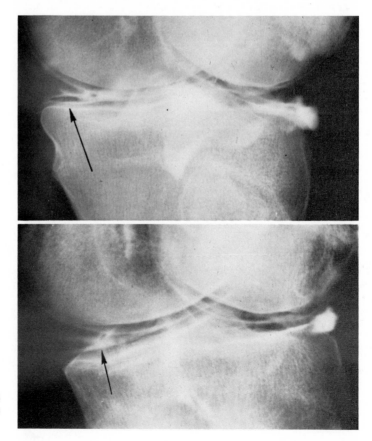

FIG. 9-8. Horizontal tears of the medial meniscus are marked by the arrows.

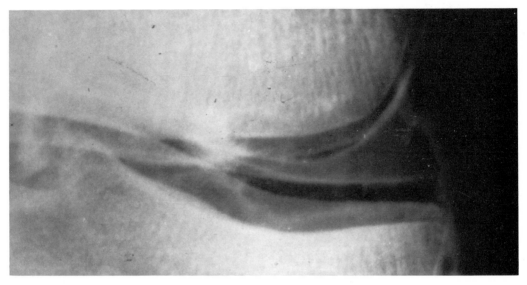

FIG. 9-9. Discoid lateral meniscus, note the abnormal width.

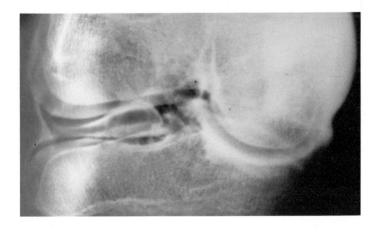

FIG. 9-10. Torn discoid lateral meniscus in a child.

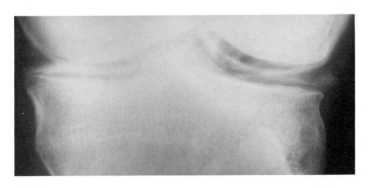

FIG. 9-11. Note the extent to which contrast agent has dispersed in a soft-tissue bulge at the periphery of the torn cystic lateral meniscus.

FIG. 9-12. Small chondral fracture of the medial femoral condyle.

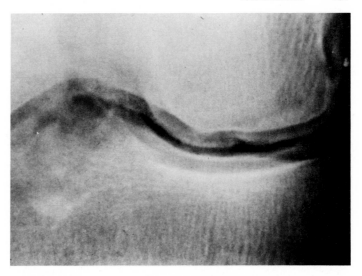

a torn cystic lateral meniscus (Fig. 9-11). When the cystic meniscus is not associated with a tear the arthrogram will appear essentially normal. However, one may be able to see a soft tissue bulge at the periphery of the meniscus.

The contrast coated articular cartilages can also be evaluated, and major cartilage erosions, chondral fractures (Fig. 9-12), or loose cartilaginous bodies can be identified. We have not been able to see the minor cartilage erosions of chondromalacia. If an arthrogram is requested specifically for the identification of loose cartilaginous bodies or for soft-tissue masses, as for instance in pigmented villonodular synovitis, we prefer to perform either an air only or contrast only arthrogram. In the double contrast study, air bubbles may form which can be confused with loose cartilaginous bodies. Capsular ruptures are detected by the extravasation of contrast agent through the ruptured portion of the capsule. Since the capsular tears heal to a watertight condition rather rapidly, usually within 3 or 4 days, the arthrogram should be performed within 3 days of an acute injury if this diagnosis is to be made.

COMPLICATIONS

One infection and five cases of mild urticaria have occurred in our series of over 7,000 patients.

REFERENCES

1. Andren, L., and Wehlin, L.: Double-contrast arthrography of the knee with horizontal roentgen ray beam. Acta Orthop. Scandinav., 29:307, 1960.
2. Butt, P., and McIntyre, J.: Double contrast arthrography of the knee. Rad., 92: 487, 1969.
3. Lindblom, K.: Arthrography of the knee. Roentgenographic and anatomic study. Acta Radiol., Suppl. 74, 1948.
4. Freiberger, R. H., Killoran, P. J., and Cardona, G.: Arthrography of the knee by double contrast method. Am. J. Roentgenol., 97:736, 1966.
5. Nicholas, J. A., Freiberger, R. H., and Killoran, P. J.: Double-contrast arthrography of the knee. Its value in the management of two hundred and twenty-five knee derangements. J. Bone Joint Surg., 52-A: 203, 1970.

10

Arthroscopy of the Knee Joint

Masaki Watanabe, M.D.

INTRODUCTION

The expression, "internal derangement of the knee," coined by William Hey in 1784, describes various lesions and disorders of the meniscus, cruciate ligaments, collateral ligaments, and other structures in the knee joint. It is a condition seen frequently in daily practice, but, owing to the complexity of the structure and biomechanics of the knee joint, accurate diagnosis is not always easy. With the progress of orthopedic surgery, however, this condition has been analyzed and classified into an increasing number of clinical components. The classification of internal derangement of the knee, in my estimation at present, is shown in the following scheme:

Classification of Internal Derangements
of the Knee

1. Lesion or disorder of the meniscus
2. Lesion or disorder of the cruciate ligament
3. Lesion or disorder of the collateral ligament
4. Others:
   a. Loose bodies, osteochondral fracture, osteochondritis dissecans, osteochondromatosis, aseptic osteochondronecrosis, chondromalacia of the patella
   b. Lesion of the infrapatellar fat pads, Hoffa's disease
   c. Lesion or disorder of plica synovialis supra-, infra-, and mediopatellaris, chorda cavi articularis genu, chorda obliqua synovialis, and popliteal tendon
   d. Tumorous conditions in the joint cavity. Pedunculate xanthomatous giant cell tumor, hemangioma, fibroma, ganglion, etc.

In the diagnosis of internal derangement of the knee, especially of the meniscus lesion, the following are essential:
1. Knowledge of the normal anatomy and biomechanics of the knee
2. A correct history, especially details of the manner of the injury
3. Clinical symptoms
4. Clinical tests based on the mechanism of knee joint motion
5. X-ray, to rule out fracture

Helfet, in this and previous publications, considers that most meniscal lesions can be diagnosed from a careful history and physical examination. Smillie reports the percentage of error reduced from 7.2 to 4.0 per cent with increasing experience.[23] But he adds, "the surgeon who states that he has never excised a normal meniscus is either departing from the truth or is missing more diagnoses than he makes." It is often difficult for a surgeon to diagnose not only the existence of rupture of a meniscus but also the detailed finding of a meniscal tear on which methods of treatment can be based.

In the diagnosis of a lesion of a collateral or cruciate ligament, examination by various maneuvers for stability of the joint, such as valgus or varus stress, drawer sign, and stress radiography, are very important. But dislocation of a piece of the ruptured medial collateral ligament into the joint space or an isolated incomplete rupture of the anterior cruciate ligament is not always easy to confirm by clinical examinations.

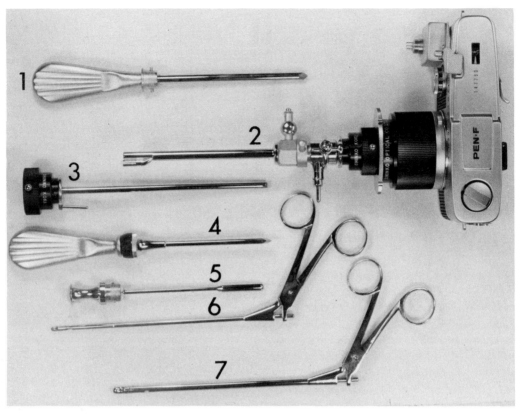

FIG. 10-1. No. 21 Arthroscope. Bulb carrier and direct viewing telescope are nested within a single sheath.

The knee joint is not a simple hinge joint. Its movement is helicoid or spiral in character which is controlled or guided mainly by a mechanism of collateral ligaments, cruciate ligaments, and menisci. As the normal spiral movement of the knee is a synchrony of extension with external rotation of the tibia and flexion with internal rotation, knee lesions that occasionally occur from a complex distortion of this pattern may lead to a resulting difficulty in diagnosis. However, accurate diagnosis is essential for successful surgery or to avoid unnecessary surgery.

More precise diagnosis of meniscal or other lesions is possible by employing three additional methods of visualization: arthrography, arthroscopy, and arthrotomy.

Arthrotomy

Arthrotomy for diagnostic purpose should be abandoned because of associated mor- bidity and quadriceps inhibition. Further, it is quite difficult to survey most parts of the menisci by arthrotomy without cutting the extensor apparatus.

Arthrography

Arthrographic diagnosis of the meniscal lesion has made great progress during the past two decades, owing mostly to the efforts of Lindblom,[13] Andren,[1] Ricklin,[21] Rüttiman,[21] and more recently, Freiberger (see Chap. 9), Nicholas, and Killoran.[3,19] It has become a routine examination, and the ratio of errors in the hands of these specialists is less than 10 or 5 per cent. Arthrography has an advantage over arthroscopy in detecting a cleavage in the undersurface of the meniscus or a parameniscal tear without dislocation. However, arthrographic diagnosis is an indirect method and therefore its interpretation is not easy, especially when the arthrogram is complicated. It is also difficult to

TABLE 10-2. Telescopes of the No. 21 Arthroscope

	Length (cm.)		Gauge of tube (mm.)	Visibility	
	Total	*Tube*		*Axis (°)*	*Angle (°)*
Direct viewing telescope	16.0	9.7	4.9	0	100
Fore-oblique viewing telescope	16.7	10.0	4.9	60	100

confirm a negative arthrogram for meniscal lesion. Arthrographic diagnosis of the cruciate ligament is still uncertain except in rare examples.

Arthroscopy

Arthroscopic examination of meniscal lesions is a direct observation, and therefore its interpretation is much easier than that by indirect methods. The most important problem in athroscopic diagnosis of a meniscal lesion is how to visualize the whole of the meniscus. For many years, visualization of the meniscus had been a very difficult problem until our No. 21 arthroscope[26] was developed for this purpose in 1959.

The use of the direct viewing telescope of the No. 21 arthroscope has made possible observation of most parts of the meniscus (with the exception of some small areas) through one puncture, the lateral infrapatellar approach. The posterior segment of the meniscus or an anomalous posterior horn of the lateral meniscus (Wrisberg's[10] or Humphrey's[6,7] ligament) is more easily observed by arthroscopy than by surgery. The major advantage of arthroscopy over arthrotomy for diagnostic purposes is the complete absence of quadriceps inhibition and the minimal morbidity following examination.

Arthroscopy also provides additional information from inspection of the synovium and articular surface. For example we know that in most cases of torn and degenerated meniscus an erosion or ulcer is found in the cartilaginous surface of the corresponding femoral condyle.

WATANABE NO. 21 ARTHROSCOPE AND TECHNIQUE FOR ITS USE

The No. 21 arthroscope was specially designed for taking color photographs of the interior of the knee joint cavity as well as for observing the meniscus. The new model of the No. 21 (1972)[29] consists of a direct and a fore-oblique viewing telescope plus accessories (Figs. 10-1, 10-2). The size and angle of vision of the telescope is presented in Table 10-2.

The main characteristics of the No. 21 arthroscope are as follows:

1. A very wide field of vision, visual angle being 100 degrees
2. A great depth of the focus, extending from 1 mm. to infinity
3. The magnification of the lens system of the direct viewing telescope is ten times at a distance of 1 mm., twice at 1 cm., equal at 2 cm., and smaller at farther distance, and therefore, the dis-

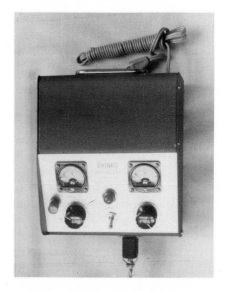

FIG. 10-2. Special transformer. (1) Cord. (2) Voltmeter for observation system. (3) Voltmeter for photo system. (4) Cord with rotating contact to bulb carrier and with synchronous exposure attachment to camera.

tortion of the image cannot be neglected

4. A small but relatively bright and long-lasting tungsten light source which is carried alongside the telescope

5. When in use, both the bulb carrier and the telescope are nested within the same trocar sheath as seen in Figure 10-1

These characteristics of the telescope, make it not so difficult for a surgeon to interpret the findings of the meniscus. In fact, when the tip of the telescope is placed in the joint, it is tantamount to saying that a human eye with extraordinary close vision is placed there.

Technique for Use

Arthroscopic procedure is performed in the following way. A needle, 18-gauge or larger, is inserted into the suprapatellar pouch, and any effusion is aspirated. The joint is then fully distended with 75 to 100 ml. of normal saline at room temperature. A rubber tube with a stopper is attached to the needle to be used as a drain pipe during arthroscopy.

There are several approaches for insertion of the arthroscope, but the best for examination of the meniscus is the lateral infrapatellar approach, in which the site of insertion is in the joint line anteriorly just lateral to the patellar tendon. The knee is flexed to 20 degrees and the anterior joint line is palpated with both thumbs of the examiner alongside the patellar tendon. The site pressed with the thumb is just the site of the lateral or medial infrapatellar approach. A 6- to 8-mm. skin incision is made for trocar puncture. The trocar puncture is made in the extended position of the knee in the following two steps.

The trocar is first inserted through the skin incision in a direction from anterolateroinferior toward posteromedioproximal into the infrapatellar fat pad. The trocar is then directed parallel with the patellar groove of the femur and introduced into the suprapatellar pouch. When the tip of the sheath is confirmed to be lying in the suprapatellar pouch, the bulb carrier, and the telescope are nested within it. Sufficient hydrostatic pressure is obtained by suspending an irrigator or bottle of saline 80 cm. or higher above the level of the knee to be examined.

The suprapatellar pouch and bursa are examined with the knee in the extended position. On withdrawing the instrument slightly and bending the knee to 20 degrees, the patellofemoral joint space can be visualized in profile. It is, however, better to use the fore-oblique viewing telescope for observation of the patella instead of the direct viewing.

The tip of the arthroscope is then directed medially and moved along the medial ridge of the medial femoral condyle downward while the knee is bent to 60 degrees imposing a slight valgus strain to the joint. The tip of the arthroscope is then situated over the anterior part of the medial meniscus. The medial compartment is examined in this position. The tip of the scope can be moved along the anteroinferior surface of the medial femoral condyle. Dropping the patient's foot over the side of the table keeps the knee bent, thus allowing gravity to assist in opening the medial joint space and providing a better view of the medial meniscus.

The joint is extended slowly as the tip of the scope is returned to the suprapatellar pouch. The knee is bent with a varus strain, while the tip of the arthroscope is directed over the medial surface of the lateral femoral condyle into the lateral compartment of the joint. To permit full observation of the lateral meniscus, the knee should be flexed to 60 to 90 degrees, and in maximum varus position.

Observation of the medial or lateral meniscus is made with gentle extension and flexion of the knee, external and internal rotation of the tibia, under valgus or varus stress, and placing pressure with the free hand on the border of the meniscus. On occasion it is useful to grasp a part of the meniscus with forceps introduced into the joint and try to pull it out under arthroscopic control. This

Fig. 10-3. Areas of the menisci hidden (shaded) and visible with the No. 21 arthroscope.

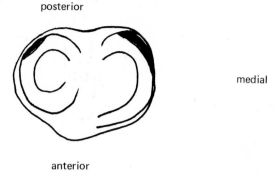

FIG. 10-3. Areas of the menisci hidden (shaded) and visible with the No. 21 arthroscope.

posterior

lateral   medial

anterior

sometimes reveals an unsuspected meniscal tear. When the field of vision with the direct viewing telescope is not wide enough for observation of some part of the meniscus, the fore-oblique viewing one should be used.

After the lateral compartment has been examined, the tip of the scope is reversed again to the suprapatellar pouch.

On conclusion of the examination including photography and punch biopsy, the joint is irrigated with 300 to 500 ml. of normal saline, and if surgery is not indicated, the skin incision is closed with a single stitch and an elastic bandage is applied. If further operative procedure is indicated, the limb is again prepared, and the surgery is carried out under the same anesthesia.

ARTHROSCOPIC DIAGNOSIS

Meniscus

As arthroscopy is a direct visualization, we can observe the form, size, location,

color, glossiness, flatness, as well as rupture, fibrillation, or tiny cleavage in the surface of the meniscus. In arthroscopy of the meniscus with the No. 21, some areas are difficult to see (Fig. 10-3). Interpretation is thus easy or difficult according to the site and type of the lesion of the meniscus.

Medial Meniscus. Arthroscopic views of the normal medial meniscus are shown in Plate 10-1A to C. The middle segment is obscured by the rounded femoral condyle, but when the tip of the arthroscope is pointed closely at it with the knee in a flexed and valgus position, a close-up view of the inner rim of the middle segment can be obtained. The inner rim here makes a few small undulant folds over the tibial plateau, due to normal laxity of the meniscus in the flexed position of the knee (Plate 10-2). The inner rim is concave; it is sharp in the young but becomes irregular and frayed with age. Loss of normal concavity of the inner rim curvature is always an important finding.

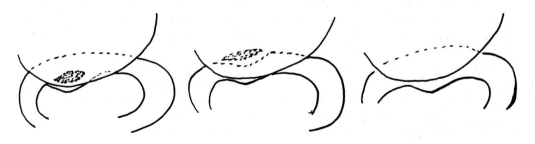

Tear in the corpus
of the meniscus
making a hole

parameniscal
tear

incomplete discoid
meniscus

FIG. 10-4. Interpretation of convex inner margin of the middle segment (see text).

If the middle segment is easily found lying under the rounded condyle, a dislocation of that part of the meniscus toward the center of the tibial plateau should be suspected. This finding of the inner rim of the middle segment may be due to a tear localized in the body of the meniscus making a hole or to a parameniscal tear in this region, or, alternatively, to a medial incomplete discoid meniscus (Fig. 10-4 and Plate 10-3).

The insertion of the anterior horn is obscured by fat. Occasionally one sees the anterior part of a normal medial meniscus lying over the anterior margin of the tibial plateau. An L-shaped tear that makes a pedunculated tag, a transverse tear, or a cross tear can be detected easily (Plates 10-4, 10-5). A bucket-handle (bowstring) tear is also easy to detect—the inner rim curvature of the dislocated part looks convex (on the contrary), and the outer margin is reduced in width (Plate 10-6). However, it is better to confirm the bucket-handle with an instrument introduced into the joint. A complete discoid medial meniscus occupies the medial side of the tibial plateau, and its inner rim looks quite thick (Plate 10-7).

The outer margin of the posterolateral part of the medial meniscus is difficult to observe with the No. 21. This part should be observed with a thin arthroscope No. 24[29] introduced through a medial posterior approach. The undersurface of the meniscus is also difficult to see. By means of the No. 24 fore-oblique viewing needlescope, some parts of the undersurface can be seen while the inner rim is held up with forceps introduced into the joint. Interpreting what is

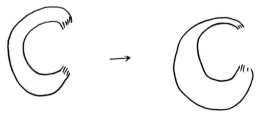

FIG. 10-5. Optical distortion of the image of the lateral meniscus: (*left*) actual form, (*right*) image.

seen on the undersurface, however, still remains a difficult problem.

The space between medial meniscus and tibial plateau is normally very narrow, and if it is too wide, rupture of the medial collateral ligament is suspected (Plate 10-8).

Arthroscopically observed, the posterior part of the medial meniscus comes into the tibiofemoral joint space when the tibia is rotated externally in flexion of the knee, and it goes out when the tibia is rotated internally. This phenomenon arthroscopically observed is considered to suggest the mechanism of McMurray's test. When a longitudinal tear is found, it is necessary to trace the tear in both directions in order to distinguish it from an L-shaped tear (Plate 10-9).

A tear of the meniscus without dislocation is often difficult to find. Observation of the meniscus, therefore, should be made carefully using the various manipulations. In cases with combined rupture of medial collateral ligament and medial meniscus, the anterior cruciate ligament must be carefully observed. On the other hand, one sees cases in which the medial collateral ligament is completely ruptured but arthroscopic view of the medial meniscus and anterior cruciate ligament appears normal. In cases of the suspected unhappy triad, the lateral meniscus must also be examined carefully.

When a suspected injury of the medial meniscus is neglected arthroscopically, it is important to observe the lateral meniscus, because occasionally pain is felt on the medial side, when the lesion exists in the lateral meniscus.

Lateral Meniscus. Observation of the lateral meniscus is begun from the posterior segment to the middle, and then to the anterior segment. the posterior horn can be traced closely to the point of its insertion, which appears red due to blood vessels lying in its surface. Often anterior and posterior segments are seen in one field of vision. Sometimes a whole view of the lateral meniscus is commanded in one field of vision (Plate 10-10). In judging the form and width of the meniscus, optical distortion of the

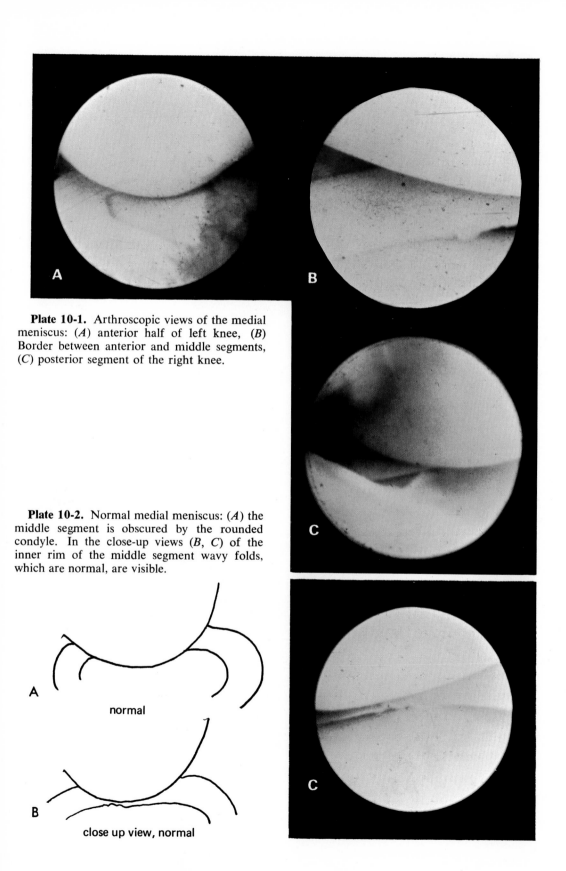

Plate 10-1. Arthroscopic views of the medial meniscus: (*A*) anterior half of left knee, (*B*) Border between anterior and middle segments, (*C*) posterior segment of the right knee.

Plate 10-2. Normal medial meniscus: (*A*) the middle segment is obscured by the rounded condyle. In the close-up views (*B, C*) of the inner rim of the middle segment wavy folds, which are normal, are visible.

normal

close up view, normal

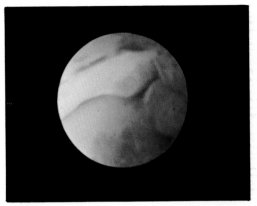

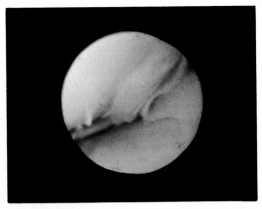

Plate 10-3. Incomplete medial discoid meniscus (right knee).

Plate 10-4. L-shaped tear of the medial meniscus of the right knee.

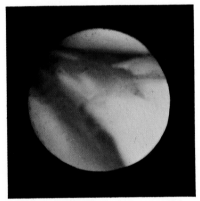

Plate 10-5. Cross tear of the medial meniscus of the right knee.

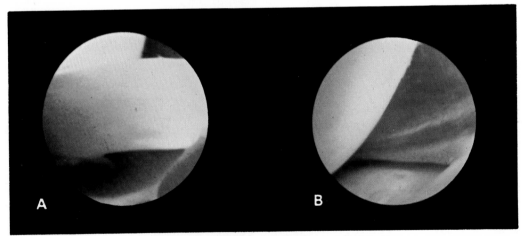

Plate 10-6. Bucket handle (bow-string) tear of the medial meniscus of the right knee: (*A*) bucket handle, (*B*) outer ridge.

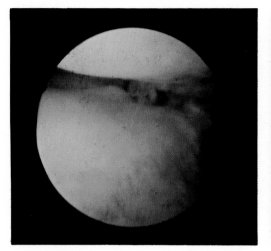

Plate 10-7. Complete medial discoid meniscus in the left knee.

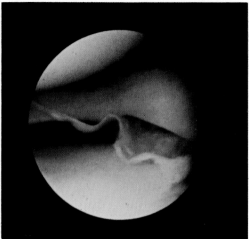

Plate 10-8. Ruptured medial collateral ligament of the right knee.

Plate 10-9. The L-shaped tear was confirmed by palpation with an instrument.

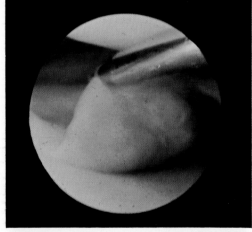

Plate 10-10. The lateral meniscus of the right knee.

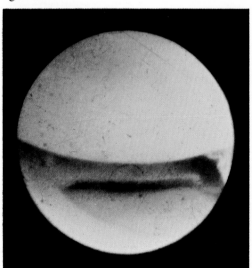

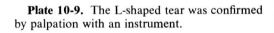

Plate 10-11. The posterior segment of the left-knee lateral meniscus shows abnormal looseness.

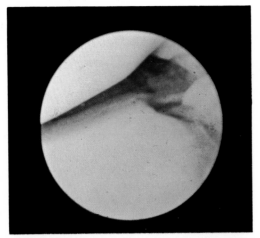

Plate 10-12. Complete lateral discoid meniscus in the right knee.

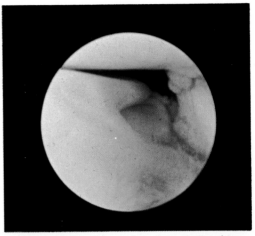

Plate 10-13. Incomplete lateral discoid meniscus in the right knee.

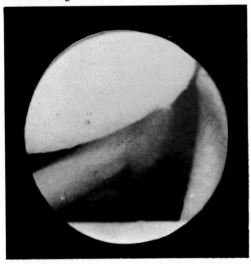

Plate 10-14. Wrisberg's ligament in the right knee.

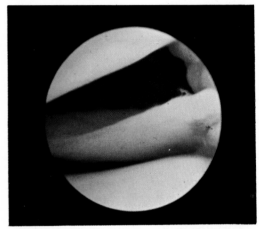

Plate 10-15. Humphry's ligament in a right knee.

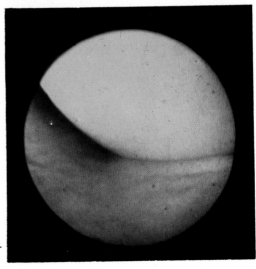

Plate 10-16. Posteromedially dislocated lateral discoid meniscus in the right knee.

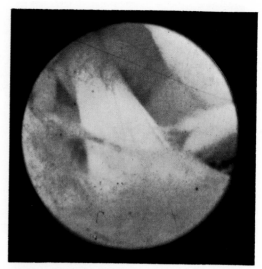

Plate 10-17. Anterior cruciate ligament in the right knee.

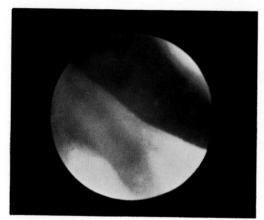

Plate 10-18. Incomplete rupture of the anterior cruciate ligament in the right knee.

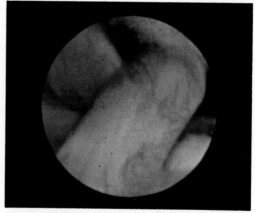

Plate 10-19. Anterior and posterior cruciate ligaments in the left knee.

Plate 10-20. This loose body in the suprapatellar pouch was removed under arthroscopic control.

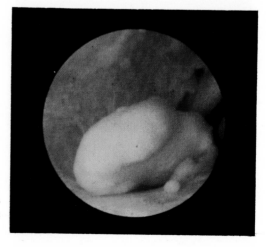

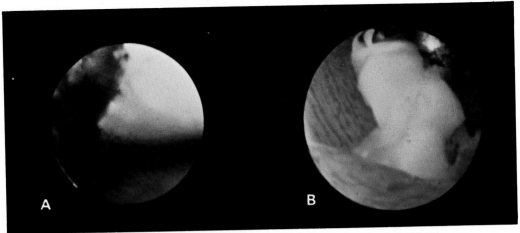

Plate 10-21. (*A*) Lateral marginal fracture of the patella. (*B*) The fragment in the lateral pouch was taken off without opening the joint.

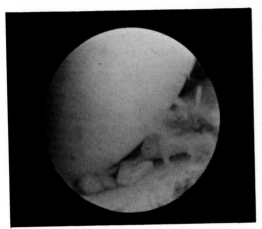

Plate 10-22. Osteochondromatosis — loose bodies in the knee.

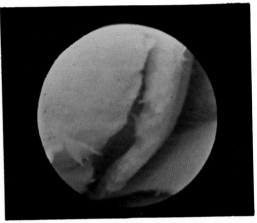

Plate 10-23. Osteochondronecrosis in the medial femoral condyle of the right knee.

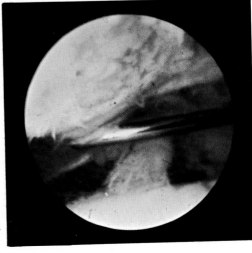

Plate 10-24. Chondromalacia of the patella seen from suprapatellar side.

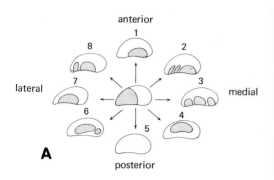

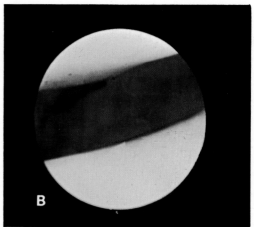

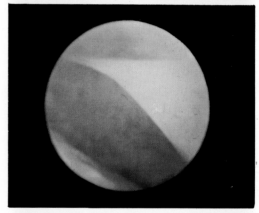

Plate 10-25. Plica synovialis suprapatellaris.
(*A*) Diagrams of normal (*center*) and variations.
(*B*) Complete left-knee septum seen from below.

Plate 10-26. Plica synovialis mediopatellaris of the right knee.

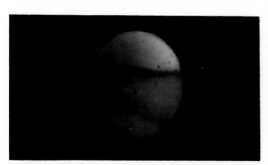

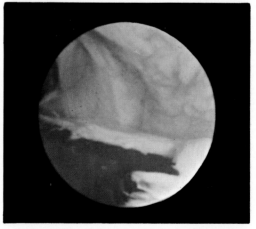

Plate 10-27. A huge shelf in the right knee of an 8-year-old boy caused some disorder of the joint. The plica was elongated by cutting it partially under arthroscopic control, and the symptoms disappeared.

Plate 10-28. Plica synovialis mediopatellaris caused a disorder of this joint. Biopsy revealed cartilagelike change of the synovium.

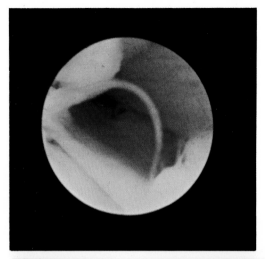

Plate 10-29. A chorda cavi articularis genu (Mayeda).

Plate 10-30. Popliteal tendon: (*A*) femoral insertion, (*B*) running obliquely behind the torn and frayed lateral discoid meniscus of the left knee.

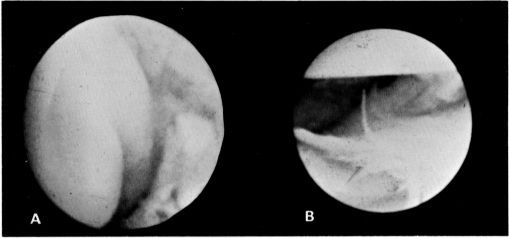

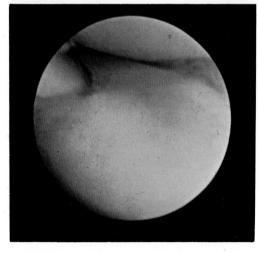

Plate 10-31. Medial meniscus of the right knee elevated by an underlying ganglion.

image must be taken into consideration (Fig. 10-5). Therefore, observation should be done by moving the tip of the arthroscope and changing the distance. The outer margin in the border between middle and posterior segments is difficult to observe with the No. 21, but can be seen with the No. 24 needlescope under maximal varus strain. The space between the posterior segment and the tibial plateau is relatively wide compared with that found on the opposite side. However, if this space is too wide due to excessive laxity, a parameniscal tear is suspected (Plate 10-11).

Lateral Discoid Meniscus. The lateral discoid meniscus is not rare among the Japanese. Smillie[23] classified it into three types: primitive, intermediate, and infantile. Kaplan[11,12] pointed out that no discoid meniscus was found in any stages of fetal development and that the discoid form develops gradually after birth and is the result of abnormal motion of the lateral meniscus with an anatomical variation which consists of the posterior horn not being attached to the tibial plateau. It is this type of discoid meniscus that Kaplan failed to find in any fetuses that he examined at Carnegie Institute and in the cases that he personally observed at Columbia University.

In Japan, Nemoto[18] examined knee joints of 70 fetuses in which he found three cases of bilateral lateral discoid meniscus. Matsushita[14] of my clinic investigated the same subject on 16 fetuses and found one case of bilateral lateral discoid meniscus. On the other hand, we see also an anomalous lateral meniscus in which the insertion of the posterior horn is defective but its size is fairly normal and which I termed "Wrisberg's ligament type."[30] I am, therefore of the opinion that among so-called lateral discoid menisci there are both congenital discoid menisci, as Smillie stated, and secondarily developed discoid menisci, as described by Kaplan.

From the viewpoint of arthroscopy, I classified the lateral discoid meniscus into the three types shown in Figure 10-6.[30]

The complete discoid meniscus occupies the lateral side of the tibial plateau and blocks the view of the tibial plateau completely (Plate 10-12). Such a discoid meniscus appears as if it were the tibial plateau itself, so that observation must be done by placing pressure with free hand on the peripheral border of the meniscus in order to distinguish it from the true tibial plateau. The incomplete discoid meniscus shows many variations in its size and form and structure. In arthroscopy of the incomplete discoid meniscus, the close-up view of its concave part of the inner rim often resembles the view of normal lateral meniscus lying on the tibial plateau (Plate 10-13). The anomalous posterior horn of the lateral meniscus shows variations in size. Wrisberg's ligament is easy to detect (Plate 10-14). Humphrey's ligament is rare in Japanese (Plate 10-15). The lateral discoid meniscus often dislocates posteromedially; it is diagnosed from its relationship to the corresponding rounded condyle (Plate 10-16). A ruptured and degenerated discoid meniscus sometimes loses its meniscal appearance.

Clinical Statistics. From 1958 to 1971, 320 knee joints suspected of internal derangement were arthroscopically examined in our clinic. Among them were 208 meniscal lesions or disorders, 18 ruptured ligaments, and 94 other disorders. Among 208 meniscus cases, surgery was performed on 153, and the results are shown in Table 10-3. The ratio of ruptured medial meniscus to the lateral is approximately 1:2 (29:54), but when discoid meniscus is excluded, the ratio should be corrected as 3:1 (27:9).

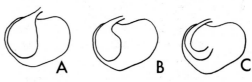

FIG. 10-6. Classification scheme for anomalous lateral meniscus: (*A*) complete discoid meniscus; (*B*) incomplete discoid meniscus; (*C*) Wrisberg's ligament type.

TABLE 10-3. Results of Surgery on 153 Menisci

Meniscus operated	Medial (torn)	Lateral (torn)	Total
Meniscus excluding discoid meniscus	32 (27)	19 (9)	51 (36)
Discoid meniscus	6 (2)	93 (45)	99 (47)
Meniscus ganglion	2	1	3
Total	40 (29)	113 (54)	153 (83)

TABLE 10-4. Types and Distribution of Discoid Meniscus in Table 10-3

Types	Medial (torn)	Lateral (torn)	Total
Complete	5 (1)	68 (38)	73 (39)
Incomplete	1 (1)	15 (7)	16 (8)
Wrisberg's ligament type	0	10	10
Total	6 (2)	93 (45)	99 (47)

Cruciate Ligaments

The anterior cruciate ligament is better observed by lateral infrapatellar approach and with the knee bent to 60 to 90 degrees (Plate 10-17). It looks like a white tendinous band coated by thin synovial membrane and contains a few blood vessels. The anterior ligament can be traced to its femoral insertion as well as to the divergent inferior part. Complete or incomplete rupture of the anterior ligament can be observed (Plate 10-18).

Behind the anterior ligament, the femoral insertion of the posterior cruciate ligament can be seen (Plate 10-19) bordered by a red, eroded areola in the cartilage of the medial condyle (Plate 10-1C). The posterior ligament is sometimes difficult to see; fat pads in this region hinder its view. When the anterior ligament is torn (and worn out) observation of the posterior ligament becomes very easy.

Collateral Ligaments

There is not much to be emphasized in arthroscopic examination for injury of col-

lateral ligaments. The diagnosis is made by clinical examination, and, from the viewpoint of arthroscopy, careful observation of any combined injuries is most important. If the medial ligament is ruptured at the level just below the meniscal attachment, a widening of the gap between medial meniscus and tibial plateau is evident arthroscopically (Plate 10-8). And if a piece of ruptured medial ligament is impacted into the joint space, it can be detected by arthroscopy.

Others

Loose bodies, osteochondral fracture, osteochondritis dissecans, osteochondromatosis, aseptic osteochondronecrosis, and chondromalacia of the patella are enumerated in this category. Some examples are shown in Plates 10-20 to 10-24.

Hoffa's disease is usually diagnosed by clinical examination. Intraarticular lesion of the infrapatellar fat pads or synovial fringe is sometimes found as a suggillation in the tissue.

Synovial pleats or chordae sometimes cause characteristic disorders of the joint. Plica synovialis supra-, infra-, and mediopatellaris are three main synovial pleats of the knee joint. Plica synovialis suprapatellaris, an incomplete septum between bursa and recessus suprapatellaris, separates them in the medial half and is a good mark for interpretation of the location of the tip of the arthroscope. However, there are many variations in its extent (Plate 10-25A). Plate 10-25B is a view of a complete septum. I have never yet encountered a single example of pathology of this plica. Plica synovialis infrapatellaris can be observed running over the anterior cruciate ligament. As the joint cavity is distended with saline during arthroscopy, this plica is somewhat stretched so that it usually looks thinner and the blood vessels running through it become visible. In some cases a membranous septum is found between the plica and the anterior ligament. It is possible to damage this plica by careless arthroscopic procedure, but its clinical significance is not clear. I have only encountered one case in which the plica synovialis infra-patellaris was thickly scarred and caused some disorder of the joint.

Plica synovialis mediopatellaris is a synovial pleat on the medial wall of the knee joint cavity starting from the medial plica alaris toward the medial part of the plica synovialis suprapatellaris.[22,28] It is very often seen in the knee joint of Japanese (nearly half), and Iino called it "the band" in his work on arthroscopy of the knee joint in 1939.[8] It is also called simply "the shelf,"[17] because of its shelflike appearance (Plate 10-26), but it shows many variations. Plica synovialis mediopatellaris is considered, as are the preceding two synovial pleats, to be a persistence of the synovial septum of the fetal stage. A considerable number of cases of internal derangement of the knee due to a certain change of the plica synovialis medio-patellaris have been reported in Japan. In my estimation, however, it causes some derangement of the joint only when it is too large (a huge shelf) or becomes too hard (Plates 10-27, 10-28).

The chorda cavi articularis genu (Mayeda, 1918)[15] is a cordlike or stringlike structure found in various sites of the joint cavity (Plate 10-29). Mayeda considered it to be a retained septum in the synovial cavity and classified it into six types according to the site of its insertion. From the viewpoint of arthroscopy, I classified it into three types, according to its relationship to the main synovial pleats.[28] Only when a chorda becomes very thick and hard does it tend to cause derangement of the joint.

Chorda obliqua synovialis[25] means a chorda in the synovial membrane which can be palpated in the extended position of the knee either medial or lateral to the patella, running obliquely toward the medial or lateral joint line (Fig. 10-7), and is not palpable when the knee is flexed to about 90 degrees. It is a special structure in the synovial membrane, and its clinical significance was investigated by Takahashi of my clinic in 1960.[24]

The lateral outer pouch consists of the lateral wall of the joint cavity and lateral synovial surface of the lateral femoral condyle. The popliteal tendon can be seen in the depth of the lateral pouch, which runs in the posteroinferior direction and disappears as it curves medially behind the lateral meniscus to its exit in the posterior capsule (Plate 10-30). I have performed arthroscopy in one case of popliteal tendon click, in which a mechanism of the click was investigated.

Pedunculate xanthomatous giant cell

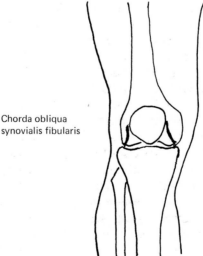

Chorda obliqua synovialis fibularis

Chorda obliqua synovialis tibialis

Chorda obliqua synovialis.

FIG. 10-7. Chorda obliqua synovialis.

tumor, hemangioma, fibroma, and ganglia, were observed. Plate 10-31 is a case of ganglion under the medial meniscus.

CONCLUSION

Through the development of the No. 21 arthroscope, arthroscopy has become a practical diagnostic measure for internal derangement of the knee. As arthroscopy is a direct visualization, its interpretation is easy. The use of arthroscopy has permitted not only diagnosis of the existence of rupture of the meniscus but also the observation of detailed findings of a meniscal tear on which methods of treatment can be based. In order to improve accuracy of arthroscopic diagnosis of the meniscus, the original technique for use of the No. 21 and full muscle relaxation throughout the examination are essential.

Arthroscopy is a procedure with minimal morbidity. It does not cause quadriceps inhibition and can be performed repeatedly. Partial meniscectomy or cutting off the posterior horn prior to surgery under arthroscopic control can be performed in selected cases. Removal of loose bodies without opening the joint is often carried out successfully by means of the arthroscope and its accessories.

Further, we are conducting research on the use of the No. 24 arthroscope for the knee joint, employed in tandem with the No. 21 in order to observe areas presently inaccessible to the No. 21 alone, such as the undersurface of the meniscus, the outer ridge of the meniscus in the border between middle and posterior segments, the tibial half of the posterior cruciate ligament, and the popliteal cavity.

BIBLIOGRAPHY

1. Andrén, L., and Wehlin, L.: Double-contrast arthrography of knee with horizontal roentgen ray beam. Acta Orthop. Scandinav., *29*:307, 1960.
2. Casscells, S. W.: Arthroscopy of the knee joint. J. Bone Joint Surg., *53A*:287, 1971.
3. Freiberger, R. H., Nicholas, J. A., and Killoran, P. J.: The value of double-contrast arthrography in the surgical management of the knee injury. J. Bone Joint Surg., *49A*:1482, 1967.
4. Helfet, A. J.: Mechanism of derangements of the medial semilunar cartilage and their management. J. Bone Joint Surg., *41B*:319, 1959.
5. ————: Management of Internal Derangements of the Knee. Philadelphia, J. B. Lippincott, 1963.
6. Heller, L., and Langman, L.: The meniscofemoral ligaments of the human knee. J. Bone Joint Surg., *46B*:307, 1964.
7. Humphrey, G. M.: A Treatise on the Human Skeleton Including the Joints. Cambridge, Macmillan, 1958.
8. Iino, S.: Normal arthroscopic findings of the knee joint in adults. J. Jap. Orthop. Assoc., *14*:467, 1939.
9. Jackson, R. W., and Abe, I.: The role of arthroscopy in the management of disorders of the knee. J. Bone Joint Surg., *54A*:310, 1972.
10. Kaplan, E. B.: The lateral meniscofemoral ligament of the knee. Bull. Hosp. of Joint Diseases, *17*:176, 1956.
11. ————: Discoid lateral meniscus of the knee joint. J. Bone Joint Surg., *39A*:77, 1957.
12. ————: Personal communication, 1961.
13. Lindblom, K.: Arthrography of the knee. Acta Radiolog. Scand., [Suppl.]:74, 1948.
14. Matsushita, A., Watanabe, M., and Takeda, S.: Investigation on so-called discoid meniscus. J. Jap. Orthop. Assoc., *35*:851, 1961.
15. Mayeda, T: Ueber das strangartige Gebilde in der Kniegelenkhöhle (Chorda cavi articularis genu). Mitt. med. Fak. Kaiserl. Univ. Tokyo, *21*:507, 1918.
16. McMurray, T. P.: The semilunar cartilages. Brit. J. Surg., *29*:407, 1940.
17. Mizumachi, S., Kawashima, W., and Okamura, T.: So-called synovial shelf in the knee joint. J. Jap. Orthop. Assoc., *22*:1, 1948.
18. Nemoto, H.: Study on discoid meniscus of the knee. Niigata Med. J., *64*:404, 1950.
19. Nicholas, J. A., Freiberger, R. H., and Killoran, P. J.: Double-contrast arthrography of the knee. J. Bone Joint Surg., *52A*:203, 1970.

20. Okazaki, H.: Clinical significance of arthrography and arthroscopy to diagnosis of internal derangement of the knee. Clin. Orthop. Surg., *3*:1046, 1968.

21. Ricklin, R. P., Rüttimann, A., und Del Buono, M. S.: Die Meniskusläsion. Stuttgart, G. Thieme, 1964.

22. Sakakibara, J.: Study on "Iino's band"–a synovial pleat in the knee joint of Japanese. J. Jap. Orthop. Assoc. *46*:846, 1972.

23. Smillie, I. S.: Injuries of the Knee Joint. ed. 4. Edinburgh and London, E. & S. Livingstone, 1970.

24. Takahashi, S.: On the chorda obliqua synovialis of the knee joint. Teishin Igaku, *12*:1, 1960.

25. Watanabe, M.: The development and present status of the arthroscope. J. Jap. Med. Instr., *25*:11, 1954.

26. ———: Arthroscopic diagnosis of internal derangement of the knee. J. Jap. Orthop. Assoc., *42*:993, 1968.

27. Watanabe, M., and Takeda, S.: The No. 21 arthroscope. J. Jap. Orthop. Assoc., *34*: 1041, 1960.

28. Watanabe, M., Takeda, S., Ikeuchi, H., and Sakakibara, J.: Chorda cavi articularis genu (Mayeda) from the viewpoint of arthroscopy. Clin. Orthop. Surg. *7*:986, 1972.

29. ———: Arthroscope—present and future. Surgical Therapy, *26*:73, 1972.

30. Watanabe, M., Takeda, S., and Ikeuchi, H.: Atlas of Arthroscopy. ed. 2. Tokyo, Igaku Shoin, 1969.

11

Management of Injuries to the Semilunar Cartilages

Arthur J. Helfet, M.D.

Since only peripheral tears of the cartilage are likely to heal, treatment of ruptured semilunar cartilages in most instances includes surgical excision. After the first accident to the knee it is impossible to determine whether the tear is peripheral or not. Therefore, it is reasonable, if successful reduction is possible, to treat the acute injury conservatively. When the cartilage has been deranged twice or more often, healing is most unlikely, and operation should be advised—the sooner the better. Surgery is necessary and urgent, also, if attempts to reduce the displacement fail. The persistently displaced or retracted cartilage inexorably produces patterns of traumatic erosion and stretching of the capsular structures. These changes are irreversible. Early operation is preventive, but removal of the offending cartilage is also advisable, as will be argued, at any stage of the resultant traumatic arthritis. Surgery should be advised also if the patient's occupation is one in which a potentially unstable knee would be especially hazardous, e.g., work on ladders or at heights. During the war it was not customary to send a soldier back to a fighting unit until the injured meniscus had been removed.

Treatment of the pain and distress of the initial incident includes rest with splinting, management of the resultant effusion and reduction of any displacements of cartilage. Relief from weight bearing and/or a Jones bandage give adequate rest. Complete immobility is not necessary, but movements which would displace the cartilage again should be avoided. Sir Robert Jones[8] described a compression bandage composed of a thick layer of cotton wool, a firm calico, flannel or crepe bandage, reinforced by a second layer of wool and a firmer bandage (Fig. 11-1). If weight bearing is urgent, the addition of a plaster-of-paris or other rigid back splint is necessary. The splint should extend from just below the buttock to 6 inches above the ankle and should be fixed to the thigh and the leg at least at three, and preferably at four, points.

Acute pain is relieved quite simply by the injection of 5 to 10 ml. of 1 per cent procaine, made up in normal saline, into the suprapatellar pouch (Fig. 11-2). With proper aseptic precautions, this is a safe "office" procedure and has value not only for relieving pain but also as a sufficient anesthetic for aspiration of the effusion or reduction of the displaced cartilage.

ASPIRATION OF THE KNEE

Mild effusion requires no more than the compression bandage, but if tense or rapidly increasing it requires aspiration. The easiest route, shown in Figure 11-2, is through the natural notch formed behind the insertion of the quadriceps into the upper pole of the patella. At this point only skin and fibrous capsule cover the synovium, and the route is relatively insensitive. The skin should be

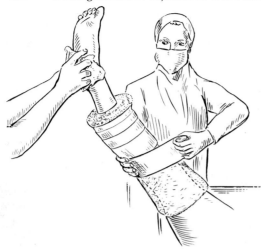

FIG. 11-1. The Jones compression bandage applied from mid-thigh to mid-calf.

cleansed with soap and water, then alcohol, and then painted with iodine or sprayed with a thin layer of one of the self-sterilizing aeroplastic solutions. The latter helps to seal the puncture wound afterward, but all that is required is the firm pressure of an iodine dab for a few seconds after the needle is removed. The skin quickly seals itself. Aspiration always should be followed by firm bandaging with either a Jones' compression bandage or a crepe bandage applied thickly and firmly but not tightly.

Hemarthrosis requires a needle of slightly thicker bore than that used for a simple effusion. The necessity for aspiration is more urgent and invariably should be followed by a compression bandage.

REDUCTION OF
THE RUPTURED MENISCUS

The essence of reduction of the displaced meniscus is reversal of the torque of the original injury. If extension and lateral rotation of the tibia are the movements blocked, attempts to overcome the block by manipulating further in these directions will aggravate the rupture and the displacement. Instead, the tibia must be unwound into flexion and medial rotation. Once the cartilage is slack, a jerk into normal extension will pull the cartilage back into line. The simplest method is to inject local anesthetic into the knee joint and show the patient how to do the maneuver himself. The patient sits on the edge of a table. The knee is flexed passively. Full medial and then lateral rotation is repeated until the full range is obtained, usually suddenly and sometimes with a click. Then the patient kicks the leg out —as if at a ball—to the limit of extension (Fig. 11-3). Sometimes a sticky knee may be helped by rocking the flexed tibia forward and backward on the femur (Fig. 11-4). If unsuccessful, the manipulation may be repeated under Pentothal anesthesia when abduction or adduction, while extending and externally rotating the leg, also may be tried. If displacement persists, i.e., the rotation signs remain, there is no alternative to operation.

Prolonged skin traction in bed is not recommended. When accompanied by regular

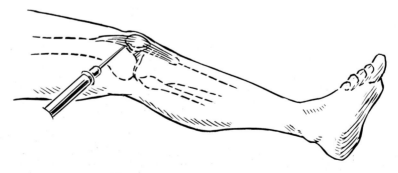

FIG. 11-2. Aspiration of the knee through the suprapatellar pouch. The needle is inserted into the natural notch formed behind the insertion of the quadriceps into the upper pole of the patella.

FIG. 11-3. Reduction of displaced meniscus. (*Top, left*) The patient sits on the edge of the table. The knee is flexed passively. (*Top, center*) Full medial rotation of the leg. (*Top, right*) Then lateral rotation is repeated until the full range is obtained. (*Bottom*) Then the leg is kicked out, as if at a ball, to the limit of extension.

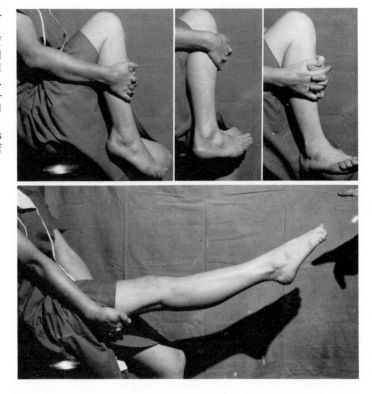

isometric thigh muscle drill (quadriceps and hamstrings) the acute symptoms do settle down and the effusion subsides. But the "rotation" signs denoting persistence of the displacement of the torn meniscus usually persist. Recurrent effusions in an aching knee, with or without locking and "giving way," eventually demand meniscectomy.

CONSERVATIVE TREATMENT

Conservative treatment for the first injury should be continued for 4 weeks by which time the peripheral tear should heal soundly. (Most ligamentous structures repair in that time.[3,9]) A compression bandage or splint is kept on for 10 days and is followed by a crepe bandage and, most important, limited activity. In other words, the knee requires protection from further injury rather than immobilization.

MUSCLE EXERCISE

As with injury to any joint, rehabilitation of the power and excursion of all muscles acting on the knee is essential. Quadriceps drill should be augmented by hamstrings drill. It is as easy to do static contractions of both together as of either separately. It is of interest to note that when these two groups are contracted, automatic contraction of the gastrocnemii and the popliteus takes place as well. The whole muscular mechanism of the knee is activated.

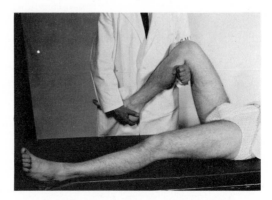

FIG. 11-4. Sometimes a sticky knee may be helped by rocking the flexed tibia forward and backward on the femur.

Wasting of the muscles associated with an injured joint is more rapid than occurs through disuse and inactivity alone. A neurotrophic reflex, it would seem, is abolished. The wasted muscles plus inactivity in turn delay the disappearance of joint effusion and swelling. The circulation of the joint and its musculature are complementary and under the same neurotrophic control, and it is probable that muscle activity acts chiefly by increasing the blood supply to the joint and, therefore, increasing absorption of fluid and the products of injury.

The patient should be instructed to contract all the thigh muscles to their full extent, to hold the contraction for a full second, and then relax as fully. The exercise is repeated 12 times per waking hour. No more is required. Overexercising often induces fatigue and a new effusion. As power improves, straight-leg raising exercises may be substituted, but not before the patient realizes that "straight-leg" means *full extension.* The value of much exercise is lost by raising the leg with the knee slightly flexed.

Full extension is even more important postoperatively. Before the cartilage is removed, the final arc of extension and lateral rotation has been absent for some time. After operation it is essential that the patient recover this final stabilizing phase of movement. There is *never* difficulty in recovery of flexion. On the contrary, the knee has the failing of finding comfort in flexion at any time of stress. In older patients whose cartilage lesions have reached a stage of traumatic arthritis, full comfort postoperatively is not attained until the knee can achieve full extension in walking. This is understandable, for only in full extension does the patella lie comfortably, with equal tension on both slopes of the trochlear groove of the femur.

Other forms of physiotherapy may be used, if it is understood that their only function is to improve circulation and, therefore, the absorption of fluid and the metabolites of injury. Heat and massage in any form cannot strengthen muscle. Only exercise can achieve this. Faradization may teach the patient how to contract the muscle and prepare it for exercise, but for restoration of power it cannot compete with active and forceful contraction.

SURGERY OF THE SEMILUNAR CARTILAGES

The requisites for successful and relatively pain-free surgery of the knee are *accurate diagnosis, gentle atraumatic surgery* and *clear visualization of each step,* associated with controlled preoperative and postoperative rehabilitation. These factors are inherent in the whole technic to be described and apply to assistant as well as surgeon. Overenthusiastic retraction results in postoperative pain and effusion. So that he can see every step, the assistant should face the side of the knee that bears the incision. The incision must be adequate but not excessive. It is never necessary to use forceful traction to reach the posterior end of the cartilage, and powerful forceps are a temptation to be resisted. Special knives that incite blind incision into the posterior end of the cartilage should not appear on the instrument tables of any but those who devise them, have trained themselves to use them safely and who, presumably, require additional reach. I have seen more damage to the synovium and the posterior capsule and more postoperative pain and hemarthrosis from these devices in the hands of the less experienced than from any other cause.

The following technic is based on that of the Liverpool school as used by Sir Robert Jones, Sir Harry Platt, T. P. McMurray, W. R. Bristow, and most of their disciples. During the last 30 years and from the study of over 2500 operations, minor modifications have been made in the incision and in the amount of posterior horn which it is necessary to excise.

SKIN PREPARATION

Forty-eight hours of skin preparation had always been a ritual, but a few hours preparation is now considered safe and sufficient. The limb from groin to toe is shaved, scrubbed with soap and water, painted with 70 per cent alcohol, and wrapped in sterile towels. After the tourniquet has been applied the skin is painted with two coats of 2 per cent iodine in 70 per cent alcohol or preferably betadyne. Operating through sterile stockinette is not advocated.

Hemostasis

In young patients the limb is exsanguinated by an Esmarch bandage. A tourniquet, preferably pneumatic, is applied well up the thigh. To avoid the use of a tourniquet in old people, the method described to me by Amnon Fried of the Beilenson Hospital in Tel Aviv is recommended. The skin and the capsule in the area of the skin incision are infiltrated with 0.5 per cent procaine or Leostessin in saline with 0.75 ml. of 1:1,000 Adrenalin per 100 ml. The rest of the 100 ml. is injected into and distends the knee joint. After 5 minutes the joint is anesthetic while the quality of hemostasis is remarkable. A sucker copes with the fluid once the joint is opened. At the end of the operation the patient is able to extend the knee actively. With the technic to be described, postoperative oozing is negligible.

Operative Technic

The leg is placed to hang over the end of the operating table at right angles to the thigh. The leg should be free of the edge by at least an inch. The draped foot is gripped by the gowned knees of the surgeon. This permits easy rotation and abduction and adduction of the bent knee and allows good vision of the intercondylar space or the back end of the cartilage as the need arises—an essential for gentle surgery. A small sandbag along the edge of the table lifts the thigh and facilitates free movement of the leg at the knee (Plate 11-1A).

The Incision. The incision that I prefer is almost horizontal, sloping very slightly downward and backward in line with the upper surface of the meniscus (Plate 11-1B).

It does not extend far enough back to injure the medial or the lateral ligament. The whole extent of the incision is over the joint and does not cross the lower border of the femur. Infrapatellar branches of the saphenous nerve (Fig. 11-5) are always cut, and the patient should be warned that there will be a patch of anesthesia in front of the knee

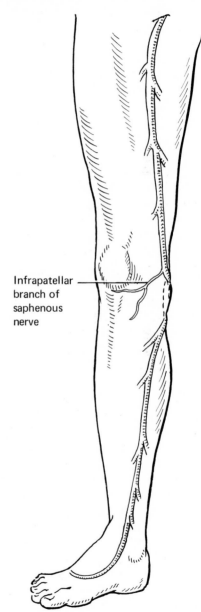

Infrapatellar branch of saphenous nerve

FIG. 11-5. Infrapatellar branches of the saphenous nerve are always cut.

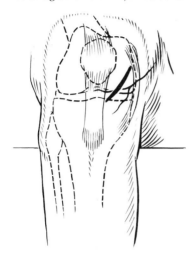

FIG. 11-6. This oblique incision may cut branches of the saphenous nerve where they cross the lower border of the femur and so give rise to a painful neuroma.

after the operation and that it may last for months. It is rarely permanent and causes no disability—when this is realized the patient feels no concern. In no instance have I seen the notorious "neuroma" form in this scar. It happens only in the scar that crosses and becomes adherent to the edge of the femur (Fig. 11-6) and causes pain

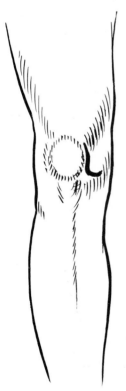

FIG. 11-7. For inspection of the patella the anterior end of the horizontal incision should be curved upward.

when the scar is tensed. Excision of the neuroma and freeing of the capsule from the bone relieves the symptoms.

When the articular surface of the patella needs inspection, the skin incision for the medial cartilage should be curved upward from the anterior end to run in the gap between the patella and the medial edge of the femoral condyle (Fig. 11-7).

The posterior compartment of the knee is explored through a vertical incision in line with the posterior border of the tibia. With the leg hanging at a right angle, the hamstrings on the medial side are well out of the way, and only the capsule and the synovium need to be traversed (Fig. 11-8). On the lateral side, the incision is above and in line with the head of the fibula. The biceps and the peroneal nerve are below the area of operation (Fig. 11-9). Skin should be sutured gently and without tension. Few minor details in surgical technic cause as much pain as tight skin sutures.

The Operation. The joint is opened in the line of the skin incision. Three layers are traversed, and each must be carefully and separately sutured when closing up. The superficial fascia contains the infrapatellar branches of the saphenous nerve, and a few stitches of fine catgut relieve tension and add to comfort. After the capsule is divided, a sweep of the knife above and below frees it from the underlying synovium. This is a useful practice, especially on the lateral side, as it facilitates sewing up. W. Rowley Bristow taught this maneuver and nominated it as his major contribution to the operative surgery of the knee joint. When opening the synovium, the incision should skirt the fat pad; care should be taken not to cut into it at all, since scars and adhesions of the fat pad are a potential cause of pain (Plate 11-1C).

Once the joint is open, the assistant retracts the synovium gently with two blunt hooks, the fat pad is pulled forward by a Langenbeck type right-angled retractor, and the interior is inspected (Plate 11-1D).

Lesions of the anterior two thirds of the semilunar cartilage are evident—the transverse tear and "parrot beak" of the free edge, the longitudinal bowstring tear in the substance of the cartilage, the peripheral detachment from the capsule, and the retracted anterior end. The last are the most interesting and are relatively common, so much so that in 1909 Sir Robert Jones reporting on 117 cases found that 53 carti-

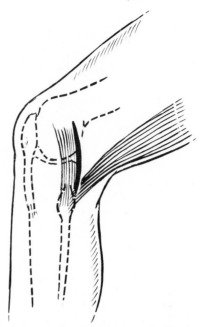

Fig. 11-9. On the lateral side the incision is above the biceps and the peroneal nerve in line with the fibula.

lages were torn from their anterior attachment, compared with 16 bowstring tears and 8 complete peripheral detachments.[7]*

Thomas Annandale of Edinburgh described the retracted cartilage for the first time.[1] On November 16, 1883, he performed not the first meniscectomy (which is to the credit of Bradhurst of St. George's Hospital, London in 1866) but the first recorded operation for displaced semilunar

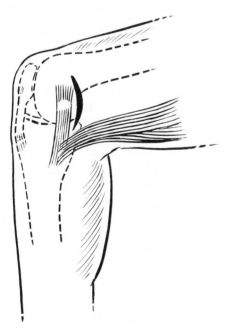

Fig. 11-8. The posterior compartment on the medial side is explored through a vertical incision.

---

* Out of 117 cases operated on (1906, 1907, 1908) for injury to the cartilage in which a lesion was found:
  53 were torn from their anterior attachment
  16 were split longitudinally
  8 were attached by the cornua and torn from the capsule
  7 were displacements of the posterior horns
  12 were fractured transversely opposite the internal lateral ligament
  8 were loosely bound circumferentially with no other appreciable abnormality
  8 had undergone changes in the loose anterior extremity of the semilunar of the nodular type, some being as lumpy and large as a pea
  3 cases exhibited no trace of the cartilage
  2 cases showed anterior part doubled and adherent to the posterior part

cartilage. He found "that the internal semilunar cartilage was completely separated from its anterior attachment to the tibia and was displaced backwards about half an inch."

He did not excise the cartilage but cured his patient by drawing the cartilage forward and stitching it to its former attachment. Ten weeks later the man was back at his work with a normally functioning knee.

If the anterior end is free, it may be picked up with a pair of dissecting forceps. Otherwise, a blunt hook is passed around the free margin, and the cartilage is dissected off near the edge of the tibia close to the synovial margin (Plate 11-1E).

There would seem to be little purpose in freeing the whole cartilage by dividing the peripheral attachments. If each incision into the substance of the cartilage is made close to the edge, there is no bleeding postoperatively, whereas dividing the vascular peripheral attachments often results in hemarthrosis. Nothing is lost by leaving a narrow rim of cartilage. It may even minimize the minor radiologic changes described by Fairbank after meniscectomy.[6] Not one of hundreds of knees with the residual rim of cartilage has developed a single detrimental symptom. On the other hand, the rim must be meticulously trimmed. No tag or fringe must be left to float frondlike into the joint. These may give rise to continued symptoms due to nipping. On the lateral side, cutting into the meniscus protects the lateral inferior geniculate artery which may be involved if the synovium is damaged (Plate 11-1F).

The freed anterior end of the meniscus is gripped in Kocher's or other forceps. Mild tension is exerted by pulling forward and toward the center of the joint, and a sharp blade splits as much as cuts the meniscus along the edge. The author prefers a fresh Bard-Parker blade, but any keen knife may be used. The strokes are gentle, and care is taken not to scratch the articular cartilage of the tibia.

The pull on the meniscus invaginates the posterior capsule into the joint, and by rotating the foot between his knees the surgeon brings more of the meniscus into view. In the laxer joint still more may be seen if the assistant pulls the whole tibia forward on the femur.

Ultimately the meniscus is dislocated into the intercondylar space. By rotating the leg in the opposite direction, the posterior attachments to the tibial spine are brought into view and divided (Plate 11-1G, H).

The stage at which the meniscus slips into the center of the joint varies. If the posterior horn is detached, it occurs early, and the operation is simple. If the posterior horn is normal and the joint tight, it is more difficult. But usually only a little patience to ensure that each incision is made under direct vision is needed to complete the operation. Charnley's retractor is most suitably angled to expose the curve of the semilunar cartilage.

Difficulties with the Posterior Horn

Without ill-advised blind dissection it is impossible to remove the whole posterior horn through an anterior incision. A small segment always remains. But as long as the rim is firmly attached to the capsule, and if its substance has not been damaged by accident or during the operation, no harm ensues. In such cases there is no necessity to open the posterior compartment to remove it. The removal of the posterior fragment through a separate incision is essential: 1) when a tear or pedicle of the residual fragment is seen from the front, 2) whenever there is a history of "giving-way" of the knee and the loose posterior horn has not been adequately removed; and 3) after accidental fracture of the meniscus during operation.

After repeated derangements of the knee, as most writers have emphasized, there is often more than one split in the posterior horn. "Giving-way" is usually associated with lesions of the posterior halves of the cartilage. Preoperatively, too, the appropriate click over the posterior horn is elicited. If there is no such history or clinical finding, it may be assumed that the back end is intact. The fragment that remains only because of the technical impossibility of removal through an anterior incision in an otherwise tight posterior horn does not merit the additional posterior arthrotomy. The number of times in which judgment based on these criteria has been wrong, and subsequent operation has been necessary, is negligible.

A second operation is usually the result of a subsequent accident to the knee in which the posterior horn has been injured. Accidental fracture of the meniscus during the operation may occur through excessive traction on the cartilage or with an unusually deep transverse or oblique tear, or when the bowstring has left too meager a margin.

Views expressed in this chapter differ from the deeply rooted surgical inclination to remove the meniscus in its entirety. But it is felt that leaving a smooth and narrow rim of cartilage makes for less complicated convalescence and more rapid recovery without detriment to the future of the knee. Also, without the indications listed above, it is unnecessary to make a second incision to remove a *stable* posterior fragment.

Operation to Remove a Separate Posterior Horn

The vertical incision (Fig. 11-8) in line with the posterior border of the tibia crosses the joint line. The synovium of the posterior compartment is entered above the level of the meniscus. The space is well displayed by a right-angled retractor. Straightening the leg a little may show up the residual fragment of meniscus to better advantage. The cartilage is divided anteriorly and posteriorly as necessary. The synovium, the capsule, and the fascia are sutured in separate layers with fine plain catgut.

The Infrapatellar Pad of Fat

The anterior end of the meniscus has intimate attachments to the fat pad, which must be meticulously protected from injury. Freeing of the cartilage must be careful and gentle. This applies particularly to the retracted cartilage, the anterior stump of which may be thickened and somewhat fibrous and involved in scar with the fat and the synovium. Presumably, the scarring is the sequel to hemorrhage at the time of the detachment of the meniscus from the cruciate ligament. The thickened stump-plus-scar leaves its mark on the articular cartilage of the condyle of the femur. If the condition has been present for any length of time, straightening the knee will show the indentation or erosion on the anterior articular surface of the condyle. It is produced during weight bearing when the knee is straight. Both the bulk of the stump and the scar should be trimmed.

The Lateral Meniscus

Lateral meniscectomy does not differ materially from excision of the medial cartilage. The joint space is smaller, but the middle segment is not attached to the capsule and once the anterior end is free, the meniscus slips more easily into the center of the joint. Care must be taken not to injure the lateral inferior genicular artery which runs outside the synovium between the lateral ligament and the posterolateral aspect of the meniscus.

For the last 10 years, the approach described by Bruser[2] has been used. The fibers of the iliotibial band (when the knee is fully flexed) are horizontal and parallel with the joint line. Splitting the fibers in this line provides an easy and atraumatic exposure of the joint. Instead of the patient supine and flexing the knee on the table as advised by Bruser, the knee is flexed over the end of the table with the foot grasped by the knees of the surgeon as for the medial meniscus. To open the joint, the knee is raised till well flexed. Bruser's horizontal incision splits the iliotibial band in line with the joint and is extended as far anteriorly as the patellar tendon. The relaxed fibular collateral ligament is at the posterior end of the incision and must not be injured. The synovium is opened in the joint line, and care is taken not to injure the fat pad, by sloping the anterior end of the incision upwards. The foot is then lowered so that the thigh rests on the flexed table. I prefer this, because gravity, aided by the weight of the suspended foot and, if necessary, traction by the knees of the surgeon, increase the joint space.

Good exposure of the meniscus is obtained and complete excision is possible. Incision into the meniscus, especially posteriorly, should leave a narrow rim to avoid incising vascular synovium and capsular attachments. A hemostatic lock stitch closes synovium. The edges of the iliotibial band are opposed by a few intermittent sutures of fine catgut.

Inspection of the Opposite Meniscus

Unless the alar folds are exceptionally voluminous, it is possible to inspect the anterior end of the opposite meniscus. A right-angled retractor or flat dissector holds the pad of fat forward, and a light is shone across the joint. Detachments of the anterior end and bowstring tears may be observed. It is also useful to examine the articular cartilage of the lateral condyle, for patterns of erosion give specific information. These and changes in the patella will be discussed in Chapter 13.

The wound is sutured in four layers—synovium, capsule, fascia and skin. A lock stitch using a small fistula needle with No. 00 plain catgut ensures hemostasis in the synovium, and the same stitch is continued to close the capsule. A few sutures to join the fascia relieves tension in this sensitive layer rich in nerve fibers (Plate 11-1L, M, N).

Postoperative Care

With the knee straight, and before the tourniquet is released, a Jones compression bandage is applied from mid-thigh to mid-calf. It is applied firmly but not tightly. No splint is necessary (Plate 11-1Q).

The nursing staff and the physiotherapists must be made to understand that the patient's objective is to recover full extension of the knee. Often this has been impossible for some time before the operation. After an uncomplicated operation, recovery of flexion is never difficult (Plate 11-1P).

The leg must lie flat on the mattress. Pillows behind the knee are forbidden, and flexion must not be attempted. A sandbag along the outer side of the leg and the foot prevents the leg rolling over and adds to comfort, as does a bolster against the sole of the foot.

Static muscle drill for the thigh is instituted as soon as possible, often on the first but usually on the second day. If the patient has learned the procedure preoperatively, there is little difficulty. Once a *complete contraction* is achieved, convalescence is comfortable. This is an interesting phenomenon. Full contraction of the thigh muscles induces a feeling of normality—really, the absence of conscious sensation—and thereafter the exercises are quite comfortable.

If the foot swells, as it does occasionally, denoting that the bandage is too tight, it should be unwound without disturbing the inner layer of wool and reapplied. A dozen full contractions an hour are sufficient. Overexercise is of no value; indeed it disposes to effusion. After a few days attempts are made to lift the straight leg, and this may be assisted by the surgeon or the physiotherapist.

On the tenth day the Jones bandage is removed, the sutures are taken out, and a crepe bandage is applied, firmly and thickly but not tightly. It should extend no more than an inch above the upper border of the patella and 2 inches below the upper surface of the tibia and be applied in figure-of-eight fashion, crossing behind the knee. Gentle, active flexion is permitted and encouraged, and 30 or 40 degrees or more is usually possible immediately. The patient is allowed to stand and to walk, the distance depending on the tone of the thigh muscles. This should be the yardstick in rehabilitation. As long as exertion is within the compass of the thigh muscles, increasing activity rapidly improves power and tone, but overexertion and re-

Plate 11-1. The technique of medial meniscectomy:

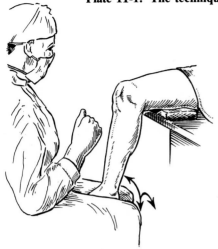
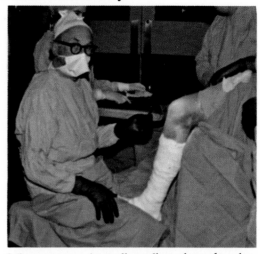

(A) The foot is gripped by the gowned knees of the surgeon. A small sandbag along the edge of the table lifts the thigh and facilitates free movement of the leg at the knee.

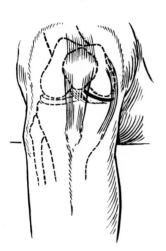
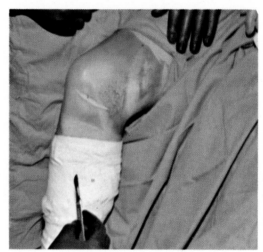

(B) The horizontal incision slopes very slightly downward and backward in line with the upper surface of the meniscus.

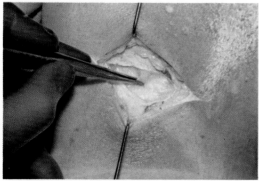
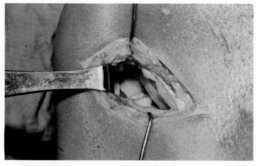

(C) The capsule is divided and the synovium is picked up preparatory to incision.

(D) The anteromedial joint space is opened. A bowstring tear is obvious, as is the erosion on the articular surface of the medial femoral condyle. The cruciate ligament is intact.

Plate 11-1. **The technique of medial meniscectomy.** (Continued)

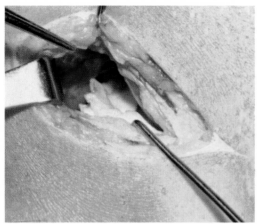

(E) The anterior horn of the meniscus is freed from the tibial spine.

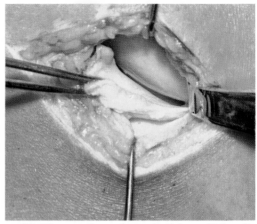

(F) The meniscus is excised by splitting its substance near the peripheral attachment.

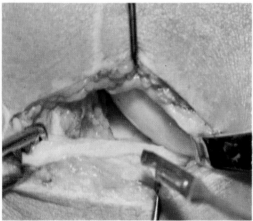

(G) As the posterior border is freed the meniscus is slipped into the intercondylar space.

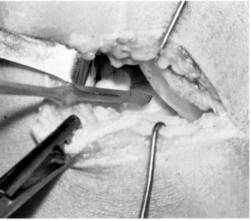

(H) The posterior end is divided from the tibial spines in the intercondylar space.

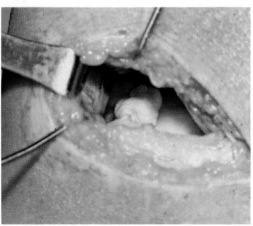

(I) The enormous bowstring of this discoid meniscus is removed as an almost separate body.

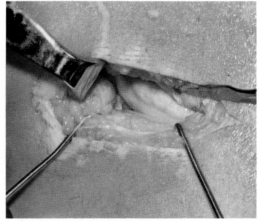

(J) Early chondrophyte formation on the edge of the medial femoral condyle.

Plate 11-1. The technique of medial meniscectomy. (Continued)

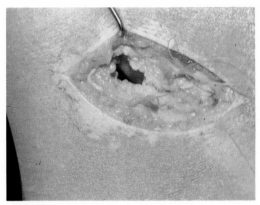

(K) The synovium is closed with a hemo-static lock-stitch suture of fine catgut.

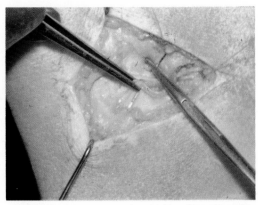

(L) The same suture is continued to close the capsule.

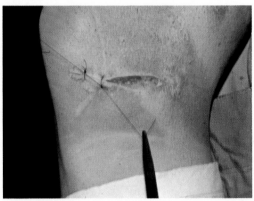

(M) Separate sutures of black silk or nylon are used to close the skin.

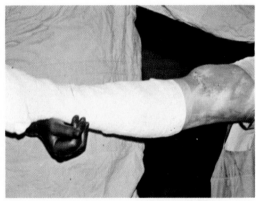

(N) Extension is complete with full external rotation.

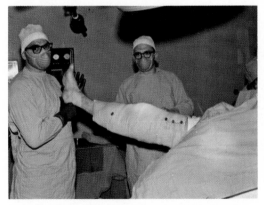

(O) A Jones compression bandage has been applied.

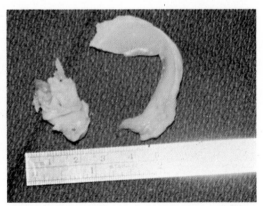

(P) The fragments of the bowstring discoid meniscus.

peated fatigue result in wasting of muscle and recurrent or persistent effusion. If this occurs, a day's rest in bed, followed by non-weight-bearing exercises is the quickest course.

The prognosis is good. The fit athlete on a guided program of exercises resumes sporting activities including football in 6 weeks. The middle-aged are fit for all normal activities in 6 to 8 weeks. The most resolute and fit patient in my experience was the regimental sergeant major of a Royal Marine Commando unit, who returned to full duty in his unit in 3 weeks. In my unit at Drymen Military Hospital during one year of the war, 120 servicemen operated on for internal derangement of the knee all were transferred to the Convalescent Depot for Scottish Command. Before returning to their units in Category A, Major Duthie and Captain Macleod[4,5] demanded that each soldier should do a physical assault course, a 3 mile cross-country run and a 15 mile route march. Of the 120, 103 or 85.8 per cent were classified as A1. The average time for all 120 from admission to the hospital to return to the unit was 63 days (W. R. Bristow, 1944*). Many rugby players have played first class ("major league") rugby in 6 weeks without harm, and two have taken their places in international teams 6 weeks after meniscectomy.

Older people return to normal activities, housework, golf and tennis. They lose their pain and no longer suffer recurrent attacks of aching and swelling after activity.

This is the group in which recovery of full extension of the knee (which includes external rotation of the tibia) is of greatest importance. Until full extension is easy and natural and the rotation signs have disappeared the knee is not always comfortable, and restoration of adequate muscle power and tone is difficult.

Postoperative Complications

Synovial Effusion. The reaction to operation is a mild effusion in most knees. Usually

---

* Personal communication.

---

it has resolved by the tenth day and does not recur if all exercise and activity is carried out progressively within the compass of the strengthening muscles. Occasionally the reaction is excessive, and tense effusion results which may require aspiration. If so, injection of 1 per cent procaine in saline simplifies the aspiration and promotes absorption. When the effusion is due to fatigue or strain, rest, followed by graduated exercise, is advocated. Forcing exercise and physiotherapy often aggravates the condition.

Hemarthrosis and Pain. Early in the Middle East Campaign in the last war, many meniscectomies were performed by young and inexperienced surgeons. The postoperative hemarthrosis rate in some military hospitals varied between 60 and 80 per cent. Three factors, not always coincident, were no doubt responsible:

1. The quality of the surgery. As anywhere else, inexperience or rough operating technics lead not only to postoperative hemorrhage, bruising, and swelling but to increased pain and delayed healing as well.

2. The prevalent teaching that the whole meniscus must be removed. This leads to damage to the vascular synovium and to the uncontrolled and untutored use of special meniscectomy knives to remove the posterior horn. It is essential that each stroke of the knife should be within the vision of the surgeon. On the lateral side, also, the vulnerability of the geniculate artery was demonstrated.

3. The cult of early movement. There is no need to flex the knee for the first 10 days, by which time the wounds are well healed. In this connection it was remarkable that even in some of these hospitals that used postoperative splinting by plaster-of-paris slab or cylinder for 2 weeks, the operation acquired the reputation of causing severe pain and rough convalescence—an accurate reflection of the surgeon's technic.

Hemarthrosis and pain are considered under one heading, for hemorrhage is associated with, and is probably the most common factor in, postoperative distress.

Smillie[10] contends, with justification, that hemarthrosis occurring as a complication of operation has more serious consequences than that resulting from simple trauma. It is more liable to be followed by protracted convalescence due to adhesions, synovial thickening and persistent effusion. He ascribes this to the presence of a large area of raw synovial membrane from which the meniscus has been dissected. This is the very factor that can be avoided by leaving a narrow rim of meniscus. Each incision should be made into the substance of the cartilage. In this way the operation is practically bloodless, and hemarthrosis becomes an exceedingly rare complication of meniscectomy.

Division of the Infrapatellar Branch of the Saphenous Nerve. The incision described and recommended invariably divides the infrapatellar branch of the saphenous nerve. Therefore, the operation is followed by a patch of anesthesia over and lateral to the lower end of the patellar tendon and the tibial tubercle. Sometimes this is permanent, but often in a few months partial or complete sensation is recovered. After explanation the patient realizes that a patch of anesthesia is no disability. In no instance has a painful neuroma complicated the scar from this incision. The only painful scars result from a more vertical incision (Fig. 11-6) which divides a branch of the nerve as it crosses the lower edge of the femur. The scar with the nerve end adheres to the bone. Irritation by repeated tension on the adhesions results in a painful neuroma. Stretching the scar reveals the neuroma, for the small segment that contains the nerve ending blanches. The finding may be confirmed by the hypersensitive reaction to tapping with a blunt point. The scar should be surgically freed from the bone, and the neuroma and the nerve isolated and divided well away from the scar.

Healing of the Wound. Great care should be exercised in assessing the condition of the skin before operation. If abraded or infected, operation should be delayed till all signs of inflammation have disappeared. With this proviso, healing is seldom delayed.

The late Professor T. P. McMurray once told me that Sir Robert Jones believed that synovial fluid delayed wound healing and that he took great care to wipe all traces of synovial fluid from the skin edges before suturing.

With modern theater and surgical technics, joint sepsis following meniscectomy is almost unknown. Routine postoperative chemotherapy or antibiotics are unnecessary and in this series have been prescribed only in a few instances when wound discomfort and a niggling temperature have suggested stitch infection. When the dressings are removed for the first time on the tenth day, the skin wound occasionally is found to be moist or inflamed around a suture.

Residual Tags. The patient with a residual posterior fragment gives the history of recurrent internal derangement of the knee in spite of previous operation. The symptoms may be similar or changed in character, but the patient remains disabled, either by recurring stabs of pain, always in the same place, or by the knee "giving-way." The incidents may or may not be followed by effusions. Examination reveals finger-point tenderness over the fragment plus an easily elicited diagnostic click and, frequently, pain on complete flexion or on squatting. Occasionally, stabs of pain in the region of the collateral ligaments are due to pedicled or frondlike tags. The pain and tenderness are always over the tag, and, with the characteristic momentary nature of the incidents, are diagnostic.

Mistaken diagnosis before the first operation, a missed cartilaginous loose body and a recurrent subluxation of the patella must all be considered in the differential diagnosis, but the detection of a residual fragment is usually simple.

Experienced surgeons using the preoperative criteria described in Chapter 7 coupled with careful inspection and assessment during the operation seldom miss an unstable posterior fragment or tag. The treatment is always excision of the fragment.

BIBLIOGRAPHY

1. Annandale, T.: An operation for displaced semilunar cartilage. Br. Med. J., *1*:779, 1885.
2. Bruser, D. M.: A direct approach to the lateral compartment of the knee joint. J. Bone Joint Surg., *42B*:348, 1960.
3. Bunnell, S.: Surgery of the Hand. Philadelphia, J. B. Lippincott, 1956.
4. Duthie, J. J. R., and Macleod, J. G.: Rehabilitation after meniscectomy. Lancet, *244*:197, 1943.
5. ———: Meniscectomy in soldiers. Lancet, *246*:182, 1944.
6. Fairbank, T. J., and Jamieson, E. S.: A complication of lateral meniscectomy. J. Bone Joint Surg., *33B*:567, 1951.
7. Jones, Sir Robert: Notes on derangements of the knee. Ann. Surg., *50*:969, 1909.
8. ———: Notes on Military Orthopaedic Surgery. London, Cassell, 1918.
9. Mayer, L.: The physiological method of tendon transplantation. III. Experimental and clinical experiences. Surg., Gynec., Obstet., *182*:472, 1916.
10. Smillie, I. S.: Injuries of the Knee Joint. Baltimore, Williams & Wilkins, 1962.

12

Primary and Secondary Osteoarthritis

Arthur J. Helfet, M.D.

Osteoarthritis is defined as primary when it occurs without any known cause, and as secondary when it can be traced to a demonstrable abnormality in the anatomy and mechanics of the joint. More and more evidence is accumulating that most osteoarthritis in the middle-aged and elderly is secondary in nature, and indeed that primary osteoarthritis is rare. Although true primary osteoarthritis can occur, as in acromegaly and in chondromalacia of the patella in the young, when degenerative arthritic change occurs in the hips and knees of older people, faulty mechanics can usually be implicated.

The realization that it is possible to "arrest" osteoarthritis in both the hip and the knee by changing mechanics of the joint has led to a reappraisal of the articular disorders that up to now have been labelled primary osteoarthritis.[12] For instance, I have been convinced for a number of years that the complex of symptoms and signs found in an osteoarthritic knee—the areas of pain, the deformity, and the patterns of erosion of articular cartilage—can usually be traced to mechanical derangement of a meniscus. The clinical picture of meniscus damage as more usually seen in the young has by now been modified by superimposed degenerative changes of aging.[6-8]

Instead of a prevailing view[3] that the primary lesion is one of patchy degeneration of articular cartilage, mainly in non-weight-bearing areas, in most instances the primary disorder is of the aging soft tissues of the joint deranged by trauma, often minimal. The effect on the articular cartilage is secondary and usually occurs in non-weight-bearing areas at the site where the affected soft tissues block the normal pattern of movement. In most instances the sites of erosion and the sequence of change may be traced to a derangement of a single meniscus and the consequent interference with normal joint movement.

AGING OF ARTICULAR AND MENISCAL CARTILAGE

It is known that, with aging, the matrix of the articular cartilage loses its resiliency,[8] and any abnormal stress, especially if repeated, results in a gradual wearing down. The patterns of erosion so formed faithfully mirror the eroding agent, the meniscus.

The changes are usually focal in character and are first confined to one or the other femoral condyle (Fig. 12-1). Later, a further area of wear occurs on the medial facet of the patella (see Fig. 6-27). This results, as described on page 89, from interference with the normally synchronous movements of the tibia, femur, and patella. X-rays show localized sclerosis and cyst formation in the subchondral bone, always opposite the responsible damaged meniscus. Bauer and Smith (1969) using a focusing collimator to study detailed isotope uptake in bone, have demonstrated local increased metabolism in the juxtaarticular bone in osteoarthritic

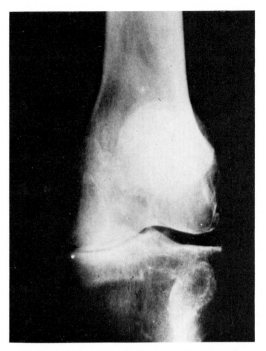

FIG. 12-1. Advanced osteoarthritis confined to the medial compartment of the knee. The X-ray shows localized sclerosis and cyst formation opposite the responsible damaged meniscus.

knees (Fig. 12-2).[2] This local increase corresponds closely to areas of irritation and erosion of articular cartilage opposite a deranged meniscus.

Indeed the evidence is that osteoarthritis of the knee seldom begins as a generalized phenomenon. At the start it is usually restricted to one compartment of the joint (Fig. 12-1), and only rarely and at a late stage does it spread to involve the whole of the articular surfaces.

The young meniscus is white, elastic, and firm but pliable (Fig. 12-3; Plate 12-2). It is avascular, except where it is attached to the capsule of the joint. When cut, it is fibrous, the fibers all running in its longitudinal axis. In cross-section it is elongated with a thin free edge extending into the joint. Microscopically it consists of fibrocartilage cells lying in a collagen matrix (Fig. 12-3B). As it ages, the meniscus becomes harder until all elasticity has been lost. It changes color, becoming yellowish and translucent, especially at its thin and free border. With time contraction occurs, until the meniscus

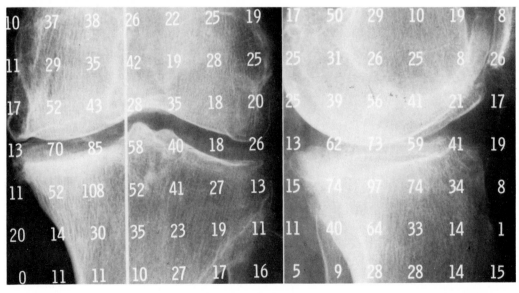

FIG. 12-2. Sr. scintimetry in a 78-year-old woman with osteoarthritis of the medial femorotibial articulation of the left knee. Note high values at involved part of knee joint. (*Left*) Frontal projection. (*Right*) Lateral projection showing low values at patellofemoral articulation in spite of presence of large osteophytes that were probably secondary to osteoarthritis of the femorotibial articulation (From Bauer, G. C. H., and Smith, E. M.: J. Nucl. Med., *10*:109, 1969).

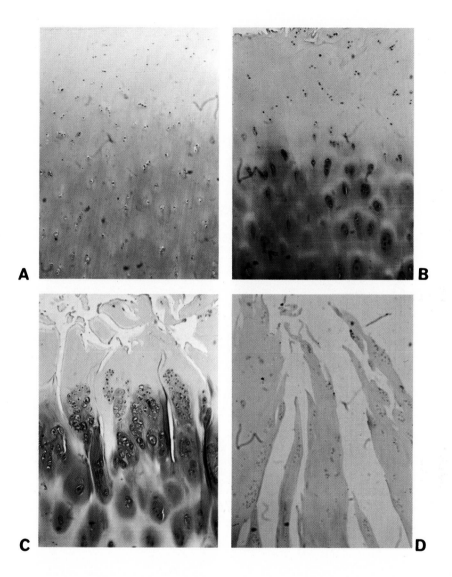

Plate 12-1. (*A*) The surface of normal human articular cartilage is smooth, and cells are regularly dispersed. The cartilage at the surface contains no mucopolysaccharide, whereas the deeper zones are positive for mucopolysaccharide. (*B*) There is a fissuring of the articular surface; clumps of chondrocytes in the deeper zones are surrounded by halos of increased mucopolysaccharide. (*C*) In human cartilage with advanced degenerative changes, the cartilage is diminished in height, and the fissures extend into the deeper zones. (*D*) Human articular cartilage with advanced degenerative changes is fissured throughout and devoid of mucopolysaccharide. Clumps of chondrocytes also lack a mucopolysaccharide halo.

The above sections are stained with a metachromatic (cationic) dye (safranin-O) and counterstained with fast green. The cationic dye forms a metachromatic compound with polyanions, such as chondroitin sulfate and keratan sulfate. Areas of the cartilage not containing anionic polysaccharide are counterstained with fast green.

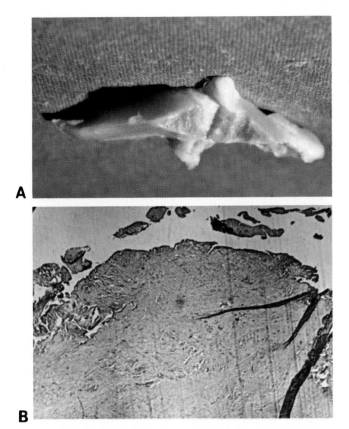

Plate 12-2. (*A*) The aging meniscus is yellowish, hard, and contracted. (*B*) When all the cells have disappeared, a mass of fibrous tissue remains, peripherally invaded by blood vessels.

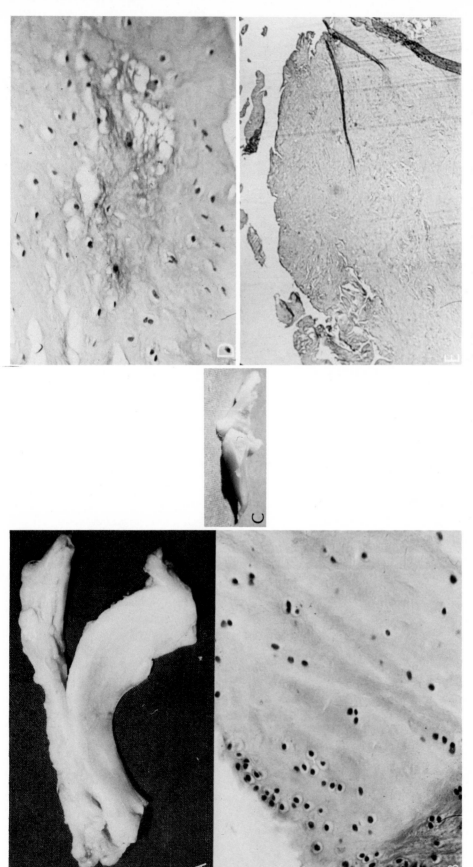

Fig. 12-3. (A) Gross specimens of young meniscus. (B) Photomicrograph showing fibrocartilage cells lying in a collagen matrix. (C) With aging the meniscus finally becomes yellowish and hard and contracted in both longitudinal and transverse directions. (See color Plate 12-2.) (D) The photomicrograph shows a loss of cellular elements, although some of the cells resemble those of true cartilage. Intercellular material is more abundant and is gradually replaced by fibrous tissue. (E) Finally the cells have disappeared and the meniscus is a mass of fibrous tissue with peripheral invasion of blood vessels. (See color Plate 12-2.)

becomes triangular in cross-section (Fig. 12-3C). Microscopically there is a gradual loss of the cellular elements. The intercellular material becomes more abundant (Fig. 12-3D) and is gradually replaced by fibrous tissues (Fig. 12-3E). Finally it is invaded by blood vessels and completes the process of degeneration. Such a degenerated meniscus is unable to stand up to the abnormal stresses to which it may be subjected. In the end the hard, inelastic lump of fibrous tissue makes one understand the complaint of some old people that "it feels as though there is a pebble in my knee."

PATHOLOGICAL DERANGEMENT OF DEGENERATIVE MENISCUS

The hardened degenerative meniscus is subject to injury in a manner different from the younger meniscus. The process of fibrosis tends to cause the meniscus to contract in shape and length and so to retract from its moorings to the anterior tibial spine. A minor injury usually in rotation and often almost unnoticed, may pull it off altogether. It forms a lump in the anterior compartment and so doing causes the typical limitations of movement—the interruption of the normal synchrony of flexion-extension and rotation of the knee joint—and initiates the process of erosion that we label osteoarthritis. In a way, just as we consider many fractures of the neck of the aged femur to be "pathological," the separation of the meniscus from its attachment to the tibial spine may also occur from insignificant stress and so may also be deemed "pathological."

If the mechanical derangement is treated surgically so that normal symptomless movement is returned, the joint will be restored and will recover comfort and function. The prognosis is not poor, it is good. The earlier the surgical correction, the better the eventual result.

Moreover the process of degeneration, which is otherwise progressive, is arrested, and X-rays eventually may show restoration of more normal juxtaarticular bone structure with solution of sclerosis and repair of tra-

beculation (Figs. 12-4; 12-5). In an osteoarthritic hip a similar arrest occurs after intertrochanteric osteotomy (Fig. 12-6).

PATHOGENESIS OF OSTEOARTHRITIS

The true incidence of any "primary" objective change in the hip has been questioned by R. O. Murray.[11] He has studied the X-rays of two hundred patients said clinically to have primary osteoarthritis of the hip. His study excluded any subject in which the arthritic changes could possibly be attributed to a disorder occurring earlier in life. The X-rays of each arthritic hip were assessed to determine three different standard measurements. These were: (1) the CE angle of Wiberg, (2) acetabular depth, and (3) the femoral head ratio (FHR) as indicated by the degree of tilt deformity of the femoral neck. These measurements were compared with those from X-rays of 100 clinically normal hips. Murray found that 65 per cent of abnormal hips had sufficient preexisting anatomical abnormalities to justify placing the arthritis in the "secondary" category. The average age of onset of symptoms in this group was 51.5 years. Normal anatomy was found in the remaining 35 per cent of patients showing arthritic change. In these patients the average age was 57.7 years at the time of onset of symptoms. Murray postulates that the presence of joint incongruity, when demonstrated even in a symptom-free hip, will indicate a potential for later development of osteoarthritis. Where the radiograph of the hip is normal, the subsequent development of osteoarthritis becomes much less likely.

Heine in 1926 demonstrated that normal articular cartilage grows throughout life, though with decreasing vigor in old age.[4] There is a constant process of absorption and replacement of bone and cartilage that leads to shaping and remodelling of the articular surfaces of the long bones. This process has a close similarity to the changes of developing osteoarthritis, as has been emphasized in the classical work of Lent

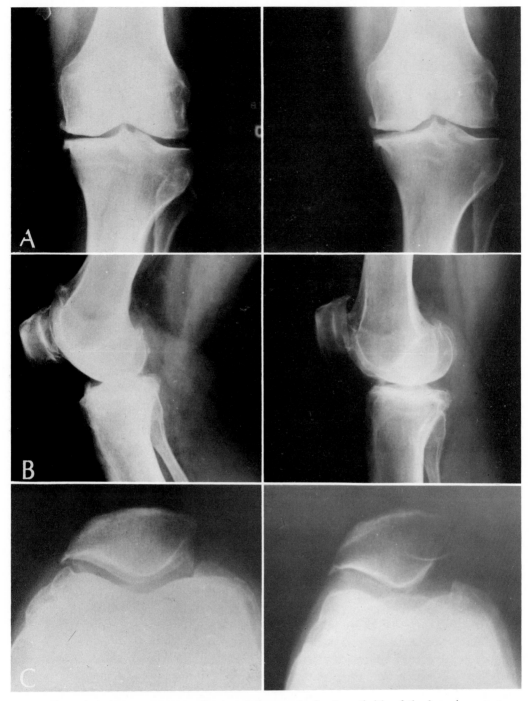

FIG. 12-4. Roentgenograms document the arrest of osteoarthritis of the knee in a man aged 72 between February 1964 and January 1966 following operative correction of mechanical derangement. (*A*) Anteroposterior view; (*B*) lateral view; (*C*) skyline view of patella. Note localization of osteoarthritis to the medial compartment, resolution of subchondral sclerosis, and recovery of normal trabeculation, and marked clarification of bone structure.

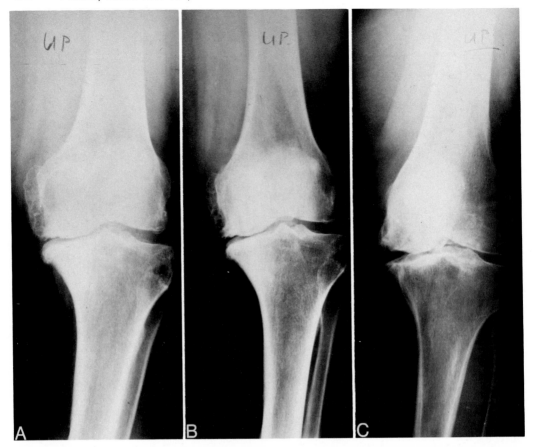

Fig. 12-5. Gross osteoarthritis, left knee in a 70-year-old patient. (*A*) Medial meniscectomy and debridement limited to the medial femoral condyle and medial facet patella
were performed—January 1963. (*B*) May 1964; the patient was walking comfortably.
There is improvement in joint space, in articular definition, and in juxtaarticular sclerosis,
and trabecular pattern. (*C*) Four and a half years later, in December 1968, the patient
can still walk comfortably. Roentgenograms show further improvement in articular
definition and in juxtaarticular bone structure. Sclerosis and cyst formation are diminished, and the trabecular pattern is more normal.

Johnson.[10] Johnson showed that joints, like
bones, remodelled to meet special stress requirements through the activity of the articular cartilage (Fig. 12-7). Use or overuse in
the normal pattern would not necessarily
produce osteoarthritis, but with aging, areas
of "tangential shear" lead to local erosive
changes which Nissen aptly calls epichondrosis. In other words, the osteoarthritis occurs
at local sites of excessive cartilage abuse. In
Johnson's own words, "any distortion of
surface contour by local overgrowth or erosion activates all of the remodelling mechanisms, and a vicious circle of accelerating

destruction and attempted repair develops,
with both repair and destruction upsetting
the lubricating wedge of function and increasing frictional damage."

We are still far from understanding the
biochemical and physiochemical processes
involved in either the osteoarthritic process
itself, or in the "arrest" that may follow
juxtaarticular osteotomy in the hip, or correction of internal derangement in the knee.

Changes in Juxtaarticular Vascularity

The role of hypervascularity in the evolution of the disease and as a cause of pain

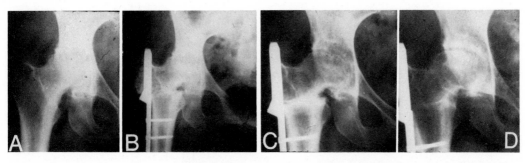

FIG. 12-6. (*A*) Severe osteoarthritis in the hip of a woman, aged 57. In March 1967, she could walk at most six blocks with a cane. Note obliteration of joint space, marked sclerosis and cyst formation. (*B*) Immediately after intertrochanteric displacement derotation realignment osteotomy using Wainwright spline. (*C*) In January 1968, 10 months later, the joint line is visible. The sclerosis is resolving with healing of the cysts. (*D*) Two and one half years after surgery, in October 1969. Note.definition of joint space and improved appearance of juxtaarticular bone. The patient was examined again in July 1972; she had no pain on any activity and could walk unlimited distances unsupported without limping.

was demonstrated by Harrison et al.[3] and Trueta[15] and convinced Nissen[12] and others that the hyperemia associated with osteoarthritis causes arterial congestion which is relieved by osteotomy. Nissen quotes the dramatic results of forage of the medullary cavity of the neck and Scaglietti's ligation of the main vessels round the upper end of the femur to support this thesis. On the other hand Wardle,[16] Helal,[8] and Apley[1] have demonstrated venous congestion in the medulla of the tibia in osteoarthritis of the knee and Hulth[9] has done similar studies on the hip joint. Helal makes another interesting observation. Sixty-seven of 100 patients with osteoarthritis of the knee were found to

FIG. 12-7. The diagram illustrates the remodelling processes that occur in an osteoarthritic knee joint. (*A*) Upward and lateral cartilage growth; (*B*) local periosteal new bone formation; (*C*) chondrification followed by ossification of a tendon or capsule. (Johnson, L. C.: Kinetics of osteoarthritis. Lab. Invest., 8:1223, 1959).

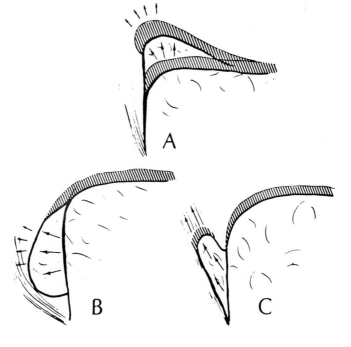

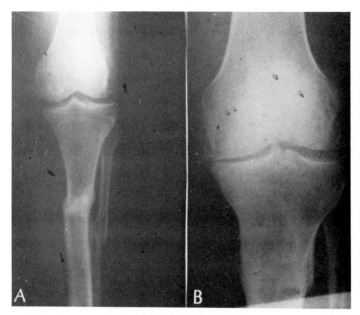

FIG. 12-8. (*A*) A dense sclerotic barrier formed in this knee after osteotomy, and the patient's pain was relieved. (*B*) When no barrier formed, this patient was not relieved. The roentgenogram, however, shows derangement of the medial compartment that should respond to intraarticular operation. (Courtesy of Alan Apley)

suffer from varicose veins of the affected leg, whereas only 22 per cent of patients in a similar age group without osteoarthritis were found to have this affliction.

Richards and Brookes[14] have investigated the changes in pH and CO_2 levels of bone blood following experimental osteotomy. An immediate intense arterial vasodilation occurs. Subsequently there is a sustained rise in local pH accompanying formation of abundant spongy bone over the next 3 months or so. This alkalinity lasts until spongy bone is replaced by compact bone. The pH then moves toward acidity. It is likely that clearance of bone sclerosis occurs during the active arterial alkaline phase, but that sclerosis itself is probably established in association with venous engorgement and a more acid environment.

Recent work by Chin and Weiss in my department has demonstrated increases in lysosomal acid phosphatase in osteoarthritic cartilage. They consider that a degenerative type of osteoarthritis may result from the acid phosphatase liberated by lysosomal activity in the chondrocytes. Other authors have previously expressed belief that the lysosomal complex has the ability to degrade cartilage.

MECHANISM OF PAIN IN OSTEOARTHRITIS

Pain in osteoarthritis has three main causes. It may be the result of hypervascularity, or it can be mechanical—associated with movement—or muscle pain. Nissen,[12] Apley,[1] Helal,[5] and Wardle[16] and others believe that bone pain after activity and night pains are due to venous congestion and that it is relieved by osteotomy. Apley showed me cases treated by himself and Helal where successful results were obtained when the union of the osteotomy is associated with formation of a sclerotic barrier across the medulla that, presumably, prevents filling of the dilated venous system. In other cases, where no such barrier was formed, the pain was not relieved. They therefore consider using an acrylic disc to act as a venous plug across the osteotomy site (Fig. 12-8). Harrison et al., Nissen, and Trueta have demonstrated and associate arterial hyperemia with pain and claim that osteotomy relieves the excessive circulation.

Most pain in osteoarthritis is felt on movement of the joint. Of all the tissues the capsule and synovium are richest in nerve supply and the pain follows the block to movement by fibrous contraction in these tissues. Sudden movement will cause a sudden pain, rapidly relieved when the attempt is over; prolonged or repeated attempts at the same movement cause longer lasting pain. Both are relieved by rest. Skeletal pain is due basically either to tension or ischemia, conditions produced by movement against resistance. *Removal of soft tissue blocks to movement by intraarticular correction or extraarticular muscle release,*[13] *or osteotomy which bypasses the fixed deformities should cause dramatic relief of pain,* and so they do. In the early stages, manipulation or stretching to overcome capsular contractions and adhesions are also helpful.

The third type of pain originates in muscles. Intraarticular lesions of joints tend to affect muscles working on the joint reflexly and adversely. They weaken and waste. Muscle spasm is painful. Besides, fixed deformity of the joint puts muscles at a mechanical disadvantage resulting in early fatigue and strain as evidenced by ache and cramp.

Relief of Pain

Correction of deformity with realignment produces a biological effect on the articular tissues and also a mechanical relief of tensions caused by the deformity. It becomes noticeably easier to restore muscle strength and bulk and to rehabilitate the patient for a wider range of activity without strain after osteotomy, a fact that again stresses the need for a judicious exercise program for all osteoarthritic joints.

In the relief of pain the sealing of a vascular channel, either arterial or venous, cannot be the sole mechanism for if so, osteotomy without displacement would be as successful as with displacement. Nor would a vascular block in one bone explain the anatomical improvement on both sides of the joint. Also, forage of the neck of the femur would be more generally helpful. Nor can it be simply relief of tension. For why does simple division of the muscles around the hip produce only temporary relief? It may be that we should consider separately the aspects of immediate relief of pain, and of long-term relief of pain plus restoration of more normal bone and joint anatomy. Then it becomes feasible that prompt relief is due to the immediate relief of tension and that the long-term relief of pain and the improvement of juxtaarticular bone structure and shape and accommodation of the joint is due to normal and stable use of the joint and the consequent development of improved and adequate, but not excessive or congested, circulation.

The dramatic results of multiple division of the muscles of the hip—the "hanging hip" operation—seldom last, except in some old people whose minimal activities make little demand on the hip. The instability or incongruity or epichondrosis that led to the osteoarthritic state in the first place remain but in a weaker and less controlled joint. The sacrifice of muscle power is justified only when it is not necessary.

ARREST OF PRIMARY OR SECONDARY OSTEOARTHRITIS

The basic manifestations of osteoarthritis are those of a *desperate, but inefficient, attempt by cartilage to repair itself.* It would seem that juxtaarticular osteotomy of the hip or knee, or correction of the soft tissue derangement in the knee, or muscle release at the hip, each in the appropriate circumstance, continue the same repair processes but in correct and profitable directions, i.e., that arrest is but a correction of a previous process of repair.

In considering our concepts of primary and secondary osteoarthritis we find, associated with even subtle abnormalities of mechanical stimuli to the normal remodelling and growth of bone ends, intense vascular metabolic changes, which include the liberation of a lysosomal enzyme complex. The resulting changes may well give rise to Johnson's condition of "tangential shear."[10] Intense vascular and metabolic changes follow both damage to the articular surface and juxtaarticular osteotomy to one side of a joint. In all these situations, the mechanics of the joint are altered.

Presumably a "primary" label would attach to osteoarthritis which results from enzymes being liberated from the deep chondrocytes without any previous mechanical injury, and so to those instances of undetermined and apparently unblemished origin that we cannot as yet explain.

REFERENCES

1. Apley, A. G.: Personal communication, 1965.
2. Bauer, G. C. H., and Smith, E. M.: 85Sr. Scintimetry in osteoarthritis of the knee. J. Nucl. Med., *10*:109, 1969.
3. Harrison, M. H. M., Schajowica, T., and Trueta, J.: Osteoarthritis of the hip. A study of the nature and evolution of the disease. J. Bone Joint Surg., *35-B*:598, 1953.
4. Heine, J.: Virchow Arch. Path. Anat., *260*: 521, 1926.
5. Helal, B.: The pain in primary osteoarthritis of the knee. Postgrad. Med. J., *41*:172, 1965.
6. Helfet, A. J.: Mechanism of derangements of the medial semilunar cartilage and their management. J. Bone Joint Surg., *41-B*: 319, 1959.
7. ———: The concept of arrest of osteoarthritis in the hip and knee. *In* Apley, A. G. (ed.): Recent Advances in Orthopedics. London, J. & A. Churchill, 1969.
8. ———: Osteoarthritis of the knee and its early arrest. AAOS Instruction Course Lectures. Vol. XX. 1971.
9. Hulth, A.: Circulatory disturbances in osteoarthritis of the hip. Acta Orthop. Scand., 28, 1958.
10. Johnson, L. E.: Kinetics of osteoarthritis. Lab. Invest., *8*:1223, 1959.
11. Murray, R. O.: The aetiology of primary osteoarthritis of the hip. Brit. J. Radiol., *38*:810, 1965.
12. Nissen, K. I.: The arrest of early primary osteoarthritis of the hip by osteotomy. Proc. Roy. Soc. Med., *56*:1051, 1963.
13. O'Malley, A. G.: J. Bone Joint Surg., *44-B*: 217, 1962.
14. Richards, D. J., and Brookes, M.: Physicochemical sequelae of experimental osteotomy. Proc. Roy. Soc. Med., *62*:435, 1969.
15. Trueta, J.: Studies on the etiopathology of osteoarthritis of the hip. Clin. Orthop., *31*:7, 1963.
16. Wardle, E. N.: Osteotomy of the tibia and fibula. Surg. Gynec. Obstet., *115*:61, 1962.

13

Management of Osteoarthritis of the Knee Joint

Arthur J. Helfet, M.D.

Traumatic arthritis is no more than localized wearing or erosion of the articular cartilaginous surfaces of joints. With age articular cartilage loses its glisten and resilience, and in the old joint is yellowish, dull and brittle. Aging in itself is not necessarily a cause of osteoarthritis but, like overweight, gout, and other maladies, renders the joint more vulnerable to and accelerates the progress of osteoarthritic changes. Toxins, whether infective or metabolic, leave the cartilage dull and soft. Hormonal disorders of the pituitary and the thyroid produce effects that are not understood as yet. The adrenals are related to rheumatoid arthritis but, as far as we know, not to the osteoarthritic process.

Articular cartilage is abraded by incongruity of joint surfaces which may be congenital, as in the hip; due to deformity, as in knock-knees; or to malalignment following fractures; or it may be caused by loose bodies during each excursion between the joint surfaces. The knee is particularly vulnerable, for the articular cartilage of the femoral condyles and the patella is injured also by derangements of the semilunar cartilages and/or the patella. Indeed, it is now the author's firm conviction that *the most common cause of traumatic arthritis of the knee in middle-aged and elderly people is injury, often unsuspected, of the semilunar cartilages.* Injury is often unnoticed or of such minor character that the degenerative changes in aging tissues which render the

meniscus so susceptible merit investigation. The menisci undergo changes similar to those of articular cartilage, becoming yellowish in color and firmer in consistency with loss of elasticity. The term meniscosis is sometimes used to denote this.[2] Collagen fibers hyalinize, and cellularity is significantly reduced. It is a reasonable surmise that as the meniscus hardens and becomes drier, it tends to contract and is the more easily pulled off its anterior moorings to the cruciate ligament. The moorings of the posterior horn to the capsule are firmer and more extensive and less likely to give. Indeed, it is feasible that in certain circumstances the anterior detachment may be spontaneous. Note that in the older age group the retracted meniscus is the common finding (see Tables 6-1 to 6-6).

The anterior horn of the medial meniscus is the most frequent culprit, but each type of meniscal injury produces its particular pattern of erosion, accompanied by its own complex of symptoms and signs. *The respective clinical features should be recognized, for, in most instances, pain, the main factor in disability, may be relieved by appropriate, simple surgery.*

The manner of development of these patterns of erosion of the articular cartilages was described in Chapter 6. They are accompanied by intermittent attacks of synovitis with gradually increasing chronic inflammatory changes in the synovium. Osteophytes form at the edges of the articular cartilage. Gradually, the capsule stretches with some laxity of the joint, chiefly in the anteroposterior direction. It is probable that, partially at least, the laxity is apparent and not real, for many a knee in incomplete extension with muscles relaxed may demonstrate mild signs. The thigh muscles waste, and the knee presents a typical picture with a prominent medial femoral condyle and a suggestion of valgus deformity. To increase comfort in walking the knee tends to flex more, with the result that fixed flexion deformity is increased and, of course, extension is lost.

The clinical symptoms have a similar sequence. The onset is mild and often unnoticed. The patient may not remember any injury or may record a simple and momentary twist or sprain. Occasionally the patient experiences an accident with dramatic dislocation of a semilunar cartilage, followed by recurrent and typical incidents and attacks. As is natural, however, medical aid is sought sooner if the early course is severe. The usual story of the osteoarthritic knee is one of mild onset and intermittent attacks of pain and swelling or "rheumatism," slowly increasing in severity and frequency. The leg becomes weaker and does less work before discomfort. The patient is inactive and puts on weight. These attacks usually are relieved by rest or by limiting activity, but, in time, relief comes more slowly and may be less complete. Eventually weight-bearing itself is painful, and, finally, there is the intolerable sensation of "walking on a stone in the knee." The ultimate phase is bone pain in bed at night, aggravated by warmth, so that the patient tends to sleep with his leg outside the bedcovers.

The first symptoms to disturb the patient may be pain on walking downstairs and later also on climbing. This indicates involvement of the patella. As a consequence of the erosive process, whenever the malaligned quadriceps muscle is contracted, the patella is tensed against the medial trochlear slope of the femur (Figs. 6-27, 6-28), so that, if these surfaces are sensitive, pain occurs.

After a twist or fall, sometimes minor in character, the knee locks and becomes acutely painful and swollen. The pain is felt on the medial side and is associated with tenderness over the back end of the cartilage. At operation one finds a retracted medial meniscus with transverse fracture of recent origin at the junction of the middle and the posterior thirds.

This type of osteoarthritic knee demonstrates the same physical signs as the displaced anterior horn of either meniscus. In time the signs are progressively exaggerated. Finally, in fact, there is more swelling and wasting and limitation of extension than would be the case with a comparable displacement of the young knee. The rotation signs—limitation of external rotation of the tibial tubercle, prominence of the medial femoral condyle, pain over the anterior end of the meniscus on forced extension, wasting of thigh muscles, etc.—are always present. Typical, too, is finger-point tenderness of the anterior horn of the meniscus and, at a later stage, of an area on the undersurface of the medial femoral condyle just in from the edge. This is detected in the flexed knee and later, when the medial femoral condyle is prominent, with the knee extended as well. The other area of tenderness is the medial border of the patella and the adjacent trochlear surface of the femur. An interesting phenomenon is that manipulation as described on page 152 usually results in an increase of movement and comfort. With thigh muscles relaxed and the knee flexed, the leg is rotated passively internally and externally until increased movement is obtained, often with a click. If an increased range of extension results, walking will be more comfortable. This phenomenon is usually temporary but confirms the presence of an unstable meniscus.

TREATMENT

The urgent and constant objectives of treatment are: (1) recovery of extension of the knee joint with (2) relief of tension

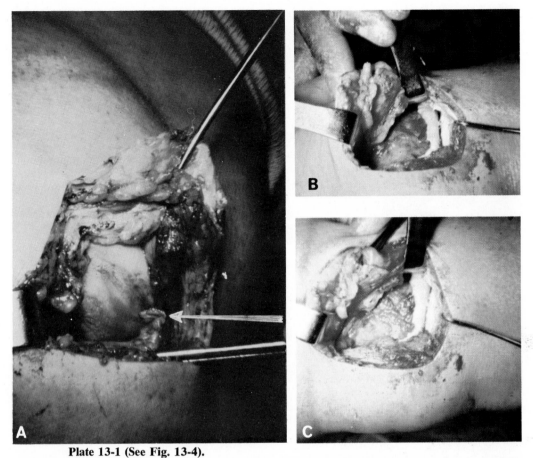

Plate 13-1 (See Fig. 13-4).

(A) Operative photograph of patient, aged 43, showing early osteoarthritic changes on the articular surface of the medial condyle of the femur due to bowstring meniscus with detached anterior horn. Chondrophyte formation is obvious on the medial edge of the femoral condyle. The erosive patterns are typical. (B) The knee is straightened before the meniscus is removed. The medial femoral condyle protrudes over the tibial margin. (C) After removal of the meniscus full extension is recovered, and the femur and tibia are in rotational alignment.

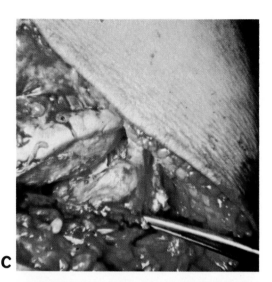

C

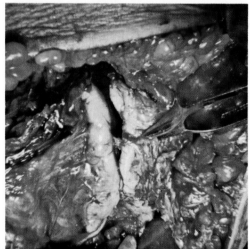

D

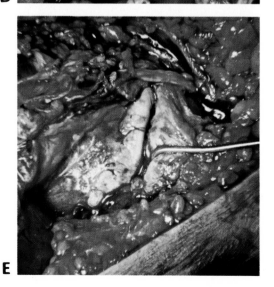

E

Plate 13-2 (See Fig. 13-5 for A, B & F).

(*A*) Patient, aged 68, with severe osteo-arthritis of the right knee. The medial meniscus had been removed 18 months earlier without significant relief. The knee is locked with limitation of external rotation of the tibial tubercle and protuberance of the medial femoral condyle. The patient had medial instability from laxness of the capsule. (*B*) The roentgenogram shows marked erosion of the medial femoral condyle with sclerosis and cyst formation. (*C*) The operative photograph shows residual posterior horn nipped in and locking the joint. The articular surface is severely eroded with marked chondrophytosis. (*D*) Before excision of the residual meniscus and obstructing chondrophytes, the femur and tibia of the extended knee were not in alignment; the femoral condyle protruded. (*E*) At the end of the operation the knee extended fully in proper rotational alignment. The semitendinosus tendon was transposed into a groove in the medial femoral condyle (see Chap. 16). The patient was able to walk in 2 weeks using a cane. Three months later she had recovered muscle power, was walking well, and could climb stairs. (*F*) She could take full weight on her bent knee.

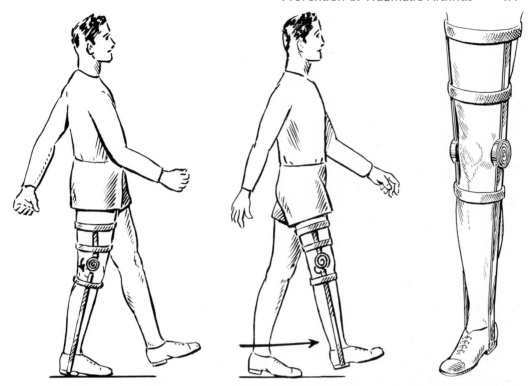

Fig. 13-1. (*Left*) the knee spring is loaded by flexion of the knee. While weight remains on this foot, the mere act of going forward on to the other leg aids in this process. (*Center*) As soon as weight is taken on the left foot and as the right leg swings through, the spring is released, aiding extension of the knee. (*Right*) Anterior view of the knee spring on the leg.

of the patella in the trochlear groove and (3) recovery of muscle power and bulk. By the time displacement or recurrent displacement of the meniscus has existed long enough to produce traumatic changes in the knee joint, the only treatment in most cases is surgical. The damaging meniscus, or, in some instances, fragments of the meniscus, must be removed.

PREVENTION OF TRAUMATIC ARTHRITIS

It is questionable whether conservative treatment is really worthwhile. Once the arthritic process is in progress, is it possible to stay further erosion without surgery? One can sometimes teach the patients to reduce displacement of the meniscus themselves, and if so, by limiting activity and by prevention of all strain, conservative treatment,

when circumstances demand it, may be practicable. The patient must exercise assiduously to maintain muscle strength and bulk, for the stronger muscles can allow greater activity and withstand more strain before discomfort and effusion result.

When operation is contraindicated, the wearing of a caliper fitted with a knee-spring is helpful. (See Figs. 13-1 and 13-2.) This is a light caliper fitted into the heel of the shoe, with an extension spring at the level of the knee joint. The spring is loaded by flexion of the knee. When the leg is raised, as weight is taken on the other foot the spring is released and reinforces the quadriceps in extending the knee. In this manner it helps the patient to maintain full extension of the knee—the important movement—and also limits untoward flexion and rotation strains.

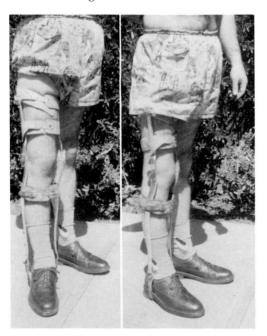

FIG. 13-2. Patient in caliper with knee spring. He has a postpolio paralysis of the right quadriceps. In a rigid caliper he felt awkward and fell several times. Wearing the knee-spring he feels more agile, and he has not fallen. The "lively" splint acts also as an *exerciser*. Several patients have recovered muscle power after using this spring.

THE USE OF INTRAARTICULAR INJECTIONS

At the end of the last war, Waugh advised intraarticular injections of a solution of lactic acid with a pH of 5.8.[17] His thesis was that as synovial fluid in osteoarthritic knees is slightly alkaline, it would be neutralized by the acid solution. The technic used is the injection, once a week, of 10 ml. of a saline solution of lactic acid with 0.5 per cent procaine into and around the joint, followed by gentle passive movements and exercise. These injections are comforting, and the effect may last for a week or more.

The injection of the latest preparations of corticosteroids into swollen and painful joints is generally regarded as a valuable measure in the treatment of rheumatoid arthritis. Hollander and his colleagues[12] and Chandler, Wright, and Hartfall,[4,5] of the University of Leeds, carried out a controlled trial of hydrocortisone tert-butyl-acetate on 24 patients whose main incapacity arose from involvement of the knees.[5] They found that significant relief of pain and tenderness and improvement in movement and walking time appeared for periods lasting from 4 to 8 weeks. However, every success carries with it potential dangers, for deterioration was observed by roentgenography in another trial in 13 of 25 knee joints despite clinical improvement in the majority of cases. Chandler and Wright[4] therefore inclined to the likely view that cortisone interferes with the normal protective processes natural to inflammatory disease. Functional improvement and the relief of pain, being the most important features, encourage a degree of activity and weight bearing that is frankly traumatic. They commented on the production of a virtual Charcot's arthropathy in an osteoarthritic hip treated over an 18-month period by monthly injections of hydrocortisone. The patient had obtained almost complete relief of pain when treatment was discontinued.

It has been the author's practice over a number of years to inject only acutely painful swollen osteoarthritic knees with a mixture of 10 ml. of 1 per cent procaine in saline and 1.0 to 1.5 ml. of prednisolone (25 to 37.5 mg.). This local injection of hydrocortisone into osteoarthritic joints is of value when there is an acute exacerbation of the chronic condition, that is, when the knee is swollen and painful. When the joint is not swollen or inflamed, the clinical condition is not significantly changed. In other words, intraarticular injections are of value for pain but not in the treatment of the underlying arthritic lesion.

Injections carry the not inconsiderable danger of increased and significant destruction of articular cartilage, for, as noted above, the pain-free joint permits undue activity without the protection of a painful inflammatory reaction.

We are now observing the long-term results of injections of hydrocortisone in the knees of adults. After a variable period of comfort, symptoms recur and the roentgenograms show erosion of articular cartilage and the separation of loose bodies. Joseph Milgram reports several instances of more acute lesions (see Chap. 21). A sudden twist of a flexed weight-bearing knee has resulted in a tangential fracture of the medial femoral condyle with separation of a disk of articular cartilage. This lesion from limited trauma would be almost impossible in any knee with normal articular cartilage.

In 1965 Jocelyn Hill in a personal communication crystallized the opinion of many that:

The use of hydrocortisone for the relief of joint pain should be stopped. Symptoms are masked, producing a local steroid honeymoon in a manner similar to that produced more often in the rheumatoids. Destruction proceeds not because of any local malignant activity on the steroid's part but simply because the weight-bearing joint, like a Charcot's, is pounded to destruction. Since many of these elderly bones are also osteoporotic, the addition of steroids to the diet can sometimes produce a central hip protrusion, for example, in a bed-ridden patient. This suggests that unguarded muscle pull is sufficient to cause this damage. Experience in the treatment of rheumatoid arthritis suggests that much joint pain and stiffness (viz., elbows, wrists, feet, and knees) can be relieved by simple surgical measures, and the more generalized symptoms relieved by less dangerous drugs.

Corticosteroids probably exert their effect by countering the deleterious enzyme reactions that are a feature of osteoarthritis, and this provides the initial benefit. But normal enzyme reactions may be affected as well leading to long-term deterioration of articular cartilage.[4]

Other protease inhibitors have been tested in the treatment of osteoarthritis of the knee, often with immediate relief of pain and improvement of movement. But in a week —or at most two—symptoms have usually recurred. After further injections, improvement tended to be less and of shorter duration simulating the course after cortico-steroids and probably for the same reason, which has led us to discontinue this as therapy.

Endre A. Balazs reports in Chapter 5 on the considerations behind the use of a pure, high-molecular-weight hyaluronic acid, the principal constituent of synovial fluid, in joint diseases. In osteoarthritis the concentration of hyaluronic acid is very often lower than in normal joints, and both the viscosity and elasticity of the synovial fluid is decreased. Clinical trials of replacement of synovial fluid by intraarticular injection of a pure pyrogen-free and sterile large polymer hyaluronic acid is giving most promising results. In principle it is an ideal form of therapy: the replacement of a natural constituent by a natural product. It is not a drug, and in no instance have we had any immediate or long-term undesirable effects.

The clinical trial of Healon,* as this high-polymer hyaluronic acid preparation has been called, produced the following preliminary results in our hands. Sixty-two injections were given to 45 patients in 22 hips and 40 knees all with varying severity of arthritis. Most were selected with fair range of movement without instability. No follow up was possible on two hips and four knees. There was immediate improvement with painless movement in all but one knee and two hips. The improvement in 14 hips and 33 knees after each injection lasted from 1 week to 12 months. The average duration of improvement after injection was 6 weeks for hips and 10 weeks for knees.

RAISED HEEL

The osteoarthritic knee finds comfort in slight flexion. Once fixed flexion has developed, attempts to force extension are painful. The patient tends to walk with the knee flexed a few degrees short of this painful extreme. Raising the heel of the shoe on the side of the injured knee eases the effort of walking, which becomes less fatiguing. How-

* Trademark, Biotrics, Inc., 24 Beck Road, Arlington, Massachusetts 02174 U.S.A.

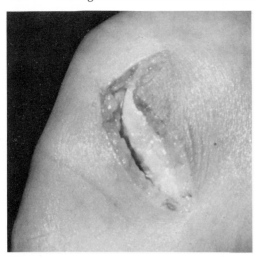

FIG. 13-3. This incision permits inspection of the articular surface of the patella as well as removal of the medial meniscus.

ever, it must be realized that raising the heel is an admission of resignation. It is always preferable to attempt the recovery of full extension by manipulation or meniscectomy.

MANIPULATION

Manipulation may be most helpful in the conservative treatment of this condition. If the displacement of the meniscus is unstable, the manipulative procedure described on page 152 frequently achieves reduction and recovery of full movement. Many a torn meniscus is unstable enough to respond to manipulation without an anesthetic, in which case it may usually be displaced as easily. Patients are taught to reduce this type of displacement themselves. They sit on the edge of a table, plinth, or high bed, with thigh muscles relaxed. First the leg is passively pulled up and fully flexed on the thigh. Then the leg is rotated in and out on the thigh until a full range is obtained, often with a feeling of "click." Finally, the foot is kicked out as if at an invisible ball, so that the knee is jerked into full extension. If the manipulation is successful, the patient can walk immediately without pain.

Manipulation for adhesions between fat pad and/or menisci and tibia following a direct blow on the front of the knee are discussed in Chapters 18 and 19.

SURGICAL "ARREST" OF OSTEOARTHRITIS OF THE KNEE JOINT

The relief sometimes achieved by gentle manipulation is, unfortunately, almost always temporary. If symptoms persist or recurrent attacks increase in frequency and severity, operation should be advised. Only by removing the torn meniscus after early diagnosis is it possible to prevent the erosion of articular cartilage and the development of the whole sequence of symptoms and signs of traumatic arthritis. The sufferer from persistent or recurrent displacement of a meniscus would be unwise to persist with palliative treatment, for each incident aggravates the intraarticular damage. Although it is usual to prescribe conservative treatment if the first manipulation is successful, the natural history of the condition and the consequences of recurrences should be explained. After further attacks, early operation should be recommended.

Meniscectomy

The technic of the operation is similar to that described in Chapter 11. When general or local circulation in some of the older patients give rise to doubt, general anesthesia and/or a tourniquet may be avoided by using the local distention anesthesia described on page 155. Modern general anesthesia is rarely contraindicated, but for an old patient a tourniquet may be unwise.

The medial end of the horizontal incision is extended upward, parallel to the patella so that the articular surface may be adequately examined see (Figs. 11-7 and 13-3). Patterns of erosion, which are evident, are a guide to the meniscal pathology. By retracting the edges of the wound and straightening the knee, the extent of erosion by the anterior horn may be followed up the femoral condyle and defined. The protrusion of the edge of the medial femoral condyle over the margin of the tibia shows well (Fig. 13-4).

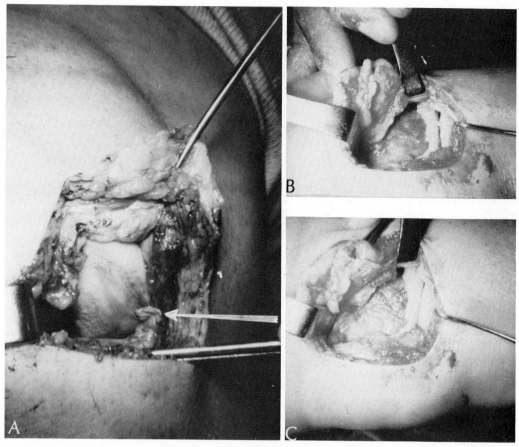

Fig. 13-4. (*A*) Operative photograph of patient, aged 43, showing early osteoarthritic changes on the articular surface of the medial condyle of the femur due to bowstring meniscus with detached anterior horn. Condrophyte formation is obvious on the medial edge of the femoral condyle. The erosive patterns are typical. (*B*) The knee is straightened before the meniscus is removed. The medial femoral condyle protrudes over the tibial margin. (*C*) After removal of the meniscus full extension is recovered, and the femur and tibia are in rotational alignment. (See color Plate 13-1.)

Moreover, it will be seen that a rim of normal articular cartilage survives between the eroded area and the bone margin (Fig. 13-6C). Removal of the meniscus is simple, for the capsule and the joint are usually rather lax. The cartilage is triangular in section and well defined. If the fat pad is adherent to the meniscus or the bone it should be freed gently. Once the meniscus is removed, it is immediately possible to extend the knee fully. The normal articular cartilage is brought into the weight-bearing area, and full rotation alignment of the femur and the tibia is recovered. An edge

of medial condyle no longer protrudes over the margin of the tibia (Fig. 13-4). If it does, it is due to condrophytes and osteophytes that have formed on the edge of the medial surface of the medial condyle of the femur and possibly on the mirror edge of the tibia. These must be carefully removed by rongeur until on extension the surfaces fit in rotational alignment (see case illustrations).

The patella is examined to assess any hindrance to free movement into the trochlear groove in extension. Only obstructing chondrophytes and osteophytes are nibbled

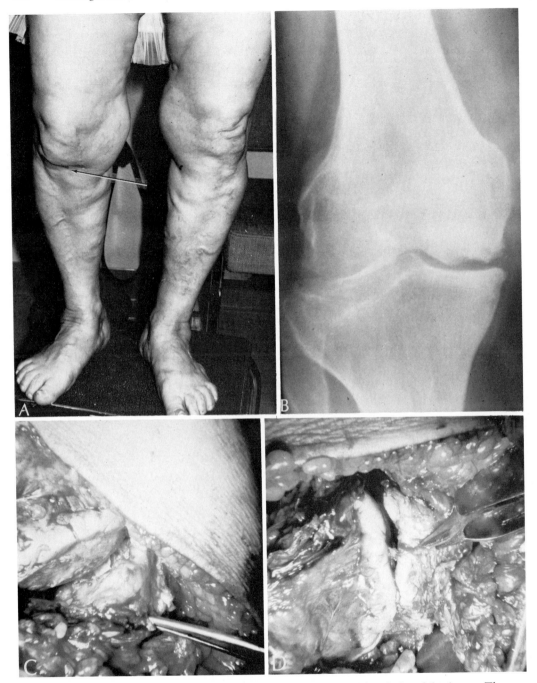

Fig. 13-5. (*A*) Patient, aged 68, with severe osteoarthritis of the right knee. The medial meniscus had been removed 10 months earlier without significant relief. The knee is locked with limitation of external rotation of the tibial tubercle and protruberance of the medial femoral condyle. The patient had medial instability from laxness of the capsule. (*B*) The roentgenogram shows marked erosion of the medial femoral condyle with sclerosis and cyst formation. (*C*) The operative photograph shows residual posterior horn nipped in and locking the joint. The articular surface is severely eroded with marked chondrophytosis. (*D*) Before excision of the residual meniscus and obstructing chondrophytes, the femur and tibia of the extended knee were not in alignment; the femoral condyle protruded. (See C, D, and E in color in Plate 13-2.)

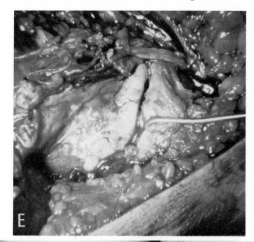

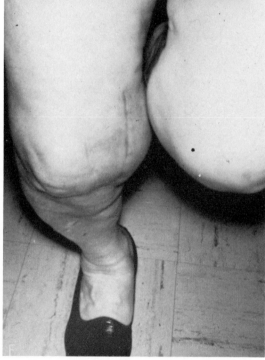

Fig. 13-5. (*E*) At the end of the operation the knee extended fully in proper rotational alignment. The semitendinous tendon was transposed into a groove in the medial femoral condyle (See C, D, and E in color in Plate 13-2.) (see Chap. 16). The patient was able to walk in 2 weeks using a cane. Three months later she had recovered muscle power, was walking well, and could climb stairs. (*F*) She could take full weight on her bent knee.

off. Eroded areas on the medial facet of the articular cartilage are carefully smoothed of abraded, fissured, and unhealthy edges. It is not necessary to remove osteophytes that do not interfere with normal movement.

TYPICAL CASE REPORTS

Case 3

Figure 13-6A shows lateral roentgenograms of the knee of a 72-year-old man with a long-standing retracted medial cartilage. The roentgenogram taken before operation shows that in the limited extension possible, the patella is squeezed against the undersurface of the medial femoral condyle, and there is erosion of the joint surfaces between the patella and the trochlear surface of the femur. In the roentgenogram taken after removal of the medial cartilage, the knee is seen to be straighter and the patella tips back into the trochlear space (see also Figs. 6-30, 6-31).

This patient had no trouble with the knee until he twisted it in January, 1957. Since then he had been unable to straighten the knee completely, and walking had been painful. These symptoms gradually worsened, and he suffered a gnawing ache in bed at night. When walking he felt as if there were a stone or lump in the medial compartment of the knee. This was relieved by bending the knee, and he tended to limp with the knee in a more and more flexed position.

On examination, extension was limited by fully 20 degrees. The anterior horn of the medial cartilage and the articular surface of the femoral condyle were acutely tender. There were signs of femoral protrusion and lack of rotation of the tibia (Figs. 7-3 and 13-6B). Roentgenograms showed erosion of the femoral articular surface and of the patella, with osteophyte formation.

At operation the medial compartment of the knee was opened. When the knee was extended, the medial condyle of the femur protruded, and lateral rotation of the tibia was restricted. After removal of the medial cartilage, rotation of the tibia was immediately restored and the knee could be ex-

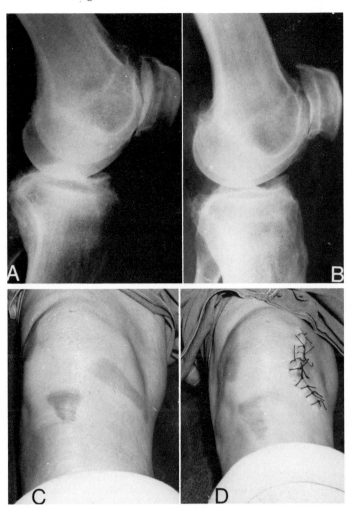

FIG. 13-6. (*A*) A preoperative roentgenogram shows that in the limited extension possible the patella is squeezed against the undersurface of the medial femoral condyle and there is erosion of the joint surface between the patella and the trochlear surface of the femur. (*B*) In the comparable roentgenogram of the knee after removal of the medial cartilage, the knee is straighter, and the patella tips back into the trochlear space. (*C*) Preoperatively, when the knee was extended the medial femoral condyle protruded, and lateral rotation of the tibial tubercle was limited. (*D*) Immediately after removal of the medial cartilage, the tibia rotates and the knee extends fully. (*E, opposite*) Compare this photograph with Figure 6-16. Note that in spite of a large area of erosion, a rim of normal articular cartilage remains. (*F*) With the knee extended and the patella retraced the eroded area on the medial slope of the trochlear surface is visible. (*G*) The unaffected lateral slope is smooth.

tended fully. There were areas of erosion on the medial femoral condyle and the medial facet of the patella. The osteophytes on the medial border of the patella were nibbled off. The findings are illustrated in Figures 13-6B-G.

Progress after operation was rapid. The knee could be extended almost completely. The gnawing ache disappeared, and 3 months after the operation the patient was able to walk and climb stairs without pain.

Comment. I have deliberately presented the history of a patient who had extensive arthritis with erosion due to a torn medial cartilage, for it shows that even at a late stage the simple excision of a cartilage is desirable. In the earlier stage not only are symptoms relieved and function restored but further degeneration is prevented. After removal of the cartilage the patient is taught to extend the knee fully. Normal articular cartilage is brought into the weight-bearing area and, once more, the contracting quadriceps allows the patella to travel in the correspondingly proportioned groove of the trochlear surface of the femur. There is no tension and no pain.

Postoperative care should be planned to

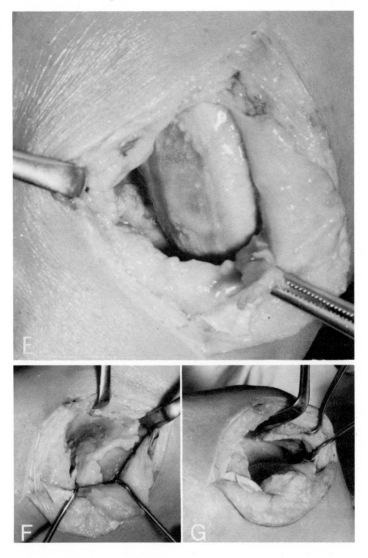

teach the patient once more to extend the knee completely. In older patients, especially, this is the main purpose of quadriceps retraining. Unless the patella shows gross degeneration it need not be excised, but the osteophytic protrusions on the medial border should be removed. Older patients are happier with than without the patella.

Case 4

Figure 13-7 illustrates the case of a man of 66. In spite of a gunshot wound of the femur during the first world war, he had enjoyed normal function and played much golf. Six months before consulting me he had fallen on the left knee. The knee was swollen and painful for 3 weeks. Thereafter he could again play golf but felt uncomfortable after a round, and in the last 2 months his knee had become progressively worse. He felt pain when he swung against the knee, and toward the end of the game his knee would ache and the leg feel lame. At first the symptoms settled down with rest, but finally the pain became constant.

On examination, the four signs that I have described were all present. The knee was tender over the articular surface of the

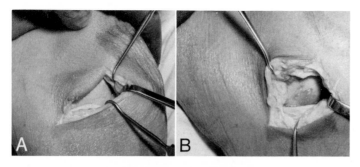

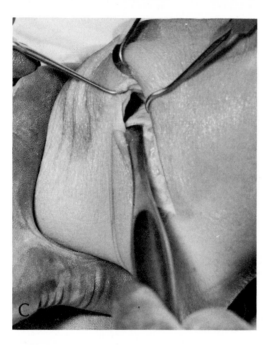

FIG. 13-7. (*A*) Linear erosion on the anterior part of the articular surface of the femoral condyle. (*B*) Erosion on the femoral condyle, linear in the anterior part and broadening out farther back. (*C*) Erosion of the medial slope of the trochlear surface of the femur caused by tension from the medial facet of the patella in the locked knee.

femoral condyle and chiefly on the medial side of the trochlear surface and the corresponding border of the patella. Figure 13-7A shows a linear erosion on the anterior part of the articular surface of the femoral condyle: the erosion broadened out farther back (Fig. 13-7A). Figure 13-7B shows the erosion of the medial slope of the trochlear surface of the femur. The erosion on the patella corresponded exactly. The lateral slopes of the articular cartilage of the femur and the patella were unmarked.

After the operation the knee straightened out completely. Convalescence was normal, and full function was recovered.

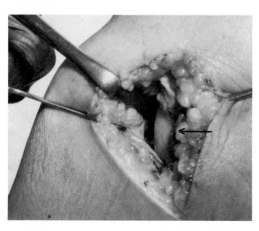

FIG. 13-8. The anterior end of the meniscus is detached, and the articular cartilage on the opposing femoral condyle is beginning to erode.

Case 5

Figure 13-8 shows the findings at operation in a 51-year-old woman. She did not recall any injury but complained of intermittent pain and swelling in the right knee for 3 months. On examination rotation of the tibia was restricted, and the femoral condyle protruded. There was tenderness over the anterior end of the medial cartilage and along the medial border of the patella. Forced passive extension caused localized pain over the anterior end of the cartilage, and forced active extension caused pain behind the patella.

Conservative treatment did not help her, and 6 weeks later the cartilage was removed. The cartilage was detached in front, the anterior two thirds were thickened, and there was an almost complete transverse fracture at the junction of the anterior two thirds and the posterior third. The fractured edge showed the typical scalloped squashed appearance (Fig. 6-20B).

Six weeks later when she had recovered good function of the quadriceps she had a full range of comfortable movement.

THE PATELLA

Intraarticular examination of the patella is required if any of the following conditions are present:

1. Postpatellar pain on walking up and down stairs or slopes
2. Tenderness of the medial border of the patella
3. Roentgenographic evidence of osteophytic or erosive changes on skyline views of the patella

The extended skin incision (Figs. 11-7 and 13-3) is necessary, and treatment is dictated by the stage and the extent of the degenerative changes in the articular cartilage of the patella.

If the changes are moderate, the release of tension with recovery of full extension after meniscectomy is sufficient to relieve pain. As soon as the patella can achieve its normal and balanced position in the trochlear groove, climbing and descending stairs is comfortable.

Débridement of the Patella

This is a helpful procedure when osteophytes are young and not too massive and desiccated, and for frayed and fissured patches of articular cartilage. If the edges of the eroded ulcers are ragged, they should be trimmed carefully. Judgment born of experience is of most value in deciding what to do in this situation. Instead of débridement, the need may be for patellectomy or patelloplasty. Débridement, when performed, should be thorough. Osteophytes and cartilage are excised gently until a smooth, almost transparent surface is obtained.

The effectiveness of the débridement may be gauged by a simple test. If the knee is flexed and extended before débridement, the impingement of the patellar osteophytes on the femoral edge is obvious. After adequate removal, movement of the patella is free and without friction or tension. Sidney Sacks of Johannesburg now does, and endorses, a partial medial patellectomy—excision of a medial strip of patella—when he finds damage or disorder of the medial articular surface.[15] Some young athletes have returned to vigorous games after this operation which is necessary only if true and localized chondromalacia is present or if osteophytosis is excessive. When erosion of articular cartilage and/or osteophytes are due to mechanical derangement, correction of the latter and débridement is all that is necessary.

Synovium and capsule are sutured. The postoperative regimen described for meniscectomy is used, with somewhat longer time periods. Compression bandage without knee flexion is maintained for 2 weeks, and thigh muscle drill may be started after 2 or 3 days.

Case 6

A patient, age 74, had injured her left knee in an accident 14 months previously. For 6 months she had suffered constantly from pain on walking, and the knee ached and kept her awake at night. Immediately after removal of the medial meniscus and débridement of the medial border of the

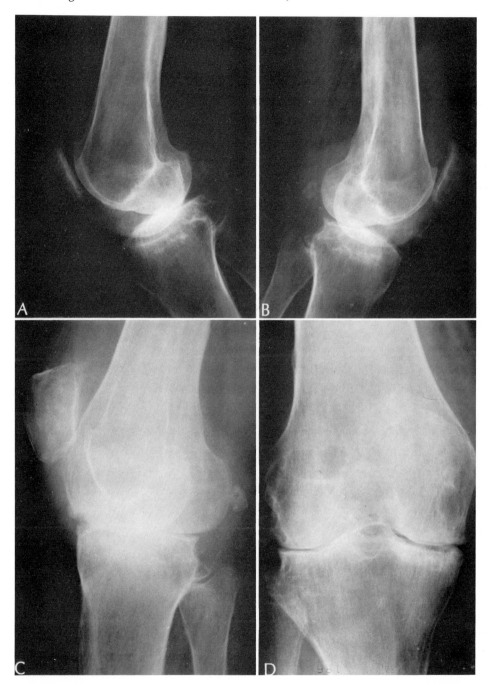

FIG. 13-9. Case 6—This patient had fixed flexor contracture in her arthritic knee. (*A*) Note the retropatellar osteoarthritis and a comparable pattern on the femur. (*B*) Ten days after meniscectomy and medial patellar debridement the patient can straighten the knee, and the patella reaches the trochlear space. (*C*) Three months later the patient is comfortable and can extend the knee fully without discomfort. (*D*) the anteroposterior view shows roentgenographic changes 3 months postoperatively, but the knee is comfortable.

patella she could sleep without discomfort. She was up on the tenth day and when examined 6 months later was walking well and could pursue her normal activities without pain (Fig. 13-9).

PATELLECTOMY

If the articular cartilage of the patella or the trochlea is widely and grossly affected, patellectomy is indicated. The skin incision is prolonged transversely (Fig. 13-10). The bone is removed subperiosteally. The synovial layer usually approximates without tension and may be closed with fine plain catgut. The repair of the capsule and the fascial and periosteal coverings of the patella must be meticulous. As in all knee surgery, the keynote is the restoration of function of the patellar mechanism and medial capsule so that complete, active extension and rotation is recovered. Therefore, the knee is extended completely with full lateral rotation of the tibia before the capsule is sutured

with #1 chromic catgut or linen thread. If necessary to achieve proper tension in the medial capsule, the edges are overlapped; and to tighten up the whole mechanism, a Bunnell-type suture of the same material is used to pull quadriceps and patellar tendons together (Fig. 13-11). Postoperatively the patient stays in bed for 2 weeks with compression bandage and a plaster-of-paris splint which includes the foot with the leg in external rotation. After removal of the skin sutures, a back splint is applied for 6 weeks; for the first 4 weeks the patient walks on crutches without bearing weight on the leg. During the last 2 weeks the back splint is removed for periodic active flexion exer-

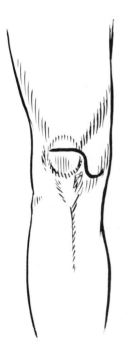

Fig. 13-10. The skin incision is prolonged transversely across the patella.

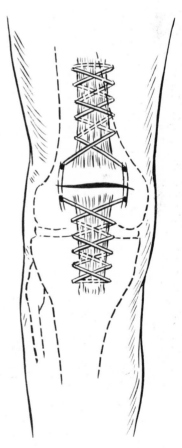

Fig. 13-11. Bunnell-type suture of chromic catgut or linen thread is used to pull the quadriceps and the patellar tendon together.

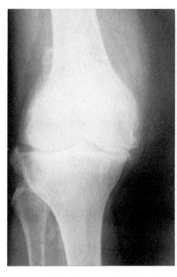
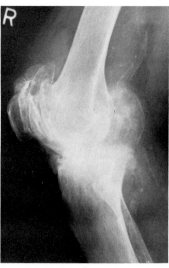

Fig. 13-12. Case 7—Preoperative anteroposterior and lateral roentgenograms of the right knee of an 82-year-old woman. After meniscectomy and patellectomy she could once more straighten the knee, and within 3 months she could walk comfortably with a cane.

cises. Thigh drill is commenced 2 weeks after operation.

Comfort is restored by this operation, and satisfactory movement is usually recovered in a few weeks. Occasionally a gentle manipulation under Pentothal is necessary to recover or accelerate recovery of movement. The manipulation should not be undertaken until the adhesions are "dry." If done too soon, the vascular adhesions bleed and the joint reacts with swelling and pain. Generally speaking, adhesions are "dry" when deep tenderness is localized, and reaction to deep heat and active use is minimal in pain and swelling. Good judgment in this regard is the criterion of success. Manipulation at the wrong time delays recovery but at the right time may result in dramatic relief.

As these older patients are happy to be without pain and do not seek violent activity, the short-term results of patellectomy are good and the long-term prognosis usually better than in younger patients.

Case 7

The oldest patient, 82 years old, had for some years given up all hope of walking without severe distress. Pain in the right knee kept her awake night after night. One day the knee gave way and she fractured the

neck of the femur near the head. The head was replaced by an Austin Moore prosthesis. Her knee was swollen with some 15 degrees of fixed flexion deformity due to a torn medial meniscus. Roentgenograms (Fig. 13-12) show the articular surface of the patella to be extensively eroded. The meniscus and the patella were removed. She recovered extension of the knee, could walk on crutches in a month and without crutches in 3 months, and she slept well at night.

SYNOVECTOMY

When the indications are sufficient, synovectomy—or rather anterior synovectomy— is a highly recommended procedure for traumatic arthritis of the type under consideration. In this series it was rarely necessary (12 cases), but the results were as happy as those reported by DePalma.[9] Most patients lost their pain completely, and all had improved significantly in comfort and recovered at least 70 degrees of flexion from full extension. The knees moved creakily but painlessly (Fig. 13-13A).

All these cases had gross articular changes with marked effusion, thickened synovium and fixed-flexion–internal-rotation deformity. Pain was felt both on walking and in bed at night.

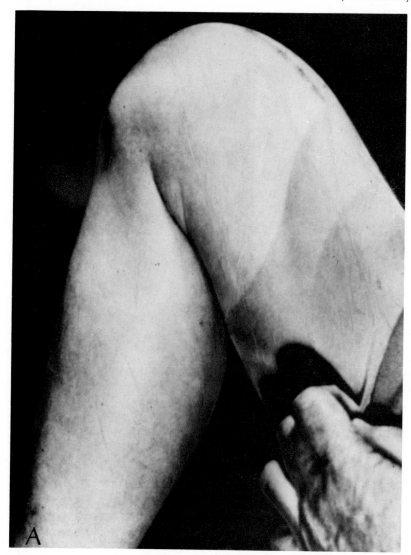

FIG. 13-13A. The widest range of flexion obtained after synovectomy in twelve knees.

The operation is performed through a long medial parapatellar wound with the leg straight, the patient lying on his back (Fig. 13-13B). The capsule is opened by a vertical incision parallel to and within ½ inch of the patellar ligament and the patella, extended upward between the medial vastus and the quadriceps tendons. The synovium bulges into the wound. The synovial effusion is syphoned off and, if the incision is adequate, it is possible to retract the patella laterally and to turn it inside out so that the articular surface points forward. By sharp dissection the thickened synovium is removed from the whole suprapatellar pouch and on each side of the femoral condyle as far back as its reflection. The menisci are usually degenerate and should be excised. The procedure for the patella depends on the state of the articular cartilage, both on the patella and the trochlear surface of the femur and has been discussed on a previous page. Diseased cartilage and osteophytes should be removed, and if possible, the patella should be preserved. The McKeever prosthesis or turning up a pedicled graft of the infrapatellar pad of fat to cover the articular surface as in the Magnuson procedure are to be considered in extreme cases in younger patients. Both have their satisfactory results. One patient preferred the knee with a McKeever prosthesis to the other from which the patella had been removed. The knee is mechanically sounder with than without its patellar pulley.

Again, the prime object of postoperative care is to restore full extension and lateral rotation of the leg. A compression bandage and extension straps are applied so that the limb can be suspended in balanced traction. For the first week a back splint is added. Thigh drill is started on the second or the third day and flexion exercises in suspension

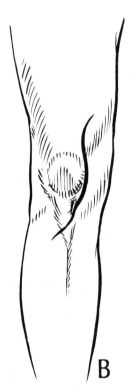

Fig. 13-13B. Long medial parapatellar incision for synovectomy.

when the back splint is removed. It is important that full extension is recovered after each act of flexion of the knee. Three weeks after the operation the patient may walk on the back splint with crutches and 3 weeks later without crutches. Sometimes when old people experience difficulty in recovering muscle power and bulk, a caliper with knee spring (Fig. 13-1) should be used until unassisted walking can be undertaken without strain. Physiotherapy consisting of massage and faradic stimulation may be used as a muscle stimulant and educator, but it is no substitute for active exercise.

UPPER TIBIAL OSTEOTOMY

The successful relief of pain in osteoarthritis of the hip by juxta-articular osteotomy has, as a natural consequence, led to the practice of high tibial osteotomy for osteoarthritis of the knee. Jackson and Waugh[14] performed the operation to correct deformity and reported all 10 patients free of pain. Wardle[16] and, later, Helal[11] and Apley[1] determined that intramedullary venous congestion, a cause of pain, could be blocked by an osteotomy below the tibial tubercle. Dramatic relief of pain was ascribed to the sclerotic barrier formed by union across the medullary canal. Apley shows a patient in whom the osteotomy healed without sclerosis and who was not relieved (see Fig. 12-9).[1] Coventry,[8] Devas,[10] and Insall[13] and others subsequently reported satisfactory results.

In 1969 Benjamin advocated double osteotomy—above and below the joint—for osteo- and rheumatoid arthritis.[3] Thirty-one of 36 patients with osteoarthritis and 17 of 21 rheumatoid knees received benefit from the operation.

Considering the results of relatively simple and limited intraarticular operation as emphasized in this chapter, especially in early osteoarthritis, the main indication for osteotomy should be correction of deformity. In determining the deformity to be corrected, it should be remembered that intra-articular derangement of the soft tissue invariably produces internal-rotation-flexion deformity of the tibia on the femur and often an apparent valgus.

This deformity with its block to movement is released by the intraarticular operation which should always be performed before residual valgus or varus is corrected by osteotomy. In many instances the correction is sufficient to obviate the bone operation. Patients have been seen who were not benefited by osteotomy because of intraarticular derangement. They were subsequently relieved by the intraarticular operation.

ARTHRODESIS OF THE KNEE

In the past, arthrodesis was the main salvage procedure for chronic disorders of the knee. The usual method used to obtain fusion was coaption of shaped raw bony surfaces aided in a number of ways by bone grafts and internal fixation. The results as a whole were unsatisfactory. Union was slow and unsound ankylosis a common sequel. The results have been improved immeasurably both in rate of union and solid fusion by the compression method of arthrodesis of the knee first described by Charnley in 1948.[6] One centimeter of the articular surfaces of both the femur and the tibia is removed by transverse saw cuts. Steinman pins are passed transversely through the lower femur and the upper tibia. Clamps are applied to the pins and tightened so that the opposing surfaces are subjected to approximately 100 pounds of compression load.

In 4 weeks the patient starts taking weight in a walking plaster cast; and in many cases the plaster splint may be discarded after another 4 weeks. Most patients have firm fusion in 12 weeks. Of 100 cases recorded by Charnley, in only two was ankylosis permanently unsound.

Arthrodesis may be indicated when injury or infection has disorganized or destroyed the weight-bearing surfaces of the knee. When arthritis is due to a derangement of the rotator mechanism, arthrodesis is indicated only in extreme cases. In spite of gross erosion of articular cartilage, most knees are comfortable when function is restored by meniscectomy, if necessary with débridement of the patella, patellectomy or partial synovectomy. Improvement in technic and design in knee replacements will also limit the indications for arthrodesis of the knee.

REFERENCES

1. Apley, A. G.: Personal communication, 1965.
2. Barnett, C. H., Davies, D. V., and MacConaill, M. A.: Synovial Joints; Their Structure and Mechanics. Springfield, Charles C Thomas, 1961.
3. Benjamin, A.: Double osteotomy for painful knee. J. Bone Joint Surg., 5B:694, 1969.
4. Chandler, G. N., Wright, V., and Hartfall, S. J.: Deleterious effect of intra-articular hydrocortisone. Lancet, 2:661, 1958.
5. ————: Intraarticular therapy in rheumatoid arthritis. Lancet, 2:659, 1958.
6. Charnley, J. C.: Positive pressure in arthrodesis of the knee joint. J. Bone Joint Surg. 30B:478, 1948.
7. Charnley, J. C., and Lowe, H. G.: A study of the end results of compression arthrodesis of the knee. J. Bone J oint Surg., 40B:633, 1958.
8. Coventry, M. B.: Osteotomy of the upper portion of the tibia for degenerative arthritis of the knee. J. Bone Joint Surg., 47A:984, 1965.
9. De Palma, A. F.: Diseases of the Knee. Philadelphia, J. B. Lippincott, 1954.
10. Devas, M. B.: High tibial osteotomy for arthritis of the knee. J. Bone Joint Surg., 51B:95, 1969.
11. Helal, B.: The pain of primary osteoarthritis of the knee. Postgraduate Med. Jour., 41:172, 1965.
12. Hollander, J. L., Brown, E. M., Jessar, R. A., and Brown, C. Y.: Hydrocortisone

and cortisone injected into arthritic joints. J.A.M.A., *147*:1629, 1951.

13. Insall, J. A., Bauer, G. C. H., and Koshino, T.: Tibial osteotomy in gonarthrosis (osteoarthritis) of the knee. J. Bone Joint Surg., *51A*:1545, 1969.

14. Jackson, J. P., and Waugh, J.: Tibial osteotomy for osteoarthritis of the knee. J. Bone Joint Surg., *43B*:746, 1961.

15. Sacks, S.: Semipatellectomy. S. Afr. Med. J., *36*:518, 1962.

16. Wardle, E. N.: Osteotomy of the tibia and fibula. Surg. Gyn., & Obstet., *115*:61, 1962.

17. Waugh, W. G.: Monoarticular osteoarthritis of the hip. Brit. Med. J., *1*:873, 1945.

14

Surgical Management of the Rheumatoid Knee

Arthur J. Helfet, M.D.

Most recent approaches to the surgical treatment of the rheumatoid joint concentrate on radical synovectomy in the early stages and on arthroplasty in reconstruction of the derelict joint. But a uniform prescription ignores the changing pathological states that characterize the disorganization of the joint. By taking regard of these changes, it is possible to correct deformity and recover comfort and movement by other surgical measures.

The rheumatoid process heals by fibrosis, which, by its nature, limits movement and leads to deformity. This is to be differentiated from early painful limitation of movement due to muscle spasm. In turn derangements and blocks to movement produce their patterns of erosion on the articular cartilage, leading to a phase of osteoarthrosis secondary to the articular derangement and in addition to the ravages by rheumatoid pannus.

The muscles acting on the joint also demand attention. In some instances, degeneration and fibrosis of muscle fibers occur and in others long-standing deformity causes malalignment, weakness, and contracture or stretching that may require surgical adjustment before reablement of the joint is possible.

THE SYNOVIUM

The immediate manifestation of rheumatoid arthritis is a uniformly inflamed red, swollen synovium (Plate 14-1). From the edges a membrane of malignant granulation tissue or pannus invades the articular cartilage causing lysis, pitting, and destruction (Plates 14-2A, 2B). The process is accelerated by a similar attack from the subchondral surface. This, the accepted view, has been questioned by Hamerman[1] who found that irreversible cartilage matrix depletion takes place within weeks of the onset of the disease, leading to loss of the normal mechanical properties of articular cartilage and impaired joint function. As the disease progresses patches of synovium fibrose, and adhesions form between folds of the membrane. They develop also around the infrapatellar pad of fat constricting its lobules and binding it to the tibia, to menisci, and via the alar ligaments to the intercondylar notch and the cruciate ligaments. Finally the joint is encompassed and practically obliterated by criss-crossing bands of white firm avascular fibrous adhesions with no residuum of inflamed synovium.

Therefore in the first stage only radical synovectomy would have an effect; in the second stage partial synovectomy and excision of adhesions is possible and advantageous; while in the final stage no synovium remains to be excised, and the problem is separation of adhesions and joint reconstruction.

The sclerosing synovium becomes adherent to the capsule proper and to its own folds where these envelop the menisci and cruciate ligaments. The coronary ligaments scar, depriving the menisci of mobility. Sometimes the undersurfaces of the latter become completely adherent to the tibia and when peeled off at operation leave a deep and exact imprint.

As articular cartilage is destroyed bands of fibrous tissue may extend from femur to tibia and from femur to patella, binding these bony surfaces to each other. In particularly severe cases bony fusion of the joint surfaces takes place.

MENISCI

As aging in itself results in a number of changes to the meniscus (described in Chapter 12) it is difficult to enumerate those peculiar to arthrosis or arthritis.

In rheumatoid arthritis meniscus is affected in one of two ways: it is gradually destroyed or absorbed so that at operation only ragged, marginal fragments are found, or the meniscus becomes flat and hard and bound down to the tibia. Calcification is not uncommon and in one case an area of ossification was found. In another an osteophyte has formed on the articular surface of the tibia and had transfixed and pierced the medial meniscus (Plate 14-3).

THE INFRAPATELLAR PAD OF FAT

The adhesions which form around the fat pad and between the lobules appear at operation as a mass of fibrous tissue binding the anterior horns of the menisci to the anterosuperior surfaces of the tibia from which bands extend to the patella and intercondylar notch of the femur.

As these adhesions are carefully excised or divided the lobules of fat appear and bulge anew to reform an apparently natural fat pad. To recover maximum function it is important to preserve the fat pad and restore its mobility.

THE DERANGEMENT OF THE KNEE JOINT AND "TRIPLE DISPLACEMENT"

The progress of derangement of the knee joint in rheumatoid arthritis follows fairly consistent patterns. As a bicondylar helicoid joint, the lateral articular surface of the tibia pivots on the roundish lateral condyle of the femur while the medial articular surface follows the longer winding course on the medial femoral condyle. In rheumatoid arthritis adhesions in the joint and adherence of the menisci or fat pad hamper rotation as well as flexion-extension, evident in the extended knee by the medial position of the tibial tubercle and *protrusion of the medial femoral condyle* i.e., the first deformity of the rheumatoid knee is fixed flexion and medial rotation of the tibia on the femur. This stage cannot be distinguished from the osteoarthritic knee in which the same deformity and limitation occurs.

Posterior Displacement of the Tibia on the Femur

The addition of posterior displacement of the tibia on the femur with lateral rotation of the leg completes the so-called triple displacement of the rheumatoid knee. This interesting development is induced by overaction of the iliotibial band on the flexed knee.

Normally the iliotibial band and biceps femoris are the stabilizers of the leg on the thigh. The tibia must rotate on the femur in flexion and extension. To do this while bearing weight would make for laveral instability, were it not for the stabilizing control of the biceps acting directly on the fibula and tibiofibular joint, and by the iliotibial band on the outer border of the tibial tuberosity, the point of pivot of the rotating tibia.

Once fixed flexion-internal rotation deformity of the knee is established, however, the iliotibial band acts as a posterior retractor of the tibia. The flexed tibia is pulled backwards leaving *both the lateral and*

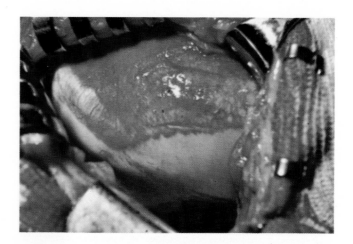

Plate 14-1. The synovium of acute rheumatoid arthritis is uniformly red and swollen.

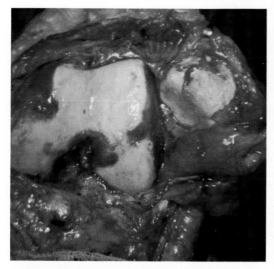

Plate 14-2. (*A*) Operative photograph of pannus invading the articular cartilage.

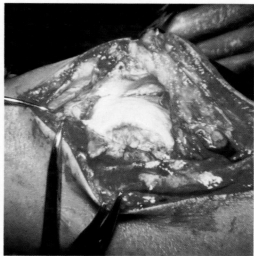

(*B*) Healing by fibrosis has commenced. Patches of articular cartilage are dull and yellow.

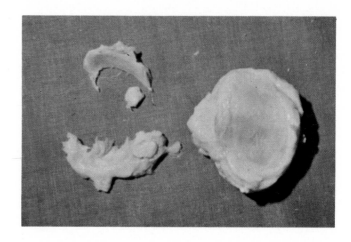

Plate 14-3. The articular cartilage of the patella has been destroyed. The menisci are degenerated, ragged and partially absorbed. The medial meniscus has been transfixed by an osteophyte.

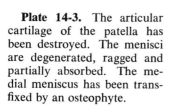

FIG. 14-1. (*A*) The swollen knees of rheumatoid arthritis with both the medial and femoral condyles protruding beyond the anterior margin of the tibia. (*B*) Lateral roentgenogram of triple displacement of the rheumatoid knee.

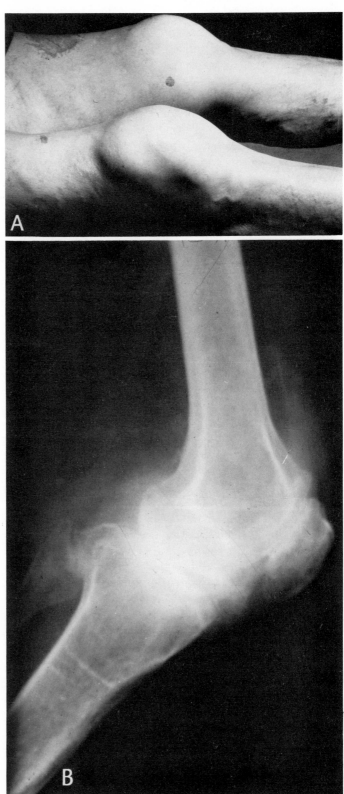

medial femoral condyles protruding beyond the anterior margin of the tibia (Fig. 14-1). This distinguishes the rheumatoid from the osteoarthritic knee, in which only the medial femoral condyle protrudes.

At the same time, since the center of the tibia is behind that of the femur, the pull of the laterally fixed iliotibial band will externally rotate the retracted tibia. The primarily internally rotated tibia is now rotated laterally but at a different point of pivot. A similar deformity and for the same reason occurs after poliomyelitis owing to unbalanced muscle action. Yount devised the simple operation of division and release of this muscle to correct the deformity.

Surgical Technique. Once these deforming forces are understood, it is possible to establish a surgical approach to reduce the deformity. Wedging plaster casts or hinged pressure devices do no more than stretch the posterior structures and change the angle of the tibia, which remains retracted in relation to the femur. Posterior capsulotomy without intraarticular and muscle release does little more although it achieves the result more quickly. The operation should make possible forward replacement of the lateral tuberosity of the tibia and rotation of the tibia on the femur.

Once the restricting tissues are released the lateral tuberosity of the tibia is pushed forward until it is aligned with the femoral condyle. Then by extending the leg on the femur with synchronous external rotation, complete reduction of the triple displacement may be effected. These maneuvers are possible after: (1) release of the iliotibial band (Yount's operation), (2) release of the rotator mechanism of the knee, particularly the menisci and fat pad and obstructing intraarticular adhesions, and (3) mobilization of, or, if inevitable, excision of the patella.

After excision of all actively inflamed synovium the particular surgery required varies. A blanket "house cleaning" is unnecessarily destructive. The infrapatellar pad of fat should be freed and preserved, not excised. The menisci, if adherent or calcified

or ossified or if replaced by fibrous remnants, should be excised. All adhesions are divided until free rotation of the tibia on the femur is possible (Fig. 14-2).

PAIN IN RHEUMATOID ARTHRITIS

The acute phase of rheumatoid arthritis is always painful. Pain is associated with the red inflammatory process and indicated by hot swelling and muscle spasm. Patients complain of a constant ache aggravated by activity with acute pain on movement. Pain is relieved by rest and support and by excision of all inflamed synovium.

As the acute phase subsides the pain and disability depends on the extent of derangement of the joint. If the rotator mechanism is tethered with limitation of the extremes of extension and flexion, the manner and type of pain is exactly the same as in comparable derangement in the osteoarthritic knee. And similarly pain is relieved by rest and support, or by excision of remaining inflamed synovium plus surgical correction of the derangement. Once the normal pattern of movement is recovered pain disappears dramatically even though the ulcers and eroded areas of articular cartilage remain, which supports the assumption that articular cartilage is relatively insensitive. Pain in the deranged joint derives from abnormal tensions in the soft tissues and not from abnormal pressures on articular cartilage.

The insensitivity of the articular cartilage is also apparent in the finally fibrosed inactive joint. Now the knee joint is stiff but not painful. As the articular surfaces are insensitive, movement recovered by division of adhesions and release of the rotator mechanism and infrapatellar pad of fat is painless. Thirty to 60 degrees of movement may be so recovered; this makes a great difference to the patient, especially in bilateral cases. The patient is able to get in and out of motor cars and to drive.

Cortisone

The role of cortisone in the management of rheumatoid arthritis is under constant re-

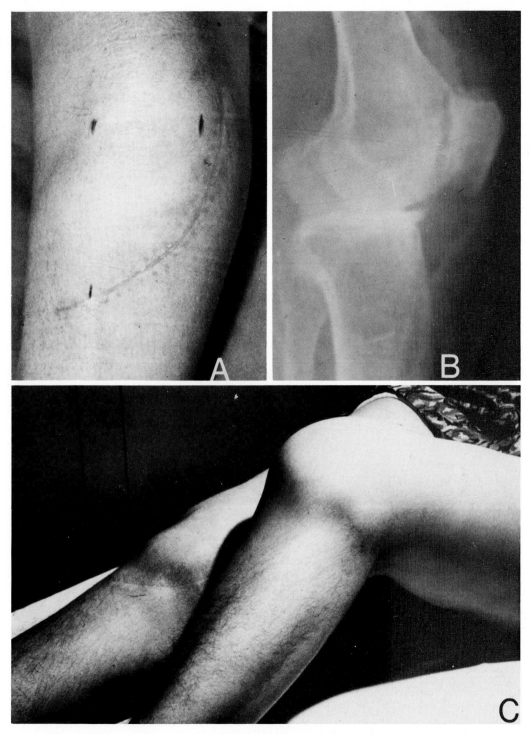

FIG. 14-2. (*A*) After release of the iliotibial band and the rotator mechanism of the right knee (including the fat pad and obstructing intraarticular adhesions) the menisci shown in Plate 14-3 were excised. The maneuver of reduction was performed. The knee is now extended. Protrusion of the femoral condyles has been minimized. (*B*) In the anterior view, the alignment of the right knee is satisfactory. Normal external rotation of the tibia on the femur is possible. (*C*) This lateral view of the knee in Figure 14-1B after operation and reduction shows that the "triple displacement" has been reduced.

view for there is little doubt that administered either parenterally or locally it often has a long-term deleterious effect on articular cartilage—especially of weightbearing joints, though the elbow has also shown change.

REABLEMENT OF THE KNEE AFTER SURGERY

An interesting and most important phase in the management of the rheumatoid knee is the restoration of power and function after surgery. A Jones compression dressing is applied with the knee fully reduced and is supported by a light plaster of Paris cast with the foot in external rotation. Isometric thigh drill with the patient consciously attempting to hold the leg in forced active extension is started next day and practiced regularly.

After the stitches have been removed, foam rubber traction is applied, and the patient begins active flexion exercises using Guthrie-Smith slings or Russell traction. Aided by the apparatus each flexion movement is followed by active full extension. Between the exercise periods the back splint is reapplied.

The main problem is recovery of full extension. Frequently intrinsic weakness, fibrosis, and stretched extensors leave an extension lag however hard the patient practices. Passive extension is full and comfortable, but active extension may lag by as much as 20 degrees. The patient has usually recovered sufficient control to walk with crutches and a back splint in 3 weeks or less. However, walking without support should not be permitted before full strong active extension is recovered. Otherwise extension lag, signalled by a feeling of insecurity or of actual "giving-way" followed by pain and swelling after effort, is not prevented. These effects are relieved by rest or support but recur with stress.

Soon after the operation the patient is usually comfortable and if the recovery of muscle power and excursion copes with carefully graduated activity, the patient is content and requests surgery for the other knee. However, if extension lag and inadequate power persist, and they may do so because of intrinsic changes in the muscle, recurrent strain obstructs recovery.

EXTENSION LAG

For patients in whom weak wasted thigh muscles after longstanding deformity denote the problem of extension lag, surgical shortening of the extensor mechanism with imbrication of the capsule of the knee must be considered, for this gives prospect of more rapid recovery of muscle control and power. The shortening required is never much and must be carefully assessed. If the extensor mechanism is overshortened, limitation of flexion and pain from patellofemoral compression develops. Transfer of the tibial tubercle with the whole patellar tendon downwards is unnecessarily elaborate and takes long to heal, when early movement is advantageous. A simpler procedure using a central tongue of patellar tendon as used for "high-riding patella" is sufficient (see p. 238). Active movements in suspension may be started 10 to 14 days postoperatively.

Once the knee is disorganized or destroyed beyond repair arthrodesis or arthroplasty are indicated. Fortunately the techniques and devices for arthroplasty have reached a stage of competence that should soon make arthrodesis a rare necessity, especially in the rheumatoid patient who is usually handicapped in other joints as well. (See Chap. 20 for a more detailed discussion of knee prostheses.)

REFERENCE

Hamerman, D.: Cartilage changes in the rheumatoid joint. Clin Orthop. Rel. Res., *64*:91, 1969.

15

Hemophilic Arthritis of the Knee

J. E. Handelsman, M.B., M.Ch. Orth.

Advances in the understanding and management of hemophilia and related inherited bleeding disorders have greatly improved the life expectancy of sufferers. As a sequel, a greater emphasis is now focused on the associated orthopedic deformities, commonly the result of repeated hemarthroses. The knees are the most frequently affected, being poorly supported weight-bearing joints susceptible to minor stresses and strains. Pain, loss of movement, and flexion contractures cause considerable disability. Hemophilic arthritis of the knee demands an energetic prophylactic and therapeutic regime.

BASIC FACTORS

A clear understanding of the etiology of the disease is recent. As late as 1932, clinicians were treating repeated hemorrhages in hemophilic patients by injecting maternal blood taken during the menstrual cycle in the belief that ovarian extract provided protection.[2] In 1937 Pohle and Taylor established that hemophilia was due to a lack of "an antihemophilic factor" in the blood clotting mechanism.[14] Deficiency in Factor IX, Christmas disease, behaves, for practical purposes, in a similar manner and will not be considered as a separate entity.

Although hemophilia is transmitted to males as a sex-linked trait by clinically normal female carriers, approximately 30 per cent of men with hemophilia have no family history of the disease. In some instances,

the defective gene has been present but not apparent because families in previous generations have produced few sons. A high mutation rate is, however, significant etiologically.

Reliable methods of assaying the deficient factor are now available, and the level is related to the clinical severity of the disease. When the circulating plasma level is under 1 per cent, the patient is severely affected, and spontaneous hemarthroses and hemorrhages are common. Moderately severely affected patients have a level of between 1 and 5 per cent, and in this category spontaneous bleeding is less frequent but may be severe after minor injuries. Mildly affected individuals have a deficient factor level of between 5 and 30 per cent and may lead normal lives, bleeding only after severe accidents or surgery. However no absolute correlation of factor level and the frequency of hemarthroses exists. With comparable factor level concentration, one patient may sustain crippling deformities following multiple joint bleeds whilst another may retain well-preserved joints. Furthermore, many experience a seasonal or phasic susceptibility to hemarthroses.[10] Additional factors thus play a part in the development of hemarthroses.

Hemophilia is not uncommon. In Scandinavia, one in 7,000 males born is a severe hemophiliac, and the incidence in the United Kingdom is probably similar.[16] There is no reason to suppose that figures are significantly different elsewhere. By including

201

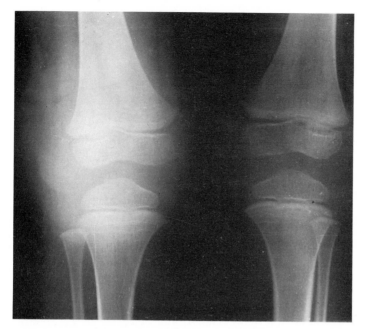

FIG. 15-1. Thickened synovium, outlined by a deposition of hemosiderin, surrounds the affected right knee in this roentgenograph.

more mildly afflicted patients and taking into account increasing survival with modern therapy, the disease assumes significant proportions. Although the victims of hemophilia are numerically few, the chronicity of the condition in hemophiliacs imposes a disproportionate strain on both patients and medical resources.

PATHOLOGY

Hemophilic blood within a joint remains fluid. The cell count is reasonably elevated, and sugar concentration drops to slightly below normal. The red cells slowly break up, hemoglobin disintegrates, and hemosiderin is released. The iron-containing pigment is phagocytosed by the superficial synovial cells and may remain in this surface layer indefinitely. Coarser aggregations of iron may be found in microphages lying in the deeper portions of the synovial membrane.[7] Repeated hemorrhages progressively increase the hemosiderosis, and ultimately the iron content may be as much as 70 per cent of the ashed weight of the synovial tissue.[17]

The actual intraarticular hemorrhage occurs from the synovial membrane. A vicious cycle is established. As the irritated synovial lining thickens and becomes more vascular with repeated hemorrhages, the potential bleeding area is increased. Ultimately a synovial lining closely resembling that found in rheumatoid arthritis may result, and it is probable that many of the chronic or rapidly recurrent "hemarthroses" are in fact irritative synovial joint effusions. Nevertheless, it is certain that once hemorrhage has occurred, that joint is predisposed to further bleeds. Apart from the increased vascularization, the joint, in particular the knee, becomes less well protected because of disuse atrophy of the associated muscles.

Ultimately the irritated synovium becomes fibrosed and contracted, and although hemarthroses and effusions may lessen, stiffness becomes increasingly severe irrespective of the condition of the articular cartilage.

Changes in the articular cartilage have been shown to occur early in the disease process. In a study of fresh postmortem specimens by van Creveld and his coworkers in 1971,[18] swollen chondrocytes were seen histologically and correlated with macroscopic cleft formation in the articular cartilage. With recurrent hemarthroses, articular cartilage eventually disappears, cystic areas develop in the subchondral bone, and ultimately this area collapses. At this stage

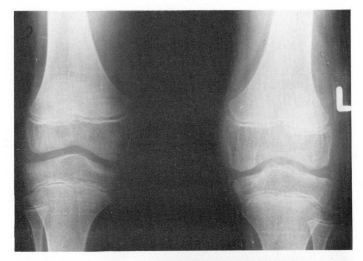

FIG. 15-2. The lower femoral and upper tibial epiphyses of the hemophilic left knee are larger than those of the normal knee because of chronic hyperemia.

gross joint disorganization is established and is associated with synovial and capsular contraction. Clinically the joint will be stiff and probably painful.

RADIOGRAPHIC APPEARANCES

Thickening of the synovium is often apparent on X-ray (Fig. 15-1). This is probably due to the deposition of hemosiderin in the synovial and capsular tissues.[8] In children, relative enlargement of the growing epiphyses of the affected knee joint is common (Fig. 15-2). This is almost certainly no more than a sign of chronic synovitis creating local hyperemia.[4]

Loss of joint space indicating damage to and disappearance of articular cartilage is associated with marked juxta-articular bone atrophy which frequently presents a lattice-like pattern. With further articular destruction, sclerosis of the articular margins occurs and subchondral cyst formation becomes apparent (Fig. 15-3). Large cysts are occasionally seen but are usually marginal and are the result of subperiosteal bleeding which may produce the pseudotumor typical of hemophilia (Fig. 15-4). Subchondral fractures ultimately lead to an appearance of gross joint destruction (Fig. 15-5).

A radiographic sign specific to the knee is deepening of the intercondylar notch (Fig. 15-3). This is seen quite early in the disease process and is said to be due to direct ero-

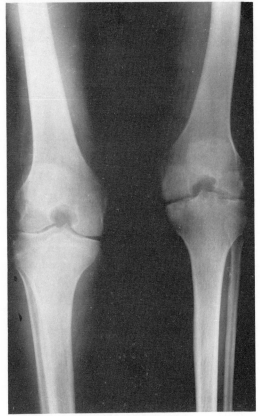

FIG. 15-3. Loss of joint space and, therefore, of articular cartilage is apparent in both knees. Subchondral cyst formation has occurred in the left knee (*at right*). Deepening of the intercondylar notch is present bilaterally. This is due only in part to erosion of the intercondylar area, as fixed flexion contracture of the knee throws the femoral condyles into greater relief on the roentgenograph.

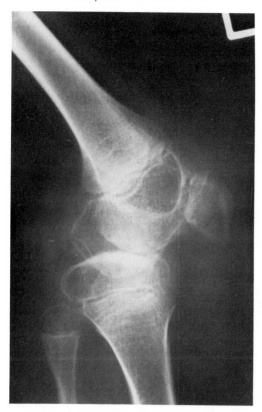

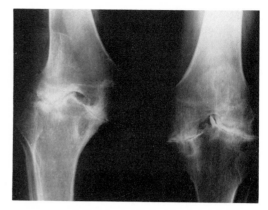

FIG. 15-5. Gross disorganization of both knees in an adult hemophiliac. Joint space is totally absent; exposed bone is eburnated and sclerotic, and some osteophyte formation suggests degenerative osteoarthritis. The deepened intercondylar notch on the left establishes the cause as hemophilia. The degree of joint disruption is illustrated by the gross subluxation of the right knee.

FIG. 15-4. Large marginal cysts are present in both femoral and tibial condyles. These probably commenced as subperiosteal hematomata and are an early stage of hemophilic "pseudotumor." This knee was painful and fixed in flexion. Arthrodesis was performed (see Fig. 15-13).

sion of the intercondylar area by hemophilic synovium.[12] Whilst this is undoubtedly true, the appearance is partly projectional because there is some degree of fixed flexion contracture in the acutely affected knee. Flexion of the femur throws the femoral condyles into greater relief and so presents the appearance of deepening of the intercondylar notch.

CLINICAL ASPECTS

Spontaneous and posttraumatic hemorrhages occur predominantly in the knee joints. The elbow, also exposed to minor trauma, is frequently affected. Other weight-bearing joints are much less commonly involved. The hip joint is well protected and torsional strains appear to be transmitted directly to the knee joint, thus often sparing the ankle.

Diagnosis

Hemarthroses of the otherwise normal knee is immediately apparent. Pain in the acute fresh bleed may be severe, and swelling is obvious. An inability to fully extend the knee is usual from the outset. However, the diagnosis of further hemorrhage in a knee that is already thickened by synovial induration and mild chronic effusion is less obvious. Pain is not always a marked feature. Furthermore, swelling may be the result of an irritative effusion rather than actual hemarthrosis, a diagnosis suggested by the rapid response of knee swelling to simple measures such as immobilization without the use of replacement therapy.

A fresh hemarthrosis in the severely disorganized knee where capsular contractions feature is usually tense and painful. Movement previously present is invariably lost.

TREATMENT PRINCIPLES

The hemophilic patient and his parents soon learn to recognize hemarthroses that require active management. It is probable that many minor bleeds are never seen by the doctor, recovery being complete after 2 or 3 days of rest. It should be stressed, however, that where swelling is accompanied by limitation of movement of the knee or pain the patient should be brought for treatment. If recurrent bleeds are neglected, rapid joint destruction will be the inevitable outcome.

Principles of management are twofold: the prevention of further hemorrhage by replacement of the deficient factor, and local treatment of the affected knee joint. Some centers withhold administration of the deficient blood factor unless conservative orthopedic techniques fail. It is our policy to institute replacement therapy whenever the patient presents at hospital, as this probably provides the best insurance against ultimate joint destruction.

REPLACEMENT OF DEFICIENT CLOTTING FACTOR

Factor VIII or IX is administered to the patient by means of an intravenous infusion of fresh plasma (FP), fresh frozen plasma (FFP) or plasma concentrates rich in the deficient factors. The administration of plasma stored at ordinary refrigerator temperatures is useless because Factor VIII in particular degrades rapidly under these conditions. The administration of fresh plasma is not always practicable, so a technique of rapidly freezing fresh plasma to −30° C soon after collection has been developed (FFP). The concentration of missing factors remains satisfactory if the FFP is administered soon after reconstitution.

In order to raise the deficient factor to 10 or 20 per cent of the normal circulating volume, it is necessary to administer 10 to 15 ml./kg. of FFP over 45 to 60 minutes.[16] However, the half-life of Factor VIII is only 12 hours so that a plasma level of 20 per cent of the normal will drop to 5 per cent some 24 hours later. It becomes obvious that during surgery, where a level of 30 per cent is necessary, so much plasma would

have to be administered that the circulation would become overloaded and the kidneys embarrassed by an excess of circulating protein. Furthermore, anemia may follow significant dilution of the red cells. Because of this methods have been sought to concentrate the antihemophilic globulin (AHG). It is possible to precipitate out the deficient factor using alcohol or ether but AHG produced in this manner is in short supply and very expensive. Animal precipitates of bovine or porcine origin are available and have the advantage of being 15 times as rich as human AHG. Unhappily these animal globulins are highly antigenic, often causing thrombocytopenia and rapid patient resistance. Their administration should be reserved for life-saving procedures.

A recent advance in replacement factor administration has been the development of cryoprecipitate. When FFP is reconstituted from −30° to +4° C, an undissolved portion remains behind. It was discovered that this "cryoprecipitate" is rich in Factor VIII and fibrinogen. Fortunately it is easy to extract and produce commercially and relatively inexpensive. Furthermore, being a concentrate, it may be given in sufficient doses during surgery to maintain the required level of the circulating Factor VIII. The dose of cryoprecipitate depends upon the concentration of the particular preparation. As there is considerable variation between the products of different blood transfusion services, blood level assays should be used as a guide.

A similar method for the extraction of Factor IX from the remnant of reconstituted FFP has recently become available.

ORTHOPEDIC MANAGEMENT OF ACUTE HEMARTHROSIS

Immediate accurate assessment of the degree of hemarthrosis is necessary in order to establish a baseline. The knee joint lends itself to exact monitoring.

The circumference of the joint at the point of maximum swelling is measured with

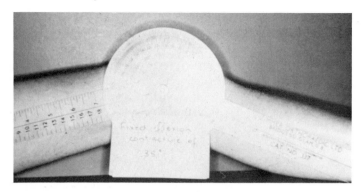

FIG. 15-6. A goniometer, used so that its axis exactly coincides with the joint line, accurately measures flexion contracture and range of movement, and records progress of the affected knee.

an ordinary tape measure and recorded on a chart. The opposite knee is used as a control, care being taken that the measurement is made with both knees at exactly the same degree of flexion.

The range of movement of the affected knee is also measured, charted and compared to the opposite knee. A goniometer is essential but must be used with care so that readings are taken with the axis of the measuring device coinciding exactly with the joint line. The standard international method of joint range measurement is followed whereby full extension of the knee is equivalent to 0°. Fixed flexion contracture is thus accurately reflected by a record of the reading. For example, a range of 35° to 100° represents a fixed flexion contracture of 35° and an actual range of movement of 65° (Fig. 15-6).

Bed rest and immobilization of the affected knee joint are essential. The Robert Jones type of pressure bandage, using two layers of wool and crepe bandages applied from the ankle to the groin, provides comfort and a degree of even compression (see Fig. 11-1). Immobilization may be assisted by incorporating four thin wooden slats situated anteriorly, posteriorly, medially, and laterally, deep to the last turn of bandage. This form of splintage allows easy removal for daily inspection and assessment of the knee joint. Furthermore, daily reapplication ensures that the compression and immobilization remain satisfactory. A well-padded plaster of paris back-slab serves a similar purpose, but our experience is that the knee tends to

flex out of the back-slab unless bandaging is made uncomfortably firm. On that account, the reinforced Robert Jones bandage is preferred.

It is essential to commence muscle rehabilitation immediately. Once the knee is held extended, a large hemarthrosis is no contraindication to static quadriceps contractions. Irritation of knee joint synovium produces reflex quadriceps inhibition, loss of protective tone, and early diminution of muscle bulk (Fig. 15-7). An immediate and energetic physiotherapeutic regime is essential to speed rehabilitation and provide joint protection.

The Role of Knee Joint Aspiration

The combination of immobilization, deficient factor replacement, and graded exercises produces rapid absorption of the hemarthrosis and speedy recovery in most instances. Some residual effusion is not uncommon and is acceptable as long as range of motion is unimpaired, pain absent and the effusion steadily diminishing. Our experience is that joint aspiration is rarely indicated and accords with the work in Oxford of Crock and Boni.[6] Aspiration should be considered when the hematoma remains very tense in spite of adequate conservative management, or where the size of the knee joint, although not tense, remains static for 10 days or more. Where regular measurement indicates that the knee joint is actually increasing in size in spite of proper treatment, aspiration must be performed.

Joint aspiration is regarded as a formal

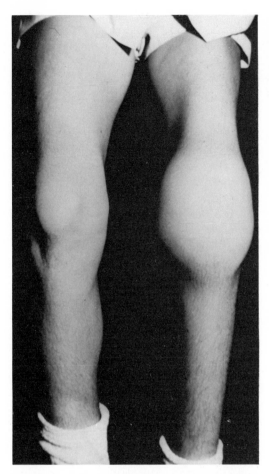

FIG. 15-7. Wasting of the quadriceps muscles is clearly shown in this patient with an acute hemarthrosis of the left knee.

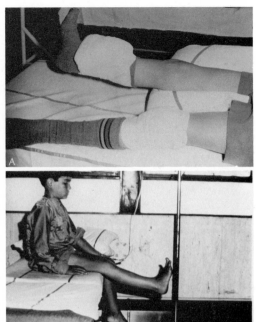

FIG. 15-8. A sandbag strapped to the patient's right leg provides resistance for isotonic exercises of the quadriceps. A small range of knee movement is obtained by elevating the thigh on a cushion (A). After recovery of the hemarthrosis, isometric quadriceps exercises are conveniently performed during a period when the patient is visiting the out-patient department for regular prophylactic plasma infusion (B).

surgical procedure and is always carried out in an operating theatre under full aseptic conditions. It is our policy to administer an infusion of FFP or cryoprecipitate just after the aspiration. Large doses of the deficient factor given prior to aspiration may lead to intraarticular clotting, making the joint difficult to aspirate.[10]

Rehabilitation

When daily joint measurements establish that the hemarthrosis is resolving, knee movement is encouraged under physiotherapeutic supervision. Isotonic exercises of both quadriceps and hamstring muscles against light resistance are now commenced (Fig. 15-8). When good muscle control has

returned, weightbearing is permitted, but only with immobilization and support. A Robert Jones bandage or light plaster back-slab is suitable, and crutches are used in the first instance.

The patient who has had recurrent bleeds needs a more protracted form of support. A long-leg caliper with a lace-up top provides a comfortable and permanent form of protection when walking. Until the knee is completely quiescent, it is advisable for these patients to use the caliper throughout the working day, or during the potentially traumatic school hours for the younger boy.

Prophylaxis for Spontaneous Hemarthroses

Patients with very low amounts of circulating antihemophilic globulin may develop

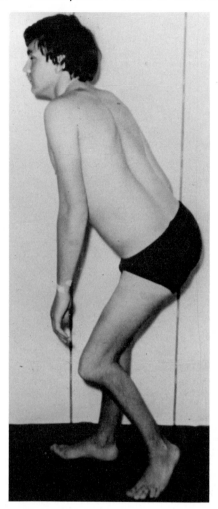

FIG. 15-9. Fixed flexion contracture of the left knee has produced a short-leg limp. The hip on that side is held flexed and the foot is in equinus. Contractions in these otherwise normal joints will ultimately develop.

spontaneous bleeds so frequently that they are almost totally incapacitated and are in danger of sustaining early joint destruction. Under these circumstances a weekly or even twice-weekly infusion of plasma prophylactically may be well worthwhile. There is considerable evidence to show that regular replacement of the deficient factor greatly lessens the number of spontaneous hemorrhages, particularly into the knee joint.[10] These infusions can be conveniently given during physiotherapy sessions which play an important part in their own right in preventing recurrent knee hemarthroses.

The Treatment of Knee Deformity

Fixed flexion contracture is the most obvious and disabling sequal to recurrent hemarthroses of the knee. Apart from pain and cosmetic deformity, the relative shortening that is produced by the flexion contracture affects both the ankle and hip joints. The foot may be held in equinus and a short-leg limp develops (Fig. 15-9).

Prevention of joint damage and capsular contraction is the fundamental aim of treatment. This depends upon early and energetic management of the acute hemarthrosis, proper physiotherapy, and the use of prophylactic FFP or cryoprecipitate when hemarthroses are multiple and recurrent.

When joint damage makes stiffness inevitable, treatment is directed at keeping the knee as straight as possible and thus in a position of function. Unfortunately many patients are referred with established knee flexion contractures. Fixity at an angle of 90° or more is not uncommon. The management depends on the patient's age and the degree of joint destruction. In children, especially where articular cartilage is present, every effort should be made to obtain correction by simple nonoperative means.

Gentle skin traction with the limb held on a padded Thomas splint can be used successfully but has definite disadvantages. The treatment necessitates hospitalization or at best a prolonged period of immobilization in bed and keeps the patient away from school or work. This consideration in the hemophiliac is of paramount importance, for half of the patient's working week may in any event be lost because of recurrent hemarthroses.[3] Furthermore, relative shortening of the collateral ligaments of the knee occurs with a severe fixed flexion contracture. These prevent the tibia from sliding forward along the femoral condyles as extension is produced by simple traction. Straightening of the limb is then accompanied by posterior subluxation of the tibia on the femur (Fig.

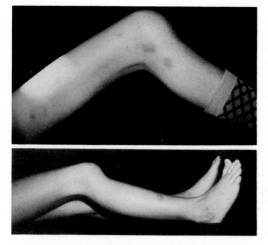

Fig. 15-10. Marked back-setting of the right tibia. A 90-degree fixed flexion contracture was corrected by a combination of traction on a Thomas splint and a hinged turnbuckle plaster cast.

15-10). (Compare The Rheumatoid Knee, Chap. 14.)

For these reasons, a special technique using serial long-leg plaster of paris casts changed weekly or fortnightly is preferred. Ordinary wedging of plaster casts or the use of a hinge and turnbuckle is not recommended, for both these methods aggravate back-setting of the tibia. Conner, studying poliomyelitis patients with fixed knee flexion contractures where a similar problem of tightness of the collateral ligaments exists, has suggested a method of overcoming the problem.[5] At each new plaster cast application, the upper tibial shaft is deliberately pulled anteriorly on the femur as gradual extension of the leg is achieved. Our experience in the hemophiliac patient has shown that this technique is applicable and is the method of choice for the management of the young patient with fixed flexion contracture of the knee. Nevertheless a degree of back-knee may be unavoidable but is of little consequence if the joint is painless, extends fully, and flexes satisfactorily (Fig. 15-11).

If carried out gently, serial plaster correction rarely requires the use of deficiency factor replacement. As correction is achieved, active mobilization must be com-

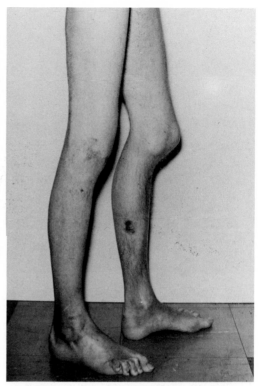

Fig. 15-11. Back-setting of the left knee does not incapacitate this young man because extension is almost full and he has a pain-free range of flexion to 90 degrees. Arthrodesis has been performed on the right knee (see Fig. 15-12).

menced and quadriceps drill emphasized. Furthermore, the correction achieved must be held by the use of a lightweight splint at night and a walking caliper during the day. As the quadriceps muscles build up, the caliper may be abandoned, but a night splint should be used until the knee is really mobile, extension virtually full, and easily maintained by quadriceps power.

Treatment of the Severely Disorganized Knee

As joint destruction progresses, both pain and stiffness usually increase. Fortunately a short, firm fibrous ankylosis is often the eventual outcome. If the knee is nearly straight and functionally satisfactory for walking, little if any treatment is required. The painful knee, on the other hand, pre-

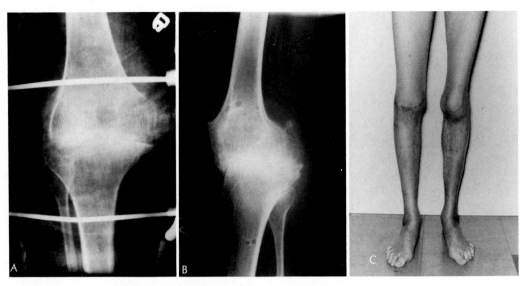

FIG. 15-12. Minimal excision of bone and the use of Charnley compression clamps (*A*) has produced sound arthrodesis in good position (*B*, *C*).

sents a serious problem because the use of analgesics such as salicylates or anti-inflammatory agents is dangerous. These may irritate the gastric mucosa or interfere with platelet function and precipitate gastro-intestinal hemorrhages.

When deformity is marked and a caliper fails to control pain, operative treatment is required. However, surgery must be under-taken in a center where adequate replace-ment factor is freely available. Any opera-tive procedure requires full liaison between the hematologist, orthopedic surgeon and physiotherapist. An AHG level of 30 per cent must be achieved and maintained dur-ing the operative procedure, and there is evidence to show that a circulating level of 5 per cent or more should be maintained until the ninth postoperative day.[13] Early muscle rehabilitation is mandatory.

The operative choice is limited. Correc-tive osteotomies for fixed flexion deformity produce unsatisfactory results because further flexion contractures after surgery often occur. Osteotomy should be used only to correct varus or valgus knee deformity in a patient with a good range of painless knee movement.

In the adult, severe pain and deformity of the knee are indications for arthrodesis. A standard technique of knee fusion using Charnley compression clamps has given gratifying results (Figs. 15-11, 15-12). In selected instances, fusion may become nec-essary in the younger patient before growth has ceased (Fig. 15-4). This can be carried out without interfering with epiphyseal bone growth by paring down articular surfaces until the underlying ossific nuclei are ex-posed. Good apposition of these bone sur-faces is achieved if the knee is held straight against the fulcrum of a tight posterior capsule. Correction of the flexion contrac-ture is in fact achieved by performing an anterior wedge resection of the knee joint. Excision of the patella is not necessary (Fig. 15-13).

Arthrodesis is performed only when a severely damaged knee joint does not re-spond to nonoperative methods. A useful range of movement often exists in spite of quite severe joint destruction and consider-able pain. In this situation, the ability to flex the knee should be preserved wherever possible, especially when extension is ade-quate. The use of the simple block-leather or plastic gaiter during the day can keep the patient comfortable at work, allow pain-free weightbearing, and still provide flexion for sitting during the leisure hours of the evening (Fig. 15-14).

MUSCLE HEMATOMATA

Knee joint deformity is not infrequently of extraarticular origin. Damage to adjoining musculature leads to replacement by fibrous tissue which slowly contracts and produces permanent shortening of overall muscle length. The calf, particularly the triceps surae muscle group, is frequently damaged by deep-seated hemorrhages (Fig. 15-15).

In the hemophiliac, a hematoma under tension within a fascial compartment may occasionally lead to occlusion of arterial inflow, producing a true muscle infarct of the Volkmann's type with subsequent muscle necrosis and contracture. This pattern is usually seen in the forearm group where damage to nerves aggravates the peripheral deformity. In our experience, a less well recognized but nevertheless severe form of muscle necrosis occurs in hemophiliacs, especially in the calf muscles. This follows a slow insidious hemorrhage deep to the fascia of a group of muscles or within an individual muscle compartment. Arterial occlusion does not occur so that the peripheral pulse is not occluded and the doctor is wooed into a sense of false security. Tension nevertheless gradually builds up within the closed compartment, and capillary blood flow becomes obstructed. Patchy necrosis of muscle fibers is produced; round cell infiltration follows; and ultimately irregular fibrous tissue replacement completes the process (Fig. 15-16). Without adequate stretching and the use of splints, this fibrous tissue steadily contracts over a period of months and if left untreated, serious shortening of the affected muscles will follow. When the gastrocnemii are affected, flexion contracture of the knee as well as equinus deformity of the foot will be the outcome (Fig. 15-17). These contractures soon become very fixed and resistant to nonoperative correction.

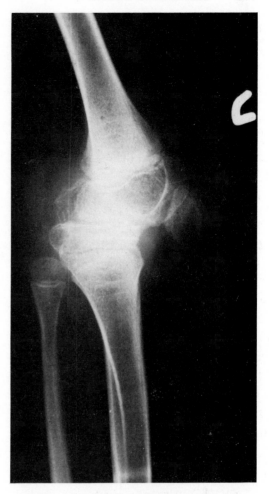

Fig. 15-13. Bony fusion has been obtained without disturbing the growing epiphyses in this 12-year-old boy's knee which was previously fixed in considerable flexion and very painful (see Fig. 15-4). Satisfactory extension of the knee has been achieved by removing more bone from the ossific nuclei anteriorly than posteriorly, straightening the knee against the contracted posterior capsule and collateral ligaments, and holding the limb for 10 weeks in a plaster cast.

The clinical importance of this insidious form of relatively painless hemorrhage cannot be overemphasized. Bleeds into the calf or other large muscle groups must be watched even more closely than the more obvious hemarthroses. During the early phase of muscle bleeds pain is a feature and should never be ignored. Later, as nerve

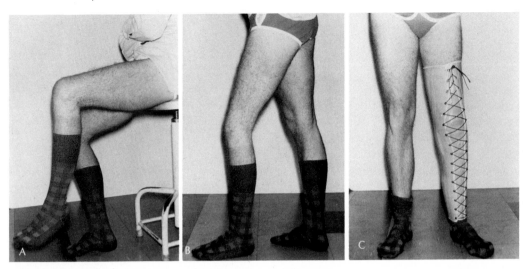

FIG. 15-14. The left knee of this 26-year-old hemophiliac patient moves through a useful but very painful range (*A, B*). A block-leather gaiter (*C*), worn only at work, provides complete relief from pain. At home, he sits with the knee comfortably flexed.

fibers become ischemic, tension may increase with little discomfort. Bleeding into calf musculature warrants hospital admission, immediate immobilization of the knee and foot in a position of function, infusion of large doses of antihemophilic concentrates

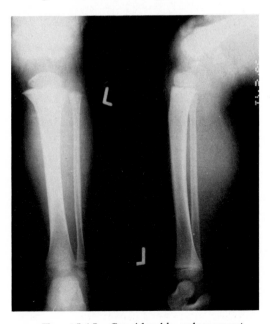

FIG. 15-15. Considerable enlargement of the calf shadow is shown by a radiograph of this 7-year-old boy's left leg. The cause is a large hematoma within muscle.

and very close observation. Circumferential measurements over the point of maximum swelling should be made at least twice and preferably three times a day, and unless this reduces rapidly and pain subsides with the administration of the deficient bleeding factor, full surgical decompression must be undertaken forthwith. This is a formal surgical procedure carried out under proper factor replacement cover. The hemotoma is completely evacuated, and tense, ischemic muscles are fully decompressed. Fascia is easily split without extensive skin incisions by engaging its edge in the slightly open tips of blunt-nosed scissors. These are then slid proximally and distally under skin, splitting the fascia as they advance. Closure of the wound over sealed suction drainage is favored. Although blood loss may be considerable through the drainage system, the surgeon may rest content that further pressure and ischemia to muscles will be obviated, and the medical team can easily assess the blood loss for replacement purposes.

Postoperative splinting in the position of function is imperative, and even when some muscle necrosis has occurred, flexion contracture of the knee and ankle can be obviated and normal function retained.

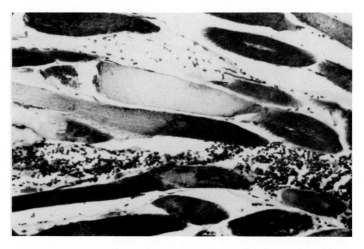

FIG. 15-16. Patchy areas of muscle fiber death and marked round cell infiltration are illustrated in this biopsy of gastrocnemius muscle obtained during decompression of a deep hemorrhage.

GENERAL CONSIDERATIONS

The regime outlined for the management of the hemophilic knee calls for an interdisciplinary team approach. The hematologist, pediatrician, orthopedic surgeon and physiotherapist all have important roles to play. Furthermore, access to a sophisticated blood transfusion service where FFP and cryoprecipitate can be manufactured is essential.

The general environment of the hemophiliac is very important. The disease lasts a lifetime, and sufferers can expect to lose a great deal of time from school or work because of recurrent episodes of bleeding, particularly into the knee joint. The possibility of progressive and permanent crippling is ever present. Besides the medical aspects, the social and economic implications of the management of hemophilia are taken into consideration. Treatment in the young patient must be aimed at ensuring that he grows into adulthood, not only without crippling deformity but also fully educated, so that he may find a useful and satisfying place in society within the limits imposed by the condition. Early diagnosis and full control before deformity occurs is thus essential. The medical team must seek collaboration with parents, teachers, and social workers so that treatment will disturb schooling as little as possible.

Unless there is a family history, hemophilia will not be suspected and rarely

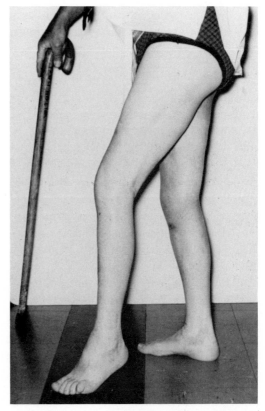

FIG. 15-17. Repeated muscle hematomata have left this patient's left calf thin and contracted. He has a fixed equinus deformity of the ankle and some flexion contracture of the knee although both joints are virtually normal.

declares itself before the age of 6 months when prolonged bleeding from cuts about the mouth or superficial hematomata suggest that something is amiss. The diagnosis can be established only by special assay techniques and when necessary, the cooperation of a hemophilia center should be sought. Once the diagnosis is established, the patient is issued a card stating that he is a hemophiliac and giving essentials such as his address, telephone number, name and address of general practitioner, blood group and deficient factor level. Any allergy—in particular to drugs—should also be noted. Some patients develop antibodies to the deficient factor and if present, this should be stated on the card. The implications of hemophilia must be made clear to the parents and to the patient when he is old enough. Their cooperation is essential, and knowledge will enable them to anticipate future problems. The criteria that demand hospital management when a joint or muscle bleed occurs should be listed in an easily understood manner.

Proper schooling arrangements are essential. In the United Kingdom, more than half a boy's educational time may be lost because of recurrent hemorrhages.[3] Although a few severely crippled children do better at schools for the physically handicapped, the average hemophiliac need not attend a special school if arrangements can be made so that he avoids periods of bustle and potential trauma.

The knee is particularly susceptible to sporting trauma, and advice about games is essential. Whilst body contact sports should be avoided, it is essential to maintain muscle tone, and certain sports should be encouraged. Usually the boy soon discovers what he may and may not do and will impose his own restrictions. Exercises such as swimming and usually cycling and running can be encouraged, and some gymnastic activities may cause no harm. A powerful quadriceps femoris muscle is the best protection against knee hemarthrosis.

THE FUTURE

A swollen, painful knee is the most disabling and time-consuming lesion in the hemophiliac. Chronic bleeds produce a thickened fleshy synovium. Effusions and further hemarthroses follow, and a vicious cycle develops.

For this reason, synovectomy has been performed for the chronically swollen hemophilic knee. Support for this enterprising concept has come from the work of Mitchell and Cruess,[11] who showed that replacement synovium contains fewer blood vessels than the synovium previously excised and is less likely to bleed. Clinical experience of synovectomy in the hemophilic patient is still small but encouraging. Pietrogrande and his coworkers[13] found that bleeding was less voluminous and severe in 23 synovectomized joints followed up for an average of 15 months. Their approach to synovectomy was cautious. Although most patients were considerably improved, the synovectomized joint did not always return to its previous range of movement. They note, however, that Storti and Askari, reporting at the 1972 International Hemophilia Meeting in Rome, reassessed 47 patients followed up for an average of 6 years after synovectomy. No further bleeds had occurred in 76 per cent of treated joints, and in the remainder, bleeds were moderate and required no substitution therapy. Joint range was usually good. Three or more bleeds in the same joint within a period of 6 months were regarded as a definite indication for the operation.

Surgical synovectomy is a major undertaking that taxes the resources of the hemophilic center. Medical synovectomy may well hold out more hope for the future than the operative approach. Encouraging work has been done on the use of radioactive gold by Ahlberg[1] and on intraarticular osmic acid by Risse and his coworkers.[15] These techniques may well provide simple treatment for the knee joint prone to recurrent hemorrhages and effusions.

At the present time, the control of hemophilia is sufficiently sophisticated for the surgeon to undertake virtually any form of orthopedic surgery indicated. Whilst arthrodesis provides the safest and most certain method of treating the grossly disorganized and painful knee joint, it is not only feasible but may well be preferable to consider total joint replacement arthroplasty, particularly when the other knee is stiff (see Chap. 20). Should the apparatus fail, arthrodesis may be easily performed.[9]

CONCLUSION

Early recognition and an energetic interdisciplinary approach to the hemophilic patient can, to a large extent, prevent knee joint destruction and deformity. When significant damage has already occurred, deficient factor replacement has enabled the surgeon to proceed confidently with the surgical procedure necessary to rehabilitate his patient.

REFERENCES

1. Ahlberg, A.: Radioactive gold in treatment of chronic synovial effusion in haemophilia. *In* Ala, F., and Denson, K. W. E. (eds.): Haemophilia. Excerpta Medica Foundation, 1973.
2. Bernstein, M. A.: The treatment of joint lesions in haemophilia by means of whole blood from menstruating women. J. Bone Joint Surg., *14*:659, 1932.
3. Britten, M. I., Spooner, R. J. D., Dormandy, K. M., and Biggs, R.: The haemophiliac boy in school. Brit. Med. J., *2*:224, 1966.
4. Boldero, J. L., and Kemp, H. S.: The early bone and joint changes in haemophilia and similar blood dyscrasias. Brit. J. Radiol., *39*:172, 1966.
5. Conner, A. N.: Treatment of flexion contracture of the knee in poliomyelitis. J. Bone Joint Surg., *52-B*:138, 1970.
6. Crock, H. V., and Boni, V.: The management of orthopaedic problems in the haemophiliac. A review of 21 cases. Brit. J. Surg., *48*:8, 1960.
7. Curtiss, P. H., Jr.: Changes produced in synovial membrane and synovial fluid by disease. J. Bone Joint Surg., *46-A*:873, 1964.
8. DePalma, A. F., and Cottler, J. N.: Arthropathy in the hemophiliac patient. J. Bone Joint Surg., *37-A*:1124, 1955.
9. Freeman, M. A. R., and Swanson, S. A. V.: Total prosthetic replacement of the knee. J. Bone Joint Surg., *54-B*:170, 1972.
10. Lurie, A., and Bailey, B. P.: The management of acute haemophiliac haemarthroses and muscle haematoma. South African Med. J., *46*:656, 1972.
11. Mitchell, N. S., and Cruess, R. L.: The effect of synovectomy on articular cartilage. J. Bone Joint Surg., *49-A*:1099, 1967.
12. Murray, R. O.: Personal communication, 1972.
13. Pietrograne, V., Dioguardi, N., and Mannucci, P. M.: Short-term evaluation of synovectomy in haemophilia. Brit. Med. J., *2*:378, 1972.
14. Pohle, F. J., and Taylor, F. H. L.: The coagulation defect in hemophilia. The effect in hemophilia of intramuscular administration of a globulin substance derived from normal plasma. J. Clin. Invest., *16*:741, 1937.
15. Risse, J. C., Menkes, C. H., Allain, J. P., and Witvoet, J.: Synoviorthesis in the treatment of chronic haemophilic arthropathy: a preliminary report. *In* Ala, F., and Denson, K. W. E. (eds.): Haemophilia. Excerpta Medica Foundation, 1973.
16. Rizza, C. R.: The management of haemophilia. Practitioner, *204*:763, 1970.
17. Rodman, G. P.: Experimental hemarthrosis: The removal of chromium-51 and iron-59 labelled erythrocytes injected into the knee joint of rabbit and man. Arthritis Rheum., *3*:195, 1962.
18. van Creveld, S., Hoedemaeker, P. J., Kingma, M. J., and Wagenvoort, C. A.: Degeneration of joints in haemophiliacs under treatment by modern methods. J. Bone Joint Surg., *53-B*:296, 1971.

16

Injuries of the
Capsular and Cruciate Ligaments

Arthur J. Helfet, M.D.

The key to successful treatment of injuries to the ligaments of the knee is accurate diagnosis. While sprains may be treated adequately by prompt and conscientious conservative means, ruptures of stabilizing ligaments invariably require surgical repair for recovery of perfect function.

H. O'Donoghue[11], who writes from an exceptionally wide experience of severe injuries of the knee joint, considers that function of the ligament depends not only on its strength but also on its length, since a ligament that is elongated does not carry out its function of preventing abnormal motion of the joint. In addition, we should maintain that *the function of the capsular ligaments* is not only to prevent abnormal movement but also to give adequate purchase to the muscles that control normal movement. The function of a cruciate ligament is that of a guide rope and not a checkstrap. The objects of treatment remain identical. Both the integrity and the length of the capsular ligaments must be restored or the function of the ligament must be replaced by static or dynamic tendon transplant.

CLINICAL FEATURES OF THE ACUTE STAGE

Ligaments are injured at their junctions with tissues of different elasticity. For the collateral ligaments these junctions are the insertions to the femur, the tibia and the meniscus on the medial side, and to the femur

and the head of the fibula on the lateral side (Fig. 16-1). Sometimes a flake of bone comes away with the ligament, or it may snap transversely, in which case the torn ends, though ragged, are well defined. At other times interstitial fibers are pulled longitudinally and rupture at different levels within the substance of the ligament, when it will appear intact though elongated.

The variations in types of tear are many. A 17-year-old high-jump champion "sprained" his left patellar ligament. It was rested by splinting for 3 weeks, after which he started training again. The first time he tried to jump, the knee gave way. At operation it was obvious that the "sprain" was a coronal rupture of the ligament with complete detachment of the upper end of the posterior half from the patella. The fresh injury had avulsed the lower end of the ligament and its expansion from the tibial tubercle and the front of the tibia. At operation the site of fresh injury is denoted by hemorrhage and ecchymosis. At the time of accident, the patient feels immediate acute pain which may subside in a few minutes—in which case the joint stiffens up and is painful again a few hours later when local swelling becomes evident. More usually, the knee remains painful, and movement and weight-bearing are difficult or intolerable. Synovial effusion always follows and is bloodstained; occasionally, a frank tense hemarthrosis develops, depending on the extent of damage to the synovium. The degree of pain and the rate of increase of effusion are proportional to the extent of the intraarticular bleeding. Severe bleeding causes severe pain.

The first distinction between sprain and rupture is in the severity of the pain. Sprains are always painful and remain so on attempted movement. After rupture of a ligament, acute pain subsides and non-weight-bearing movement, though weak and unstable, is relatively painless. Locally, the point of sprain is more tender and sensitive, though local swelling is grosser when the ligament has ruptured. This may be due to the dispersion of synovial effusion through the torn capsule which prevents the painful distention of the knee seen in closed injuries. After sprain the patient may be able to take weight, albeit very painfully, but after severe rupture of capsular ligaments the patient has a subjective fear regarding the stability of the knee and will not venture to put weight on it at all.

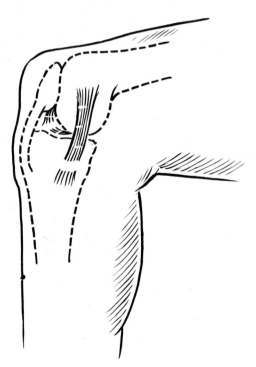

FIG. 16-1. Ligaments usually rupture at their bony attachments to the femur or the tibia.

To test lateral instability the leg must be almost straight. The word "almost" is used deliberately, for when the leg is forced into the extreme of extension and lateral rotation, even if both cruciate and medial collateral ligament are ruptured, instability cannot always be determined, i.e., in the so-called screwed home position, the knee is stable. Only after more extensive tears of the capsule can clinical instability be detected with the knee quite straight. The leg must be just off the straight when abduction and adduction strain are applied. Many knees in this position allow an impression of slight laxity, but there is no mistaking the "opening" of the side of the joint when the ligaments have ruptured. The palpating finger seems to slip between the femur and the tibia.

Doubt may arise when the capsule is strained or partially torn anterior or posterior to the ligament. In such a case attempted movement is painful, and abnormal abduction or adduction cannot be elicited with certainty. When any doubt exists, the knee should be examined under general or local anesthesia. For the latter, 10 to 15 ml. of 1 per cent procaine in saline is injected intraarticularly, and locally into the tender area.

Anteroposterior roentgenograms of the knee at the extremes of forced abduction or adduction confirm the abnormal separation of the femur and the tibia (Fig. 16-2). Arthrograms are useful in establishing the diagnosis. (See Fig. 16-3 and Chap. 9.)

ASSOCIATED LESIONS OF THE SEMILUNAR CARTILAGES

By careful examination it is often possible to diagnose an associated derangement of a meniscus—usually retraction of the anterior horn of the medial meniscus. In this case, external rotation of the knee is restricted, and protrusion of the medial condyle of the femur and other rotation signs are present. The torn anterior end of the meniscus is tender. The diagnosis is confirmed if during examination the cartilage reduces and the

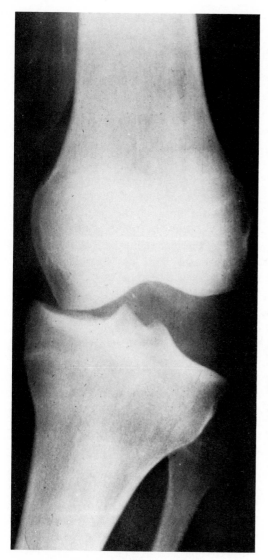

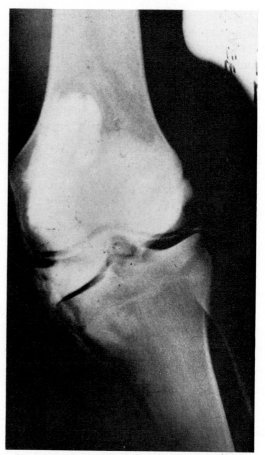

FIG. 16-3. The arthrogram shows that the medial capsule is ruptured. The medial meniscus has been separated from the tibia.

FIG. 16-2. Anteroposterior roentgenogram of the knee in forced adduction showing abnormal separation of femur and tibia. The lateral ligament has been wrenched off the head of the fibula with a flake of bone.

knee suddenly straightens completely. In such as case it is often possible to displace the meniscus again by straightening the knee while forcibly holding the tibia in internal rotation.

CHRONIC OR RECURRENT SPRAINS

Mild sprains may clear up completely even without treatment. Swelling and tenderness disappear and movement recovers. More severe sprains tend to leave a legacy of adhesions which manifest themselves by twinges or stabs of pain on certain movements. These stabs may be accompanied by a sensation of momentary weakness, that simulates the "giving way" or "buckling" experienced in internal derangement of the knee. Occasionally these attacks are followed by swelling and stiffness and local tenderness, and as the pain is felt in the same place, the history given by the patient suggests a torn meniscus. (Once the knee is examined, the differential diagnosis is easy, for extension is not limited and rotation is not blocked.) The patient feels the pain always in the same place on the same movement, and tenderness is localized to the ligamentous attachment.

Reference has already been made to the difficulty in diagnosing rotation sprains of the medial semilunar cartilage due to injury to the coronary ligaments (p. 128). This applies also to sprains of the attachments of the semilunar cartilage to the deep part of the medial collateral ligament.

RUPTURES OF THE COLLATERAL LIGAMENTS

As it has elastic components, ligament retracts after rupture or detachment from its insertion. The wrenched ends curl up and leave a gap. Rupture of a ligament is never an isolated lesion but is accompanied by damage of varying degree to adjacent capsular structures where similar changes occur. After complete rupture, therefore, it would seem unreasonable to expect the tissues to recover normal integrity and length merely by splinting the limb. The gap is crossed quickly enough by fibrous scar, but the structure as a whole is longer than previously, and the joint on that side remains lax.

The medial ligament and capsule are the important structures. The knee with a lax medial capsule is weak. The patient complains of weakness and of "giving way" under strain or from sudden rotary movements. These symptoms are more severe when the cruciate ligaments also have ruptured. The attacks may be accompanied by pain and followed by swelling. The diagnosis is usually simpler than in the acute stage, for pain, swelling, and guarding muscle spasm are mild.

Rupture of the lateral ligament causes little disability, unless associated with disruption of the iliotibial band and further capsular damage, and rupture of the cruciate, when a particularly unstable knee results.

INJURIES OF THE CRUCIATE LIGAMENTS

Sprains of the cruciate ligaments are difficult to interpret clinically, except perhaps when they have been stretched by the medial condyle of the femur in a knee locked for some length of time by a bowstring or anterior horn tear of the cartilage (Fig. 1-21, p. 16). In this case not only the cruciate but also the capsule is stretched, for laxity of the joint as a whole develops.

However, either cruciate may repture from its femoral or tibial attachment. The cruciate may take with it part of a tibial spine, and quite often the anterior ligament tear includes rupture of its attachments to the anterior horn of the medial meniscus, which retracts. In other words, the distracting force tears both the anterior cruciate and the medial meniscus from their attachments to each other and to the tibia.

If the medial capsular structures remain intact, the clinical picture is that of the retracted meniscus with typical rotation signs, restriction of movement and site of tenderness. The torn cruciate is discovered only at the operation. The knee is not unstable, and repair of the cruciate is not important, although if the injury is recent the ligament should be sutured firmly to its soft tissue insertions.

Combinations of cruciate and capsular damage give rise to major disabilities of the knee. They are, of course, usually the result of gross injuries caused by lateral hinging or subluxation or actual dislocation of the joint (see Chap. 16). If the knee is examined soon after the accident, diagnosis of the wrenched unstable knee is obvious. The patient is in shock and in great pain. Swelling is rapid. Once the leg is splinted pain may subside quickly.

Injuries of this type are always associated with tears of the synovium, often with displacements of semilunar cartilage, occasionally with tibial plateau fractures, and rarely with injuries to nerves. If the popliteal vessels are damaged, the vascular problem is predominant and demands immediate assessment and treatment. However, it is not intended to bring the management of injuries to blood vessels within the compass of this monograph.

Broadly speaking, widespread damage treated conservatively results in either a stiff or an unstable knee. The patient presents for treatment months later with a knee that "gives way" or is restricted in movement or which suffers from both defects. Dense adhesions limit movement and cause pain if movement is forced. After undue strain the knee tends to swell and ache. Musculature is poor and difficult to improve.

With lesser damage, instability is the disabling symptom, though extremes of movement also may be restricted.

The patient complains that the knee gives way chiefly on slopes and stairs. It seems that the tibia does not remain on the helicoid track on the medial condyle of the femur but slides straight forward. The incidents are painful and may be followed by swelling, with muscle spasm and pain. On the other hand, for a while at a later stage the derangements may become relatively nonpainful, and the patient is able to carry on straight away.

With the patient either sitting or lying down with muscles relaxed, these abnormal movements may be elicited passively. The classic test is the demonstration of "anteroposterior glide." With the knee flexed, it is possible to slide the tibia forward and backward on the femur (Fig. 16-4). Sometimes the patient while sitting with knee flexed can actively subluxate and reduce the tibia on the femur. However, it should be appreciated that if the leg is extended fully with full outward rotation of the tibia, the knee is locked, and anteroposterior glide can no longer be demonstrated.

The patient may simulate this action in order to stabilize the knee when walking. The foot is fixed on the ground in external rotation and, as the leg straightens, the femur is internally rotated on the tibia (see Fig. 6-34).

The articular cartilage of the unstable knee deteriorates after repeated derangements, and traumatic arthritis inevitably develops in untreated knees.

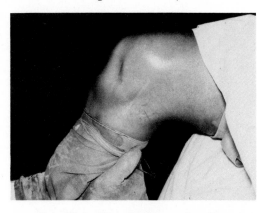

FIG. 16-4. The classic test for disruption of the cruciate ligaments is the demonstration of anteroposterior glide. With the knee flexed it is possible to slide the tibia forward and backward on the femur.

TREATMENT OF LIGAMENTOUS INJURIES

ACUTE SPRAINS

If acute sprains are untreated traumatic exudate tends to organize by depositing fibrin which is replaced by fibroblasts and then by fibrous tissue. These links of fibrous tissue, or adhesions, between components of varying elasticity lead to the troubles and the discomforts of chronic sprains. Therefore, treatment for the fresh injury should aim to relieve pain and to promote the absorption of exudate to prevent this organization of fibrous tissue. In the early stages pain is relieved fairly quickly by rest obtained through a compression bandage and, depending on the severity, bed or splinting. Hot and cold compresses or local heat and light massage promote the rapid absorption of exudate, chiefly by stimulating local circulation. Deep massage is traumatic and at this stage aggravates the condition. The best agent of all is static muscle drill. The muscle is contracted fully, held in contraction for a second, and then relaxed. This is repeated 12 times at intervals of 1 hour. Exercise against gravity and against resistance follows. Faradization is of value, as an educational aid only, when the patient finds difficulty in actively contracting the thigh muscles.

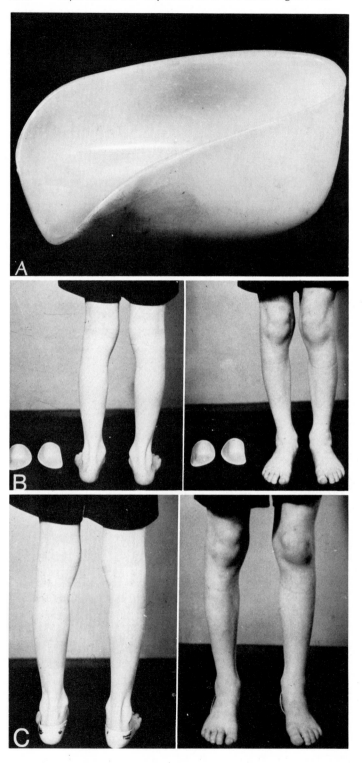

FIG. 16-5. (*A*) The heel seat molded of plastic. (*B*) The everted feet. (*C*) Complete correction in the heelseats. (From Myron Medical Products Ltd. Maidenhead, Berks, England)

Some 30 years ago, LeRiche advocated the treatment of sprains by the immediate local injection of procaine. He contended that the traumatic exudate contains metabolites that irritate the local sensory nerve endings; this initiates a reflex that causes further exudation of metabolites. A vicious circle is established and the process is prolonged. The procaine breaks the reflex by anesthetizing the nerve endings, and the swelling resolves. The patient is allowed to bear weight immediately. Whether LeRiche's theory is right or not, the local injection of procaine in saline undoubtedly does relieve pain and accelerates recovery. After the injection a crepe or a compression bandage is applied. If the injury is mild, the patient is allowed to walk with full weight-bearing; if the sprain is severe, on crutches. Tilting the medial side of the heel of the shoe on the injured side, or a heelseat inside the shoe, is an aid to comfort and recovery, for it takes stress off the medial ligament. The heelseat is a device that holds the os calcis vertically. In this way, by preventing the heel's rolling over into eversion, it controls the arch.[6] The shape and the agility of the foot are preserved, and the heelseat is effective in correcting flatfoot, in relieving foot strain, and incidentally, therefore, in preventing strain on the medial side of the knee (Fig. 16-5).

CHRONIC AND RECURRING STRAINS

Once the symptoms and signs of chronic strain are established, the condition is treated by manipulation under either local or general anesthesia. By this time tenderness is localized and the movements that cause pain are known. Manipulation under local anesthesia is more effective than that under general anesthesia when muscle strains are involved, e.g., the insertion of quadriceps to the patella. It is also effective for minor strains. A solution of procaine is injected into the tender area. As soon as the anesthetic is effective, the patient performs the previously painful movements against resistance. If flexion is painful, sitting on the haunches would rupture the adhesions, etc. For capsular and more extensive adhesions, manipulation under Pentothal anesthesia is advisable and effective.

Wasting of the thigh muscles and chronic or recurrent synovitis associated with chronic strain of the knee are treated by a regular and conscientious program of static and active exercises. There is no doubt that recovery of normal muscle power is the prime requisite in the restoration of stable function of the knee and its ability to withstand the demands of sustained effort.

RUPTURES OF CAPSULAR AND CRUCIATE LIGAMENTS

These have been grouped under one heading, since injury is rarely confined to one ligament. Moreover, the broad principles of treatment are the same for all.

The objects of treatment are recovery of function with full active movement, the most important being full extension of the knee with outward rotation of the tibia.

It is essential when ligaments are sutured that the femur and the tibia should be in their correct rotational alignment. This rule applies equally to splinting during conservative treatment and after operation.

The author is convinced, as are other writers, that the *best results are obtained not by conservative treatment but by prompt and meticulous suture of ruptured ligaments.* Most patients who suffer disability later and require further treatment are those who have been treated by splinting without surgical repair.

One hears of isolated cases in which after complete rupture of the medial collateral ligament, the patient recovered a knee strong enough to stand up to the strain of violent games. These patients naturally do not seek further orthopedic opinion. However, many knees, after excellent conservative treatment with an initial 8 to 12 weeks of splinting, break down under strain. Indeed, although the author can report two patients who gained international rugby football caps and a number who play first class (major league) club football after suture of the medial ligament, he has not seen any patient stand up to the rigors of first class football after conservative treatment. O'Donoghue[11] and DePalma[2], in reviews of their experience, record similar conclusions.

There is no doubt, also, that the main bastions of stability in the knee are the medial ligament and the medial capsule. Rupture of the lateral ligament in itself is not markedly disabling. However, when associated with cruciate plus iliotibial band and capsular damage, a particularly unstable knee is produced. The muscles probably cannot compensate for capsular weakness while bearing weight without the stabilizing effect that the lateral ligament and the biceps exercise on the leg through the fibula.

When the anatomic disturbances produced by the injury are considered, one is more convinced of the desirability of operative reconstruction of the capsular structures of the joint. The torn fibers of the ligaments tend to retract and curl up, and moreover, flaps of ligament and synovium may turn in between the joint surfaces. After conservative treatment, the probabilities are that the extraarticular ligamentous tears will be replaced by scar or fibrous tissue and that the intraarticular fringes will be absorbed or replaced by intraarticular fibrous adhesions. The result is instability and/or restriction of movement–the common sequelae.

Conservative Treatment

Mild sprains are easily distinguished from complete ruptures of ligament. Difficulties arise when the signs of complete rupture are cloaked by partial rupture and sprain of the adjacent capsule. When doubt exists, the knee must be examined under anesthesia. If skin abrasion and infection preclude open operation, or if the age or the general condition of the patient contraindicates it, or when the extent of the rupture is small enough to warrant the gamble, conservative treatment is prescribed. If the skin heals cleanly within 2 or 3 weeks, suture of the ligament still should be considered. O'Donoghue is prepared to plan incisions that bypass clean abrasions, as he considers early operation to be of urgent importance. The author's experience upholds this view.

Any displacement of the meniscus must be reduced by manipulation before the limb is splinted. The knee is held with the joint closed on the side of the rupture and with the femur and the tibia in correct rotational alignment. This means that the tibia is rotated outward; to hold it in this position the foot must be included in a plaster-of-paris splint extending from the fold of the buttock. If manipulation is necessary, or after any severe injury, it is well to administer a general anesthetic. Tense synovial effusion or hemarthrosis is aspirated. The knee is maneuvered gently to ensure that movement is not restricted by a displaced meniscus or interposed soft tissues, and a compression bandage plus the plaster-of-paris splint are applied with the knee in the corrected position.

Thigh muscle drill should be started next day, and the patient is up and walking on crutches. When swelling subsides it may be necessary to change the plaster splint. After 4 weeks the boot of the splint is removed and the patient may take weight, protected by the back splint. In the treatment of a medial ligament injury, a heelseat is worn or the heel of the shoe is tilted on the inner side. The back splint should be removed at regular intervals for gentle non-weight-bearing flexion-extension exercises. If power and stability are adequate, the patient may indulge in slowly increasing unprotected weight bearing after 8 to 12 weeks.

However, if the knee is still weak, a caliper with extension spring should be used to reeducate the thigh muscle and to add stability (Fig. 13-1). If movement remains restricted by adhesions, these are broken

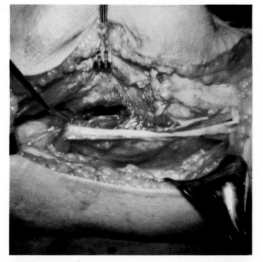

A

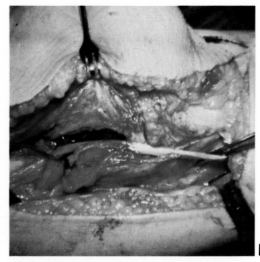

B

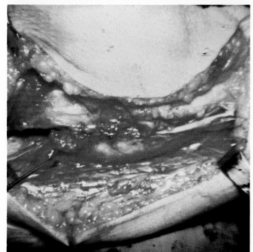

C

Plate 16-1. (*A*) The semitendinosus tendon has been mobilized and a groove has been cut in medial femoral condyle. (*B*) The tendon has been hooked into the groove. (*C*) The groove is converted into a tunnel by suturing periosteum and deep fascia.

Plate 16-2. (*A*) The normal configuration of the femoral condyles can be seen in this cadaveric knee. The trochlear walls are equal in depth, but the lateral condyle is longer than the medial. (*B*) In a patient with habitual dislocation of the patella, the trochlear groove is of adequate depth, but the lateral condyle is short —in this instance, shorter than the medial.

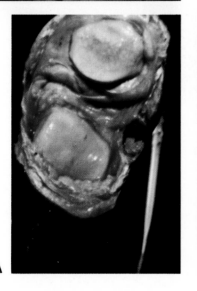

A

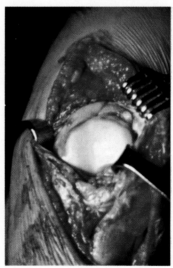

B

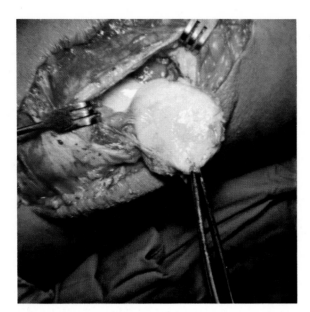

Plate 16-3. Erosion on the medial articular facet of the patella.

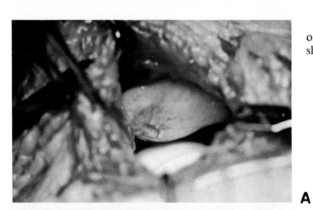

A

Plate 16-4. Abrasions and disruptions of the articular cartilage of the patella should be trimmed.

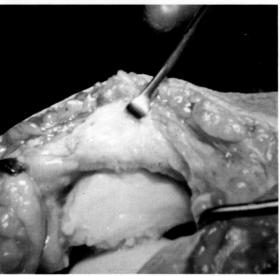

B

down at the appropriate time by gentle manipulation under local or general anesthesia.

Surgical Repair

The presence of clean abrasions does not preclude early operation. After adequate preparation with medicated soap and hibitane or 2 per cent iodine in 70 per cent alcohol, the leg is toweled and the operative area coated with an aeroplastic self-sterilizing spray. Clean abrasions are excluded by the plastic skin that is formed, and the incision is planned to avoid the affected area. Of course, if the skin is infected, open operation is absolutely contraindicated. When abrasion is present, surgery must be planned and performed under an "umbrella" of chemotherapy or antibiotics.

The operation should be performed with the patient lying on his back with leg extended and a small sandbag behind the knee. Before starting, adduction, abduction, rotation and anteroposterior movements of the tibia on the femur are tested. The incision will depend on the ligament or ligaments to be repaired. The medial collateral ligament and capsule are explored through a longitudinal incision in line with the anterior fibers of the ligament, extending from the upper border of the femoral condyle to some 3 inches below the joint line. Points of maximum hemorrhage give a lead to the site of rupture, which varies in type and degree. The full extent of the lesion should be ascertained carefully before deciding on what sort of repair is necessary.

If the ligament with part of the capsule is completely ruptured, or the ligament with the adjacent capsule is avulsed from the femur or the tibia, it is usually possible to examine the interior of the knee joint without further incision. If this is not possible and preoperative examination has suggested derangement of the medial meniscus, the knee joint should be opened by the usual anterior horizontal incision to explore the anteromedial compartment or a vertical incision in line with the posterior border of the tibia to expose the posterior horn of the cartilage. It is not always necessary to remove the cartilage. The decision depends on the type of damage. Transverse or longitudinal tears in the substance demand excision of the meniscus, as would complete detachment. If the anterior horn has been disrupted from the anterior cruciate, or the anterior cruciate and the meniscus both have been detached cleanly from their tibial anchorage, repair may be feasible. Both ends may be sutured back to the stump of soft tissue or are attached to the tibia in the manner of O'Donoghue (see p. 227). Limited peripheral tears will also reunite to torn coronary ligament. Operations to remove or reattach the semilunar cartilage are performed with the knee flexed. When completed, the knee is straightened. If the cartilage has been retained, complete extention and lateral rotation of the tibia are tested. Only if these movements are free and unrestricted can the suture be considered satisfactory. If not, the knee should be flexed again and the meniscus removed. It is important during the operation to protect the fat pad from injury.

While the ligament and the capsule are repaired, the knee should be straight, with careful adjustment of the rotational alignment of the femur and the tibia. Various technics for the repair of torn ligaments are available, and one or more of these may be necessary in a particular case. If a flake of bone has been avulsed with the ligament, it should be replaced carefully and held with a boatnail or staple. If the lower end has avulsed from the tibia, it also may be fastened to the roughened bone surface by these metal appliances, or by suture to the surrounding periosteum and soft tissue with linen or fine wire. Or small drill holes in the tibia may be used to anchor the ligament with wire or linen sutures. Defined ruptures of ligament or capsule may be repaired by interrupted sutures with imbrication or by a modification of the Bunnell type of suture. If the ligament is lax through ill-defined interstitial ruptures of fibers, darning from one end to the other using catgut with enough tension to tighten it up is a worthwhile procedure. The essential features are careful and complete repair of the damage so that, finally, tension and length of the capsule are as near normal as is possible. If the damage has been so extensive or of such ragged character that this cannot be achieved, immediate reinforcement by the semitendinosus tendon in the manner described on page 230 or of the lateral by half the biceps tendon, described on page 231, should be added. The type of suture material is not really important. Fine chromic catgut or linen or Bunnell pullout wire sutures may be used. My own preference is for linen, except when the ligament needs shortening by darning, in which case catgut is used.

THE LATERAL LIGAMENT

Interstitial ruptures of the lateral ligament are extremely rare. Disruption occurs either from the femoral attachment or, more commonly, from the head of the fibula, when the insertion of the biceps tendon also is damaged. Avulsion with a flake of bone is fairly common, for the lateral ligament is compact and firmly attached to bone. More extensive injury involves the iliotibial band where the tear may be ragged and irregular. The same principles of repair apply on the lateral as on the medial side. It is as important before deciding on the method of suture to examine each structure separately and to define the exact extent of injury but only after the popliteal nerve has been defined, isolated and protected. The injury may have displaced the nerve from its normal track. Repair of each structure must be meticulous and separate, for, as explained in chapter 1, adherence of the lateral ligament to the popliteus tendon or to any point of the joint line, or malalignment between the lateral ligament and the iliotibial band acts as a brake to flexion.

CRUCIATE LIGAMENTS

The importance of the cruciates in stability of the knee joint in the presence of an intact capsule is not as great as is generally thought. When the integrity and the length of the capsular ligaments have been restored, patients are able to do arduous work demanding strength and stability in the knee joint and even to play football in spite of an unsutured cruciate ligament. This may not apply to the athlete who demands a knee capable also of the higher flights of speed. O'Donoghue, who has unrivaled experience in treating athletes, prescribes synchronous repair of these ligaments. From the present series, instances can be reported in which patients have returned to strenuous occupations after restoration of the capsular ligaments only, in the acute stage, or after replacement of function by extraarticular tendon transfer in the later phases. One patient had ruptured the upper end of the lateral ligament, the iliotibial band and the anterior cruciate in an underground accident in a gold mine. In spite of a long period of conservative treatment, his knee was so unstable that he could walk only in a caliper. He had to give up his employment. After repair of the lateral ligament by biceps tendon transfer and imbrication of the iliotibial band and capsule, he was able to return to his work as a miner underground. Another, a bricklayer, young and powerful, tore all the medial capsular attachments and the anterior cruciate ligament. He reported for examination a year later, able to walk only in a caliper. After transfer of the tibial tubercle and transposition of the semitendinosus tendon, he was able to return to normal work, including carrying hods full of bricks up ladders.

If during the operation for the acute injury, the anterior cruciate is found to be detached from its inferior insertion, the opportunity of suturing it back to the bone ought to be taken. However, in the usual run of cases, except in most expert hands, I doubt the propriety of transarticular and intraarticular procedures for suture of the upper end of either cruciate. The lower end of the posterior cruciate is sutured only when an extensive tear necessitates exposure and repair also of the posterior capsule of the joint. Unless there is unhealed capsular damage, it is doubtful whether an isolated tear of the posterior cruciate disorganizes function materially.

Both O'Donoghue and Smillie[12] have described a technic of practically extraarticular suture of the inferior end of the anterior cruciate ligament. Two drill holes pass through the tibial tubercle, being aligned to emerge in the joint at the site of attachment of the anterior cruciate ligament. The suture is passed up one track, is darned into the lower end of the ligament and then emerges through the parallel track to be tied in front of the bone. O'Donoghue describes a similar simple suture for the lower end of the posterior cruciate. Two parallel holes are drilled from the front to the back of the tibia. The suture goes through one drill hole, emerges posteriorly, is plicated through the tibial stump of the posterior cruciate and goes back out the other hole.

The length of time before the patient is allowed to bear weight on the limb after the operation depends on the extent of the injury. If it has been severe, crutches should be used for at least 6 weeks. After the operation, a compression bandage is applied with a plaster-of-paris cylinder extending from buttock fold to toes with the foot at right angles. The knee is held just off the straight with full external rotation of the tibia. This position of splinting is always important, and its significance wll be realized when we remember the effect of the locked knee on the normal cruciate ligament. If external rotation of the tibia is prevented, the cruciate is stretched by the medial condyle of the femur. After the plaster splint has set, it should be split anteriorly in case of swelling. If constriction threatens, the bandage also should be divided through the opening. After 2 weeks, the sutures are removed and the splint is changed. While

this is being done, the position of the knee should be maintained carefully by a trained assistant. The patient is allowed to walk with crutches. After another 4 weeks, the cylinder is replaced by a back splint without including the foot. At this time, the knee is clinically stable, and periodic gentle flexion exercises are prescribed with the proviso that each time the knee is flexed, it should be fully extended before the next knee bend. Thigh muscle drill is started from the first postoperative day, and the patient may graduate to straight-leg raising, first without and then with an added weight.

After 6 weeks the patient learns to take weight first with a backsplint and then, when strong enough, with a crepe bandage. He should not return to strenuous sport for 4 months.

Substitution Operations for the Cruciate Ligaments. Operations for anatomic intraarticular replacement of the cruciate ligaments have not been included in this volume. Since 1942 when extraarticular transposition of patellar and semitendinosus tendons was first used, intraarticular procedures have had no special indication or merit.

COMPLICATIONS

Such complications as ensue are controlled by careful and timely after-care. Effusion may require aspiration and swelling, specific therapy. Slow recovery of movement is accelerated by intraarticular injections of procaine, followed, while the joint is anesthetized, by active and gentle passive stretching. Occasionally, adhesions prevent certain movements or arcs of movement, and when these movements are attempted, pain results. In such cases, gentle manipulation under Pentothal anesthesia is helpful. Calcification of the injured ligament of painless or painful character (Pellegrieni-Stieda) is relatively uncommon. Injections of procain, and hydrocortisone locally into the tender area usually relieve the symptoms. The development of late osteoarthritis depends on the damage caused to articular cartilage at the time of the accident.

Residual laxity of the capsule with weakness or instability of the knee joint is a possible sequel, the result of inadequate suture or faulty after-care. The regimen for untreated ruptures of ligaments discussed in the following paragraphs then would be applicable.

Treatment of Old Ruptures of the Cruciate and the Collateral Ligaments

Over the years a variety of operations have been designed to correct the instability due to old ruptures of the collateral ligaments of the knee joint. Most of these have relied on grafts of fascia lata or tendon to substitute for the ruptured structures. A number of these reconstructive operations have permitted comfortable use of the knee over the years but only if not exposed to prolonged and undue strain. It is rare that the grafted tissues stand up both to time and

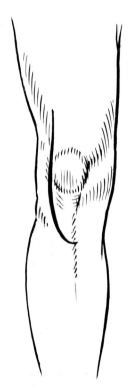

FIG. 16-6. A long lateral incision curving across the tibial crest below the level of the tibial tubercle.

stress, without stretching of the capsule with recurrence of laxity and weakness. More successful were McMurray who used the semitendinosus as a fixed graft to replace the medial ligament and Hauser who pedicled the inner half of the patellar ligament as two cross strips to replace the medial ligament and capsule. DePalma describes an admirable operation in which the anterior half of the biceps tendon is pedicled from its lower attachment to replace the fibular collateral ligament. The author uses the semitendinosus and the biceps tendons as active ligaments respectively for medial and lateral repair in the manner to be described.

If we consider that the cruciate ligaments act as check-straps which prevent anteroposterior movement of the tibia on the femur and that the resulting instability after rupture of these ligaments is due to absence of these check-straps, then the only logical course of treatment is anatomic replacement of the check-straps. On the other hand, if the cruciate ligaments are guide ropes that keep the tibia on its normal helicoid track on the medial condyle of the femur, it is possible to replace this function by extraarticular tendon transplants. This prinicple is applied:

1. by transfer of the tibial tubercle medially to ensure lateral rotation of the tibia while the knee is extending, and
2. by transposition of the semitendinosus tendon to preserve synchrony of excursion of the femur and the tibia during flexion of the knee.

In this way the guiding mechanism, of which the cruciates are a part, and the motor mechanism represented by the thigh muscles are both reinforced and the muscles are given better purchase on the tibia.

A series of 40 patients successfully stabilized by these methods has convinced the author of the advantages of replacing the function rather than the anatomy of these ligaments. In every case stability has been improved, and most patients recovered the ability and the confidence to undertake normal activities, even when strenuous. None of them has been permitted violent games such as football in which sudden abnormal, unexpected strains are probable. But strains that are foreseen and taken deliberately can be withstood after adequate retraining of the leg muscles. All the patients recovered confidence on rough ground. Two do work on ladders, and several ride horses without qualm. DePalma, who uses these methods, reports similar satisfaction with his results.

An interesting facet is that postoperatively the knee remains unstable when examined passively. When the muscles are relaxed, anteroposterior and lateral laxity still may be elicited. When the muscles are properly conditioned, active movements are stable.

Transposition of the Tibial Tubercle to the Medial Surface of the Tibia

This operation has been performed with success in a number of ways for recurring dislocation of the patella. The writer described a "slot" method in 1948. Since then one patient in this series developed a complication that has necessitated a minor modification. The patellar tendon had been overtautened and, consequently, full flexion was not recovered; years later retropatellar arthritis developed. Unfortunately, in a way, the limitation of flexion of some 15 degrees remained painless so that the excessive tight-

ness of the quadriceps mechanism was not relieved. The technic has now been modified by cutting the medial groove slightly upward and inward instead of transversely. This maintains normal tension in the quadriceps mechanism in its new alignment. The operation allows the patellar tendon a more medial purchase on the tibia and therefore ensures earlier and increased lateral rotation of the tibia during extension.

The operation is performed through a long lateral incision that starts at the level of the upper border of the patella and ends by hooking medially across the tibial crest below the level of the tibial tubercle (Fig. 16-6). The flap of skin and deep fascia is reflected to expose the patellar ligament and the tibial tubercle. Lateral and medial incisions free the patellar tendon. Care must be taken that this is complete on the lateral side. Leo Mayer reports a case that required a revision operation, for tension from the inadequately separated lateral capsule caused pain when the knee was flexed.[10] A block of bone of the same width as, and including, the insertion of the tendon plus ⅓ inch proximally and distally beyond the insertion is removed using small sharp osteotomes (Fig. 16-7). Care must be taken not to injure the fat pad with its synovial

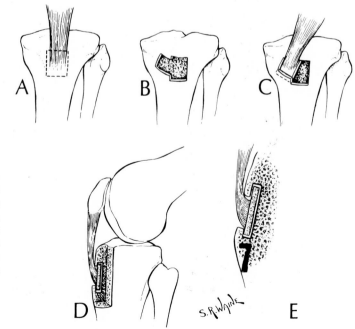

FIG. 16-7. Stages in transplantation of the tibial tubercle by the slot method: (A) The tubercle is removed. (B) A gutter is prepared to receive the tubercle. (C) The tubercle is transplanted. (D, E) Lateral views of the tubercle slotted home.

protection which lies between the ligament and the tibia. A groove the same width as the insertion of the tendon and at the exact level of the insertion is cut medially and slightly upward on the medial surface of the tibia (Fig. 16-7, *top, left*). The direction should be that of the circumference of a circle of which the patellar tendon forms the radius. It extends approximately ½ inch. The cortical block of bone is kept for use as a plug to prevent the insertion's slipping out of the slot at the end of the operation. A sharp curette or gauge is used to scoop out cancellous bone from beneath the cortex both proximally and distally until enough room is cleared beneath it to slide in the oblong of bone to which the insertion is attached (Fig. 16-7, *top, right*). Once this is tapped home, it is held securely, and contraction of the quadriceps can only lock it more firmly. To prevent any medial slip, the block of bone removed from the slot is packed into the donor site at the tibial tubercle. The medial capsule is now sutured to

the medial edge of the patellar ligament, and fascia is sutured over the raw bone surfaces (Fig. 16-7, *bottom left and right*).

Transposition of the Semitendinosus Tendon

T. P. McMurray originally described an operation in which he used the semitendinosus tendon to replace the anatomy of the medial collateral ligament.[8] He anchored the tendon by suture in two grooves cut in the line of the ligament in the femur and the tibia. The operation I use also substitutes the tendon for the medial ligament, but by permitting the semitendinosus to run free in a groove in the femur, instability is prevented in abduction by active contraction of the muscle. In addition, the muscle helps to restore the function of the cruciate ligament, for, by contracting when the knee flexes, it ensures synchrony of movement between the femur and the tibia. In other words, it prevents the tibia's running away from the femur. It has been my practice to transplant the tibial tubercle and to defer the operation for transposition of the semitendinosus to a second stage 4 weeks later. It is felt that

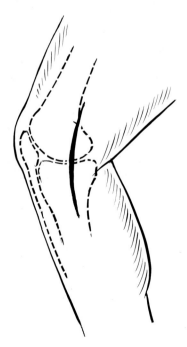

Fig. 16-8. A long slightly curved incision in line with the medial collateral ligament.

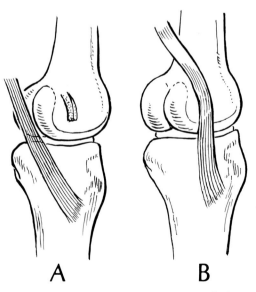

A   B

Fig. 16-9. Lively replacement of the medial ligament by transposition of the semitendinosus tendon. A groove (*A*) is made in the medial condyle into which the tendon is transplanted (*B*).

while the transplanted tibial tubercle should be splinted for approximately 6 weeks, it is desirable to start active movements of the knee joint 3 weeks after the transposition of tendon. The stage of union reached by the tibial tubercle should be firm enough after 4 weeks to permit the gentle maneuvers and movements required during the operation for transposition of the semitendinosus tendon. On one occasion the semitendinosus was transposed first and movement was initiated after 3 weeks. Six weeks from the time of the original operation the tibial tubercle was transplanted. At the operation opportunity was taken to examine the semitendinosus. It was gliding smoothly in a well-lined groove. More recently both operations are performed at the same sitting. After 3 weeks the splint is removed for gentle active movements but is reapplied for weight bearing.

With the patent supine and almost straight the operation is performed through a long slightly curved incision in line with the medial collateral ligament (Fig. 16-8). By sharp dissection the upper femoral condyle is gently cleared in line with the posterior border of the shaft of the femur and down to the reflection of the synovium of the joint. A gutter is cut, inclining posteromedially and wide enough to accept the tendon comfortably (Fig. 16-9). The maximum depth is approximately ½ inch. The proximal and the distal edges of the gutter must not be sharp. The semitendinosus, which runs most posteriorly of all the hamstrings, is identified. The tendon is freed down to its insertion and sufficiently far up the thigh to release enough length to bring it forward between the other hamstrings and slip it into the gutter. Gentle flexion of the knee and a

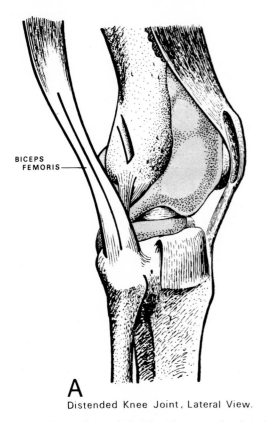

BICEPS FEMORIS—

A

Distended Knee Joint, Lateral View.

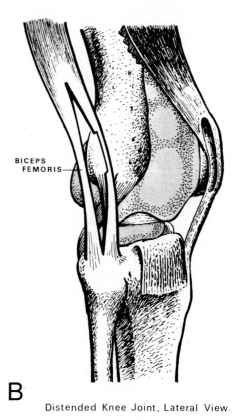

BICEPS FEMORIS—

B

Distended Knee Joint, Lateral View.

FIG. 16-10. (*A*) The biceps tendon is split in its length leaving both ends attached. A groove or hook is cut in the surface of the lateral condyle. (*B*) The anterior half of the split biceps tendon is hooked in the groove in the femur.

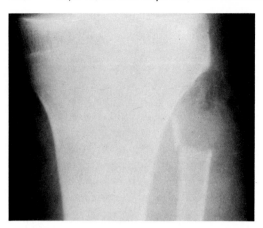

Fig. 16-11. X-ray photograph after subperiosteal excision of the head of the fibula and suture of soft tissues.

dissector to lever or shoehorn the tendon into the groove facilitates this maneuver. Because of the inclination of the groove, the tendon, once settled, is quite stable and does not tend to slip out. The groove is converted into a tunnel by interrupted linen suture of periosteum and capsule. Postoperative conditioning of the hamstring muscles is an important feature of this operation. Thigh drill is started the day after operation, and when movements are commenced 3 weeks later the patient is taught to contract the hamstrings consciously every time the knee is flexed. This should develop into a habit to give him permanent control of the knee.

Replacement of the Lateral Ligament of the Knee

The same principle may be used on the lateral side of the knee. At first the whole biceps tendon was transposed into a groove in the lateral condyle of the femur in the same way as the semitendinosus in the medial condyle, and worked well. In another operation the biceps tendon was anchored in a groove on the femur by suture. In this way, also, satisfactory stability was regained and retained. It is now found sufficient and preferable to use the anterior half of the biceps tendon (see Fig. 16-10).

A longitudinal incision is made in the line of the biceps extending below the head of the fibula. The popliteal nerve is defined and retracted. The tendon is split longitudinally leaving both ends attached. The outer surface of the lateral femoral condyle in line with the posterior border of the shaft is cleared as far down as the reflection of the synovium of the joint. A groove or "hook" is cut directed medially and posteriorly in the same way as that on the medial side for the semitendinosus. The anterior half of the biceps is then slipped into this groove which is converted into a tunnel by suturing periosteum and fascia. Care is taken to prevent injury to the capsule of the joint and the popliteus tendon. Adherence between the new ligament and these structures would cause restriction of flexion.

The replacement of a torn ligament by an active tendon or "dynamic ligament" is particularly effective. It is more powerful and longlasting than tenodesis.

I have used no other method since this one was devised during World War II. It is important to start isometric contractions soon after operation to prevent adherence in the bony groove. Postoperative stiffness of the knee has not been a significant problem. Very occasionally transient tenosynovitis of the semitendinosus has required a few days of splinting and an injection of a corticosteroid.

POSTOPERATIVE CARE

After each of these operations the wound is closed in layers. A compression bandage followed by a posterior gutter plaster splint is applied from mid-thigh to the lower third of the calf. After 2 weeks the sutures are removed, and the patient is allowed to walk on a back splint with crutches. Thigh drill is started on the second or the third day, increasing in frequency and in intensity as the weeks go by. Three weeks after semitendinosus transposition the splint is removed periodically for gentle active flexion exercises. After 6 weeks the patient may take weight, still wearing the back splint which is not finally removed for another 2 weeks. After tibial tubercle transplant, a back splint is worn until the insertion of the patellar ligament is no longer tender. Normal activities should not be permitted until the thigh muscles have recovered normal power.

TREATMENT OF RECURRENT SUBLUXATION AND DISLOCATION OF THE TIBIOFIBULAR JOINT

Subperiosteal excision of the head of the fibula was an early operation for the unstable joint (Fig. 16-11). Patients lost their pain and functioned satisfactorily, but we were uncertain that full power and stability would always be restored and would be retained. More recently arthrodesis is preferred.

The joint is exposed through an incision curved anteriorly and extending some 2 inches down the fibula. The peroneal nerve is isolated and retracted. The articular surfaces are exposed, denuded of cartilage, and apposed. A lag screw is inserted through the head of the fibula to hold it to the tibial surface. Usually tension of soft tissues resists firm apposition and may prevent sound

ankylosis. Oblique osteotomy of the neck of the fibula releases these tensions and by the time the arthrodesis is sound the osteotomy site has united (Fig. 16-12).

A long plaster cast is applied from midthigh to toes. After 4 weeks the patient may discard crutches and take weight on a rubber heel. The cast should be worn till fusion is sound, usually in 8 weeks.

INJURIES OF THE PATELLAR LIGAMENT

Contusions and sprains are discussed in Chapter 18. Rupture or avulsion of the ligament has been an infrequent injury in the experience of this practice. Clinically whereas after contusion or sprain attempted extension of the leg on the thigh against resistance is painful, after complete rupture it is not possible and the attempt is relatively painless. Early active or passive flexion is also painless, but may become uncomfortable as the range increases. The gap in the patellar ligament may be felt, especially when the quadriceps are contracted.

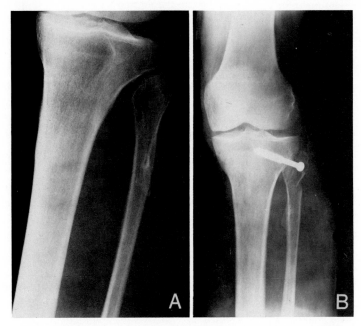

Fig. 16-12. Pre- and postoperative roentgenograms: excision of the joint and apposition of the head of fibula to the tibia by means of a lag screw. Oblique osteotomy of the neck of the fibula has been performed.

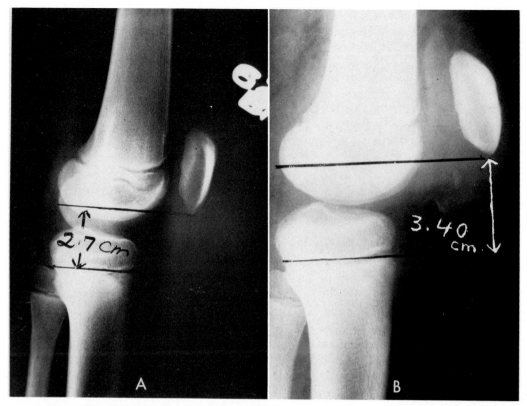

Fig. 16-13. (*A*) The distance from the epiphyseal line of the tibia to the lower pole of the patella in the normal knee is 2.7 cm. (*B*) In the injured knee with ruptured patellar ligament, the distance is 3.4 cm., an increase of 0.7 cm. Both roentgenograms are taken with the quadriceps contracted.

Precise diagnosis may be established by measurements (Fig. 16-13) of the increased distance between patella and tibial tubercle in the injured as compared with the normal knee. These measurements are useful also at operation to determine exact tension when pulling the patella down for suture. After suture, the patient should walk with a back splint and crutches for the first 3 weeks and a back splint alone for 3 more.

ACUTE TRAUMATIC DISLOCATION OF THE PATELLA

It has been customary to treat acute dislocation conservatively. While the patella is displaced—always laterally—the knee is slightly flexed, and it is usually reduced as the muscles relax, merely by straightening the leg. Anesthesia is rarely required. A compression bandage and back splint give comfort and permit weight bearing. Aspiration of the point is seldom necessary. Thigh muscle drill is initiated. The splint should be worn for 4 weeks after which movement and function return rapidly.

RECURRING TRAUMATIC DISLOCATION OF THE PATELLA

Prevention

Recurrence of the acute dislocation may follow if the capsule heals with loss of integrity and increased width; or it may follow ill-planned and poorly repaired long medial parapatellar incisions or after inflammatory or infective processes that have distended the joint.

Realization of the true pathology leads to

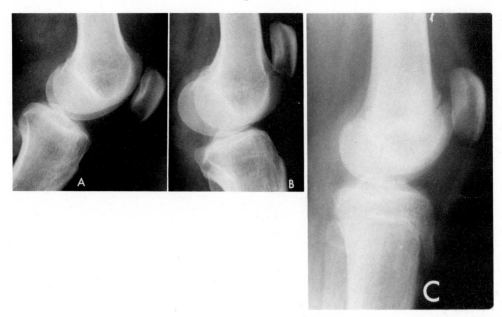

Fig. 16-14. In a normal knee the patella rests against the medial condyle of the femur when the knee is flexed (*A*); when the knee is extended with the quadriceps contracted, the patella reaches the apex of the trochlear fossa (*B*); and with the knee straight and the quadriceps relaxed, it rests comfortably in the trochlear groove (*C*).

the conviction that *immediate repair of the split synovium and capsule is necessary in all cases of acute dislocation of the patella.* It is as important as immediate repair of ruptures of the medial collateral or the patellar ligaments (see p. 59).

Treatment

Recurring dislocation of the patella has been attributed to genuvalgum, flattening of the lateral femoral condyle, laxity of the medial joint capsule, excessive length of the patellar ligament, high-riding patella, abnormally lateral insertion of the patellar ligament on the tibia, and muscular hypotonia. In addition the lateral capsule is usually abnormally tight.

Diagrams showing lateral stress on the patella by the angle of the genuvalgum are often misleading. With growth, the tibial tubercle tends to align itself in the direction of muscle action.

The importance of joint laxity, aplasia of the lateral condyle, and the high-riding patella in the genesis of patellofemoral in-

stability has been emphasized also by both McNab and Heywood.[7] Heywood, evaluating 76 patients, was able to define trauma as the sole significant factor in only 5 per cent. Most initial dislocations occurred when a relatively trivial injury was superimposed on a congenital defect. In the author's practice the most common anatomical abnormalities have been laxity of the medial with tightness of the lateral capsule, the high-riding patella, and a short rather than a flat lateral condyle (Figs. 16-14, 16-15).

The lateral condyle normally acts as a buttress for the patella against lateral slip when the quadriceps are fully contracted. Both a short condyle and genu recurvatum allow the contracting extensors to pull the patella out of this groove at a lower level. The patella becomes "high-riding" and vulnerable.

This may be determined by lateral X-rays taken with the knee held in the extreme of possible extension with the quadriceps fully contracted (Fig. 16-15). Hyperextension or genu recurvatum is also present in a good

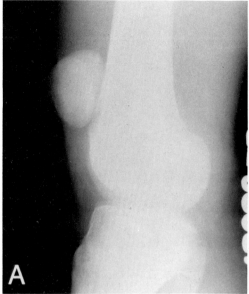

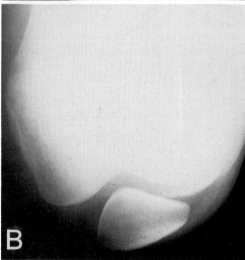

FIG. 16-15. This patient suffered recurrent dislocation at age 16 having had the first two incidents only a few months previously. (*A*) Note that in extension the patella lies above the trochlear ridge, which is short. The quadriceps is fully contracted. (*B*) In the tangential view it can be seen that the lateral ridge is not shallow. The patella dislocates because it is short.

average of hyperextension, in the dislocating group the mean angle of recurvatum was just over 9 degrees.

Mostly initial dislocation occurred when a relatively trivial injury was superimposed on a congenital diathesis. It has already been indicated that to prevent recurrence after acute traumatic dislocation it is most important to repair the vertical tears in synovium and capsule.

In contradistinction to habitual dislocation, traumatic dislocation invariably occurs in adolescent or adult patients. The resulting transverse weakness of the medial capsule of the knee joint is the basic fault to be repaired. Only surgery can effect a cure. The precise operation depends on the presence or absence of coincident anatomical or biomechanical weaknesses. Poor results are the consequences, usually, not of poor technique but of poor choice of operation.

An essential factor in sucessful long-term surgery is the appreciation in the particular patient of the track followed by the patella in its excursion from full flexion to full extension. The patella follows a sinous path (see Chap. 1) and any interference, as seen, for example, when meniscal injuries lock rotation of the tibia on the femur, or by malalignment through medial transfer of the tibial tubercle and patellar ligament, leads inevitably to articular surface damage.

For "high-riding" patella the medial capsule must be tightened both longitudinally and transversely. (Invariably the lateral capsule is tight and should as an initial stage be released by longitudinal parapatellar division.) The transfer of the tibial tubercle medially with imbrication of the medial capsule, a frequent practice, carries dangers, for, more often than not, the medial slope of the articular surface of the patella is tensed against the adjacent medial femoral condyle and leads to slow erosion and retropatellar pain. Moving the tibial tubercle lower as well as more medially (Hauser) to correct high-riding has a poor prognosis. In our experience it invariable leads to an eroded patella and retropatellar arthritis,

proportion of cases with high-riding. With L. Alaia eight consecutive cases of recurring dislocation were compared with eight clinically and radiographically normal knees.[1] Whereas the normal knees had a 5-degree

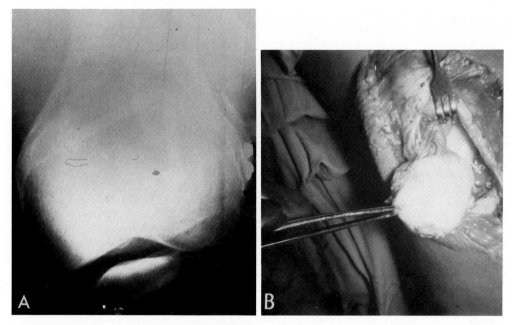

FIG. 16-16. (*A*) Tangential view of the patella after Hauser tibial tubercle transplant shows the patella to be twisted as well as displaced medially. (*B*) There is marked erosion on the medial articular facet of the patella. (See Plate 16-3 for color photo.)

and we no longer use this method. Besides disturbing the excursion of the patella, it often actually produces a twist on tendon and patella as shown in Figure 16-16 and Plate 16-3.

The effect is not the same when performed as advocated for rupture of the cruciates with medial ligament laxity (see p. 228). Then it takes up capsular slack and ensures lateral rotation of the tibia, the normal function of the anterior cruciate ligament during active extension of the knee, and a necessary safeguard when a lax medial ligament threatens a potential of weakness and instability. The additional rotation provided just aligns the patella so that in full extension it reaches its normal position in the trochlear groove.

On the other hand, if there is no transverse weakness of the capsule, medial transfer of the tibial tubercle may prevent the patella from reaching its position of comfort in the trochlear groove in full extension. Tension between the patella and the medial trochlear slope would result and lead to traumatic erosion of articular cartilage, a frequent cause of long-term disability after this operation. Medial transfer of the whole tibial tubercle should be performed only if longitudinal laxity of the capsule with or without a high-riding patella is a complicating factor.

The high-riding patella, lying as it does in the upper part or above the trochlear groove, is in its most vulnerable position for lateral dislocation. The operation described in Figure 16-17 is advised instead of the transfer of the tibial tubercle distally. A proximal central tongue of the patellar ligament is freed and buttonholed into the distal part. The shortening required is small, a centimeter at most. Overshortening is a common error. Postoperatively the patient wears a back splint for 6 weeks, but for the last 2 weeks the splint may be removed for active nonweight-bearing movement.

When only transverse laxity of the medial capsule is at fault, the Roux-Goldthwait operation, which prevents abnormal lateral excursion of the patella without altering the

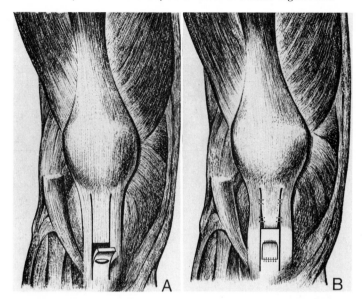

FIG. 16-17. (*A*) The patellar tendon is exposed through lateral parapatellar incision and division of the sheath. A guard is placed behind the tendon. Parallel incisions in the tendon release a central tongue which is divided at the junction of the middle and distal thirds. The proximal portion is buttonholed into the distal part and fixed with sutures. (*B*) The shortening need rarely be more than 1 cm. After the repair is completed the knee should be tested for an adequate range of flexion.

mechanics, is indicated. In addition, the relaxed capsule should be reefed or imbricated longitudinally. The Campbell procedure, a simple operation, should be used as an alternative to imbrication for gross medial capsular laxity.

Complications

Complications may result from injury, poor technique, or choice of the wrong operation.

When recurrence is due solely to the effects of the longitudinal tear of the medial capsule, the edges tend to retract and, treated conservatively, may heal with a gap and consequent weakness and further dislocation.

Arthrotomy should be used to detect osteochondral fractures or damage with fragmentation of the articular surface of the patella or femur. A lateral parapatellar approach is needed to release the lateral

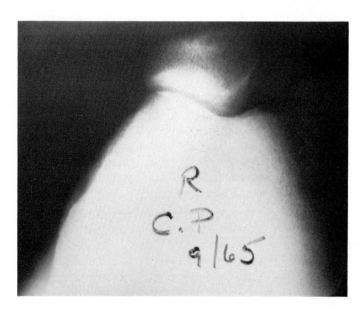

FIG. 16-18. If the lateral capsule is not released, the patella may remain tensed against the lateral trochlear slope.

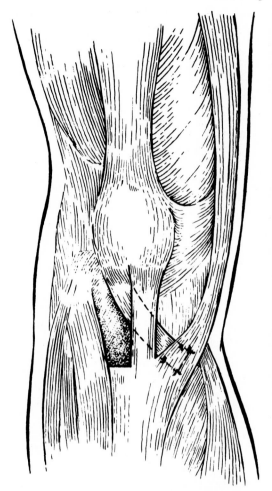

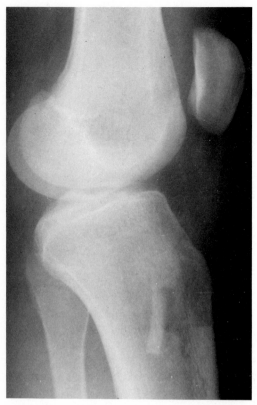

Fig. 16-20. Compare this postoperative roentgenogram with those of the patient's knee before the Roux-Goldthwait operation (Fig. 16-15). The knee is extended and the quadriceps contracted.

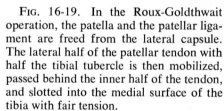

Fig. 16-19. In the Roux-Goldthwait operation, the patella and the patellar ligament are freed from the lateral capsule. The lateral half of the patellar tendon with half the tibial tubercle is then mobilized, passed behind the inner half of the tendon, and slotted into the medial surface of the tibia with fair tension.

capsule. At the same time the synovium is opened. Condylar fragments are removed and the articular abrasions trimmed (Plate 16-4). Associated ruptures of the menisci should be determined by careful preoperative diagnosis.

Two errors in technique are failure to release the lateral capsule which may lead to recurrent subluxation or even dislocation and secondly pulling the patella and the patellar ligament too far distally and/or medially (Fig. 16-18). This leads to restriction of flexion and compression of the patella in the trochlear groove and so to retropatellar arthritis, a frequent sequel of the Hauser operation.

In choosing the operation, careful regard must be taken of the customary track used by the patella from flexion to extension. In the very young, rerouting may be successful because the pliable adaptable growing articular structures may mold a new channel. In the adolescent or adult this is no longer possible, and painful osteoarthritis and patellectomy become inevitable. Unfortunately only in the relatively inactive is the long-term prognosis after patellectomy satisfactory. A fibrous or fibrocartilaginous pseudo-patella forms and in time develops its own painful

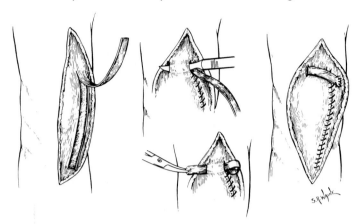

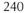

FIG. 16-21. The Campbell operation: Beginning at a level with the articular surface of the tibia, a strip of capsule 5 inches long and ½ to 1 inch wide is dissected, leaving the base attached proximally. The cut margins of the capsule are closed, thus taking up transverse slack. Through 2 slits on either side of the quadriceps tendon the strap is passed around the tendon and sutured to the soft tissues in the region of the adductor tubercle.

relationships with the articular surface of the femur.

For the Roux-Goldthwait operation (Fig. 16-19) the patella and the patellar ligament are freed from the lateral capsule. The lateral half of the patellar tendon with half the tibial tubercule then is mobilized, passed behind the inner half of the tendon and slotted into the medial surface of the tibia with fair tension.

A boy of 17, roentgenograms of whose patella were shown in Figures 16-15A and B and whose patella was quite unstable, was treated by this operation. Figure 16-20 shows the level of the patella after the operation. The lateral half of the tibial tubercle has been slotted into the medial surface of the tibia. The patella lies in the trochlear groove with normal tension, and the patient is comfortable.

The Campbell operation (Fig. 16-21) plans a medial checkstrap to lateral mobility of the quadriceps tendon.

Beginning at a level with the articular surface of the tibia, a strip of capsule 5 inches long and ½ to 1 inch wide is dissected leaving the base attached proximally. The cut margins of the capsule are closed thus taking up transverse slack. Through two slits on either side of the quadriceps tendon the strap is passed round the tendon and sutured to the soft tissues in the region of the adductor tubercle.[13] The operation has the virtues of both taking up transverse slack and of stabilizing the patellar mechanism.

SUMMARY

1. Recurring dislocation of the patella may be prevented by suture of the capsule immediately after the first acute incident.

2. Transfer of the tibial tubercle medially and distally, is infrequently indicated for recurring dislocation due to transverse laxity of the medial capsule with high-riding patella. The operation for shortening the patellar ligament described on page 238 combined with the Campbell procedure has a better prognosis.

3. Recurring dislocation due to uncomplicated transverse laxity of the medial capsule is cured by release of the lateral capsule followed by the Roux-Goldthwait operation plus Campbell's procedure or imbrication of the medial capsule.

If significant erosion of the articular surface of the patella and trochlear groove has developed, debridement or patelloplasty or patellectomy may be necessary in addition to the reconstructive procedures (see Chap. 13).

REFERENCES

1. Alaia, L., and Helfet, A. J.: Short Trochlear Groove in Recurrent Dislocation of the Knee. Report of N.Y. Academy of Orthopaedic Surgery, April, 1963.
2. DePalma, A. F.: Diseases of the Knee. Philadelphia, J. B. Lippincott, 1954.

3. Goldthwait, J. E.: Slipping or recurrent dislocation of the patella. Med. Surg. J., *150*: 169, 1904.

4. Hauser, Emil D. W.: Total tendon transplant for slipping patella. Surg. Gynec. Obstet., *66*:199, 1938.

5. Helfet, A. J.: Function of the cruciate ligaments of the knee joint. Lancet, *254*:665, 1948.

6. ———: A new way of treating flat feet in children. Lancet, *270*:1, 262, 1956.

7. Heywood, A. W.: Recurrent dislocation of the patella. J. Bone Joint Surg., *43B*:508, 1961.

8. McMurray, T. P.: The operative treatment of ruptured internal lateral ligament of the knee. Br. J. Surg., *6*:377, 1918.

9. Macnab, Ian: Recurrent dislocation of the patella. J. Bone Joint Surg., *34A*:957, 1952.

10. Mayer, L.: Personal communication.

11. D'Donoghue, D. H.: Surgical treatment of injuries to the knee. Clin. Orthop., *18*:11, 1960.

12. Smillie, I. S.: Injuries of the Knee Joint. Baltimore, Williams & Wilkins, 1962.

13. Speed, J. S., and Knight, R. A.: Campbell's Operative Orthopaedics. ed. 3. St. Louis, C. V. Mosby, 1956.

17

Major Athletic Injuries to the Knee

James A. Nicholas, M.D.

Athletic injuries to the knee are different from those that occur in daily living. As one ages, the knee changes in its quality of motion, power, and stability. In adolescence movement is usually greater although power is less, whereas in the young adult power increases, only to taper off again in later life. Also normal stability tends to increase with age. Hence athletic injury in the young differs in its effects from those in middle age.

There are other factors to consider. Previous injuries may have produced loss of movement or power. Instability, which might have been germane to the particular sport, may be aggravated by recurrent injury. The somatotype of individuals, such as the degree of looseness or tightness, may make the joint more vulnerable to injury.

Another problem depends on whether the injury occurred in contact or noncontact sports. $MV^2 \times$ loss of power (mass $\times$ velocity $\times$ loss of power) is a simple measure of the degree of load on an athlete's leg, and these forces vary in different sports. In football, lacrosse, soccer, hockey, skiing, basketball, and less in baseball, considerable forces are imposed. Whereas, in noncontact endurance sports, such as tennis, water skiing, handball, paddle ball and other active sports, as well as track and field events, primarily in running, the knee is not exposed as much to the shearing forces that test its stability. Treatment of professional athletes must aim at returning them to the sport and their livelihood. It is not acceptable to treat the medial compartment ligament injury in a cast if the ligaments are better repaired by surgery. Competitive tennis, an important life-long activity, for example, cannot be performed well with a chronically painful instable knee.

TYPES OF INJURIES

Injuries of the knee produced by athletics can be classified anatomically: to the bones by fracture or dislocation; to intraarticular soft parts; to extraarticular soft parts.

INJURIES OF THE BONES OF THE KNEE JOINTS

The basic injuries are fractures of the patella, femoral or tibial condyles, or those involving the epiphyseal plate. These are produced by direct blows. Landing on the knee in a vulnerable position can produce severe late loss of joint movement, particularly of flexion. Fractures of the patella usually result from a direct blow on the flexed knee. Some degree of rotation of the tibia on the femur may cause, in addition, a subluxated or dislocated kneecap. If the kneecap is *low,* direct injury is likely to result in fracture whereas dislocation, with or without chondral fracture, is more apt to occur in those individuals who have a *high-riding* kneecap or shallow trochlea. Falling on a knee flexed at a right angle with the kneecap riding high on the trochlea is apt to produce a different type of injury than falling

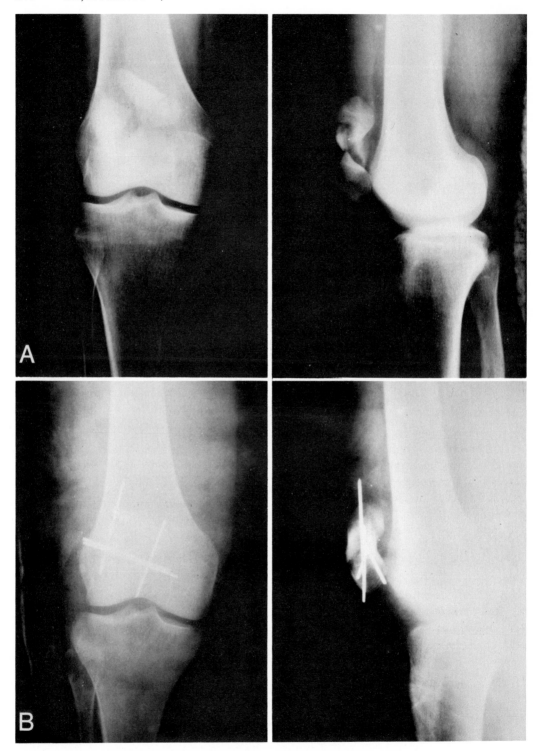

F IG. 17-1. Treatment of comminuted fracture of patella by K wires rather than excision may prevent knee instability and protect power.

on a knee in which the burden of the blow is born on the patella.

Comminuted fracture of the patella (Fig. 17-1) should be treated in athletes, especially carefully, with accurate reposition. There is no place for patellectomy. Fixation of the patella by circumferential wires, by compression fixation or by multiple Kirschner wires with restoration of a relatively normal surface can be achieved, although it may be necessary to remove incongruent fragments. Injury of this type is often seen in basketball players who hit the wall in a small gym, in football and soccer players, and in motorcyclists who land on a knee in a fall.

Displaced fractures of the lower end of the femur and upper tibia are serious, and the same rigid rules apply in treatment. Precise reposition and realignment as well as attention to minor incongruities under the patella and in the tibiofemoral joint are important. For example, a slight anterior offset after condylar fracture will usually result in terminal loss of flexion. These fractures can often be treated by closed reduction, but in many cases, especially in the young, open reduction for the lower end of the femur is indicated. Restoration of adequate motion after intraarticular supracondylar fractures is difficult to achieve. Tibial plateau fractures are rare, except in the older athelete.

To enable return to participation in sport, careful treatment is imperative. To minimize the instability characteristic of such fractures, sufficient elevation of the lateral tibial plateau with bone graft is necessary to correct a knock-knee deformity, although such malalignment is sometimes acceptable in nonathletes.

It is important to recognize articular or chondral fractures of the lateral facet of the patella or trochlear surface of the femur. (The mechanism is described in Chap. 21.) Chondral fractures are frequently seen in individuals with high-riding patellae. X-rays may be negative. Clicks, loss of movement, and rapid onset of severe hemarthrosis with occasionally free fat globules strongly sug-

gest the diagnosis. The fragments should be removed even if they are small.

DISLOCATION

Dislocation of the knee in athletes is infrequent but occurs in automobile or snowmobile racing, bobsledding, skiing and in motorcycle racing. It is a major injury, requiring urgent hospitalization, immediate diagnosis and reduction. Most dislocations are easily reduced and the sooner the better, sometimes even on the playing field. Careful examination to exclude popliteal artery laceration or peroneal nerve injury is imperative. If the foot is cold, pale, or pulseless, immediate vascular consultation should be obtained.

Management of the Acute Dislocation with no Arterial or Nerve Injury

In most cases, after reduction no lasting nerve, artery, or vein damage ensues. Instability is the problem. Unless the posterior cruciate ligament is intact it is most unlikely that instability, treated conservatively with a cast, will be compatible with good athletic performance. Reconstruction will be necessary.

For this reason, if there is a ligamentous instability of the complexes in the medial-lateral-anteroposterior compartments, the author believes that dislocated knees should be operated upon at once. The prime purpose of surgery is repair of the posterior capsule, and its attachments to the medial and lateral tibial and femoral midaxial planes. The posterior cruciate ligament demands top priority, and every attempt should be made to repair it. The anterior cruciate is usually so attenuated as to be irreparable.

Tears of the posterior cruciate ligament and posterior capsule are repaired at the some time. The medial and lateral compartments may be dealt with later.

Neurolysis of the peroneal nerve, or transfer with enveloping fat away from the lateral complex tear, should be performed lest later scarring constrict the nerve.

Dislocations of the knee are associated with so much ligamentous damage that one should try to repair the following structures, in order of importance:

1. Posterior cruciate ligament
2. Posterior capsule
3. Posterolateral corner
4. Posteromedial corner
5. Patelloquadriceps tendon tears
6. Anterior cruciate ligament

In all cases some loss of motion should be expected. Athletes can function with slight loss of motion but should be carefully rehabilitated to prevent contractures. After casts are removed bracing is necessary until power is restored.

INJURIES OF INTRAARTICULAR SOFT TISSUES

Besides the patella, the structures susceptible to major athletic injuries are the menisci, the ligaments, and the articular surfaces of the femoral and tibial condyles. Injuries to the menisci are the most frequent. Rotary forces imposed upon the posteromedial corner by the externally rotated valgus knee tend to produce tears of the posterior horn. In time, such injuries, trivial at first, continue to tear the cartilage and finally displace it into the joint, causing a locked knee. Careful diagnostic evaluation is required. A locked knee may be due to loose bodies from patellar subluxation with chondral fracture or, on occasion, to contracture of the hamstrings secondary to extensor weakness. The most common cause is the displaced meniscus. Diagnosis is based on the history, the absence of instability, the restriction of motion, the local sites of tenderness directly over the meniscus, as well as other signs described in Chapter 7, and if necessary aided by arthrography or arthroscopy (see Chaps. 9 and 10).

If a knee is locked, reduction should be attempted. This may be difficult but is possible by flexing the knee while rotating and drawing the tibia forward. The knee may unlock with an audible snap (compare the "reducing click," p. 108). However generally the knee, once locked, is not apt to recover complete extension or flexion, and reduction is basically done not as a cure, but for relief.

In some cases the infrapatellar fat pad may lock a knee because of bruising and hematoma without actual meniscus displacement. Such injuries may be accompanied by partial tears of intraarticular synovial folds or ligamentum mucosum. It should be pointed out that the cruciate ligaments are extrasynovial. The fat pad swells and may be associated with an infrapatellar tendinitis

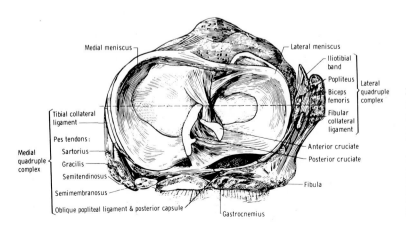

FIG. 17-2. The "quadruple complexes." There are three: one medial, one posterior and central, and one lateral. They constitute the regulating function of the posterior capsule on knee stability. (Nicholas, J. A.: J. Bone Joint Surg., *55A*:899, 1973)

with thickening and tenderness, so causing a block to motion.

Other intraarticular lesions are posterior or anterior cruciate avulsions of a small piece of bone, or osteochondritis. For large osteochondral avulsions, although accurate reduction is not always possible, operation and screw fixation may produce satisfactory results. The internal fixation should later be removed.

INJURIES TO CAPSULAR STRUCTURES ABOUT THE KNEE— "THE QUADRUPLE COMPLEXES"

The anatomy of the knee joint must be appreciated to establish a rationale for treatment of capsular-ligamentous injuries. The knee joint is invested by a large, flexible sleeve and tissues representing the quadriceps tendon, the patellar retinacula and the patellar tendon. Posteriorly, the capsule becomes thick and in some areas fairly rigid, and is characterized by condensations that the author calls quadruple complexes (Figs. 17-2 and 3). There are four structures on the medial side, four central structures, and on the lateral side four additional structures. The posteromedial corner is controlled by the semimembranosus tendon insertion into the tibia posteriorly, by the pes tendons, the medial collateral ligament and the oblique popliteal ligament of the posterior capsule.

The central portion of the capsule is reinforced within the joint by the two cruciate ligaments as well as both menisci, which are attached to the capsule through the ligaments of Humphrey and Wrisberg. On the lateral side, the capsule is reinforced by the biceps tendon, the iliotibial band, the popliteal tendon and the lateral ligament. These connect to form the arcuate ligament. Therefore, the posterior capsule controls a large part of the stability of the knee when the knee is forced into eccentric rotation.[2]

INJURIES TO THE QUADRICEPS AND EXTENSOR APPARATUS

Injuries to the quadriceps and patellar tendon occur quite commonly in athletics, particularly in the middle-aged. In basketball, hockey, and in high-jumping sports the Achilles tendon or the patellar ligament may be ruptured. Inability to extend the knee, with rapidly increasing swelling, with a gap below the kneecap leads to the diagnosis. This injury should be repaired surgically with a pull-out wire technique. The fat pad should be preserved where possible. Avulsion injuries of the quadriceps mechanism at the upper pole of the patella may occur in a forward jumping individual, usually someone over the age of 35. Here too, reattachment of the quadriceps by pull-out wire technique is important. In some cases,

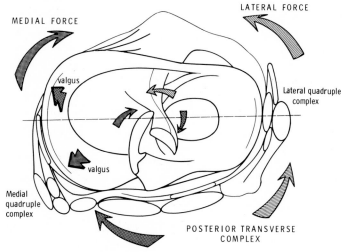

FIG. 17-3. The effect of rotation on the posterior capsular complexes of the knee. The medial quadruple complex resists external rotation and valgus. The lateral quadruple complex resists internal rotation and varus. (Nicholas, J. A.: J. Bone Joint Surg., *55A*: 899, 1973)

the lateral and especially the medial patello-femoral retinaculum are ruptured without any other signs (see also Chap. 16). Arthrography is useful in diagnosis for it will show leakage of the dye out of the joint. In the adolescent athlete, the tibial tubercle or the tibial spine may avulse instead and require surgical repair.

INJURIES TO THE CAPSULAR LIGAMENTS

The most serious major athletic injuries are those that involve stability. Forceful over-rotation of the flexed knee with the leg fixed may disrupt many component parts of the knee. It is necessary to describe the result-ing instabilities to understand both mecha-nism and the rationale of management.

Simple Instability

The author uses the term simple instability to denote that only one compartment is in-volved. For example, the medial complex structures such as the medial collateral liga-ment, can be torn without involving the posterior capsule, to produce valgus deform-ity, or one plane laxity. This can result from a blow from the side or a fall from a height. Immediate pain, a feeling of weakness, and valgus laxity are the cardinal signs. The medial collateral ligament usually tears at its upper pole. Motion may not be particularly affected over the first 12 hours, but later it may be impeded by hemarthroses. Clinically medial laxity gives the diagnosis, confirmed if necessary by arthrography. The medial meniscus may or may not be torn.

These ligamentous tears are repaired with the leg flexed and internally rotated, by re-advancement of the torn medial collateral ligament to the adductor tubercle. A cast will work occasionally, providing the menis-cus and posterior capsule are otherwise intact. The tibia should be held in varus and internal rotation.

Lateral Instability

Lateral instability of the simple type, is primarily varus rather than rotational laxity. Pure lateral instability, however, is unusual.

When present, the lateral ligament and usually the iliotibial band and/or the pop-liteal tendon are torn. In both instances, the patient feels the pop; the knee becomes quite wobbly. Pain on flexion is localized to the upper end of the fibula and over the joint line. It should be noted that the lateral side of the knee is normally slightly lax in flexion.

Simple Anterior Instability

Simple anterior instability without medial-lateral compartment signs is, in the author's experience, quite rare but has been described as a result of isolated anterior cruciate rup-ture. The patient may have a posterior-anterior drawer sign of perhaps ½ inch without medial and lateral laxity.

Posterior Instability

Posterior instability from pure posterior cruciate ligament injury is also rare, but occurs from a blow on the front of the knee with the leg hyperextending so that the cru-ciate ligament is torn off the intercondylar notch. Usually this is associated with cap-sular tear as well. Debate continues whether a cast is better than surgery. Except in cases with moderate laxity in athletes, the author advocates immediate repair even to age 50 or 60. However, casts are useful for partial tears where only one axis of joint motion is affected (simple instability).

Complex Instability

This type of instability is more common. Two or three axes of knee motion are affected. O'Donoghue's triad is the classical type. It should be realized that anteromedial is not the only direction of instability. The author describes four types of complex in-stability that, if recognized and repaired early, lead to satisfactory recovery.

Anteromedial Instability

The most common type follows anterior cruciate and medial collateral ligament rup-ture, often with derangement of the medial meniscus. This is caused by violent external rotation and abduction, the posterior medial corner rotating forward. The hamstrings and the posterior capsule restrain this movement, with the medial meniscus and collateral ligaments bearing the brunt anteriorly and medially. Marked laxity in flexion at about 15 degrees results. Pain may not be very great. Indeed, it may be possible to walk after the immediate symptoms are relieved. The patient often feels a pop. Anterior as well as external rotation laxity is diagnosed by migration of the tibial tubercle lateral to a vertical projection of the lateral edge of the patella. Arthrography stress studies, or, if the patient cannot relax, examination under anesthesia establish the diagnosis.

Treatment. The author does not feel that this injury should be treated conservatively. Operation as soon as possible is indicated, even within the first 12 hours, for this is the best time to repair the anterior cruciate ligament which has lost some of its blood supply. Many techniques are available, but the author advises removal of the meniscus and refixation of the anterior cruciate ligament. However, if the ligament has been torn in its central portion, or if the tear is "mop end" and hence irreparable, the anterior cruciate ligament should be excised. Treatment of the medial capsular structures depends on whether the residual medial collateral ligament is suitable and sufficient to anchor to the posteromedial corner and medial posterior complex.

An S-shaped incision is used. The pes anserinus tendons are exposed and turned up to see whether the medial ligament is torn underneath. Usually it is torn above the joint line. The intact part of the capsule posterior to the tear is identified. The knee is flexed, internally rotated and displaced backward, with varus stress. Volsellum clamps are used to bring the posterior capsule forward, covering the side of the tear. The capsule is brought distally as well and fixed either with a barbed staple or by sutures. If the anterior cruciate ligament is to be repaired a distal tear is anchored by drill holes to the tibia, a proximal tear to the lateral femur. It is of utmost importance to ensure firm fixation of the posterior medial corner behind the tibia as well as to the femur.

After this operation, a long-leg plaster cast is applied for 6 weeks with the tibia internally rotated, adducted on the femur to produce a varus attitude, and displaced backward. The cast remains in place for a long rehabilitation period. If it loosens it should be changed immediately.

Acute Anterolateral Instability

Acute anterolateral instability occurs when the leg is hit from the back or side while the foot is planted with the tibia internally rotated and the strain placed on the lateral side. Some part of the lateral quadruple complex, the anterior cruciate, and the lateral meniscus tear. Internal-external rotation is increased but an intact posterior cruciate ligament prevents backward tibial displacement. An anterior drawer sign and lateral laxity are present.

Repair is effected through a lateral approach to bring the part of the posterior lateral capsule behind the tear along with the lateral head of the gastrocnemius forward to the popliteus. After meniscectomy the transferred capsule and advanced lateral ligament are stapled to the posterior part of the lateral femoral condyle. The posterior capsule and iliotibial band are brought over the lateral ligament and popliteus and fixed to them. The operation is done while the tibia is bent outward with external rotation and backward displacement.

Acute Posterolateral Laxity

Acute posterolateral laxity, a third form of instability, results from rupture of the posterolateral compartment as well as the posterior cruciate ligament. It is caused by a forcible blow against the front of the tibia with the leg externally rotated and planted in varus position. Instead of the posterior medial and medial compartments tearing, the posterolateral corner tears, usually somewhere along the course of the lateral ligament and popliteus tendon. Sometimes the biceps is avulsed. In such instances, since the posterior cruciate has been torn, the lateral plateau of the tibia drops back with lateral posterior rotation and varus. In athletes operative repair is mandatory to obtain a good result. Unfortunately, the importance of this injury is frequently neglected as a surgical emergency. The diagnosis can be made from the presence of a posterior drawer sign and, on stress, laxity in varus and posterolateral rotation plus the local signs of tenderness. The medial compartment is quite stable.

Posterolateral repair is performed with the tibia internally rotated and displaced forward with the leg in valgus position. The posterior cruciate ligament should be repaired, and this may require a second medial incision. The posterolateral corner is repaired as in anterolateral instability, except that pes plasty is added to help check external tibial rotation.

Posteromedial Instability

Another type of instability that may be missed is posteromedial instability. In this instance, a blow from the front with the leg partially flexed, and in external rotation will tear the medial complex somewhere behind the medial collateral ligament below as well as above the joint line, and often both menisci. The knee, having been driven backwards, tears off the posterior cruciate ligament at its tibial attachment. Indeed, the author has seen both ends of the ligament torn in such cases. A large saccular defect will be seen in the posterior compartment and can be appreciated clinically under anesthesia by severe recurvatum as well as valgus laxity and increased internal rotation, the lateral compartment being uninvolved. Frequently the patella's medial facet is also injured by direct blow on the bone.

Surgical repair is most difficult. Essential is restoration of the posterior cruciate ligament, by drill holes and sutures to the tibia or medial femoral condyle, whichever is necessary. If it is irreparable, the semitendinosus can be transposed from back of the tibia to the medial femoral condyle (see Chap. 16). The tears in the posterior capsule are repaired, and with the knee flexed the entire capsule is mobilized forward to cover the medial ligament. The final position of the cast used in this situation is with the tibia displaced forward and the leg in varus and external rotation. It is possible, if one wishes, to transfer the biceps to the lateral side of the tibial crest. The author has had no experience with this but, just as in injury to the posterolateral compartment where internal rotation of the posterolateral corner is augmented by pes plasty, one may use the biceps on the lateral side to increase lateral-femoral or decrease medial-tibial rotation.

Results of this rare operation have sometimes been surprisingly good, but the key to success is to restore a stable posterior cruciate ligament. The author removes the menisci in this type of repair for the capsule must be mobilized.

Combined Complex Instability

When both medial and lateral or both anterior and posterior, as well as medial and lateral compartments are torn, *combined complex instability* exists. It is the author's opinion that transitory dislocation, or at least subluxation is a preliminary. In many instances the peroneal nerve has been injured. The defects on both sides should be repaired in two stages through bilateral incisions. Operations for intraarticular transposition of the iliotibial band or semitendinosus have been disappointing; they should be considered "last ditch" reconstructive salvage measures.

Rehabilitation, including a brace and an active rehabilitation program, is an extremely important part of the treatment. This is stressed in the chapter on rehabilitation.

Only those skilled in reconstructive surgery, and conversant with the limitations should undertake these operations, which are primarily for people with continuing instability despite restoration of power and the use of a brace.

REFERENCES

1. Nicholas, J. A.: J.A.M.A., *212*:22, 36, 1970.
2. ———: J. Bone Joint Surg., *55A*:899, 1973.

18

The "Dashboard Knee"

Arthur J. Helfet, M.D.

A blow on the front of the bent knee is a frequent consequence of automobile and motorcycle collisions (Fig. 18-1). The sufferer is usually the passenger on the front seat, who is thrown forward and upward and strikes a knee against the dashboard. Fracture of the upper end of the tibia, or of the patella, or backward dislocation of the tibia on the femur may result. But a lesion that might be called "the dashboard knee" merits discussion. It is less serious in its immediate consequence than frank fractures or dislocations but tends to cause protracted and troublesome disability unless the exact nature of the damage sustained is appreciated and adequately and specifically treated.

The site and the extent of the contusion depends on the position of the knee when struck, e.g., if pointing forward or if the medial or the lateral side of the flexed knee receives the direct blow. The structures involved are: the patellar ligament, the infrapatellar pad of fat, the anterior horns of the two semilunar cartilages, and the presenting articular surfaces of the femoral condyles.

The lesion is characterized by swelling and bruising of the tissues in front of the knee. There may be associated abrasions or skin wounds, and synovial effusion or hemarthrosis may develop. Unless the patella or the tibia has been involved, tenderness and pain in the early stages may not be severe. It is important to assess the exact extent of the injury and the tissues involved and to initiate treatment immediately. The formation of scar and adhesions should be prevented, for these are the main disabling factors when hemorrhage and swelling are given time to organize. A compression bandage, a back splint, no weight-bearing, heat, compresses, all should be considered. The injury is a contusion that affects each tissue characteristically.

PATELLAR LIGAMENT

Oddly enough, patellar ligament injury does not cause the most trouble, although it is in the van of the accident. When it does, a scar has formed in the ensheathing tissues and/or in the substance of the tendon. Pain is felt whenever the ligament is tensed or strained as in climbing stairs or kicking a football. Kneeling on the tender knee is avoided. Active extension of the knee is painful, whereas passive extension is painless. Conversely, active flexion tends to be symptomless, whereas passive flexion may be uncomfortable. The injured part of the ligament is always tender on pressure. Injection of the tender area with procaine and hydrocortisone should be followed by "manipulation under local anesthetic." In other words, while the anesthetic effect of the procaine lasts, the patient is asked to do those movements that normally are painful. This would tend to break down the peritendinous and the intratendinous adhesions. Physiotherapy, including heat and deep massage or ultrasound, are useful in aiding resolution. Occasionally, manipulation under general anesthetic and even excision of the scar is necessary. The injury to the ligament is seldom isolated and is usually associated with damage to the infrapatellar pad of fat.

INFRAPATELLAR PAD OF FAT

Scar and adhesion formation in and around the fat pad not only interfere with function but cause disability through pain as well. The pad is a mobile structure, but following this injury it tends to become adherent to the tibia and to be tied by adhesions to the anterior horn of the nearest meniscus, most often, the medial meniscus (Fig. 18-2). The full range of functions of the fat pad are not clearly understood. It contains a high proportion of elastic fibers, and these, plus its synovial attachments, enable the mobile structure to adapt itself to and cushion the front of the knee joint as it opens and closes in flexion and extension. It is also thought that it adjusts the intraarticular space in the knee joint to allow proper lubrication of the surfaces during movement. Adhesions at any point affect the mobility necessary for these functions.

In addition, when adhesions anchor the anterior horn of the meniscus, the rotator mechanism of the knee joint is affected. Extension and lateral rotation of the tibia

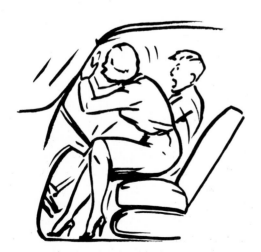

Fig. 18-1. As the passenger is thrown forward and upward the knee strikes the dashboard.

are limited, with all the signs and symptoms of a retracted anterior horn.

Swelling of the fat pad as a whole simulates Hoffa's disease.[1] It is tender. The knee aches after activity and suffers recurring or persistent effusion. Forced extension is painful and aggravates the condition. When the semilunar cartilage is involved, rotation of the tibia is limited. There is specific tenderness over the anterior horn, and the patient may complain of pseudo-giving-way due to stabs of pain on certain movements.

Adequate physiotherapy is useful and important in the early stages. If the residual adhesions are mild, manipulation under general anesthetic is advisable. In those cases in which rotation is limited, but painful when forced, manipulation may be dramatically successful, for the adherent meniscus is mobilized. For the more heavily scarred fat pad, which does not respond to treatment by these methods, surgical excision of the scar and careful mobilization should be performed. It will be found that the fat pad is adherent above and anterior to the edge of the tibia. These adhesions must all be dissected carefully. Removal of the fat pad should be avoided. The knee without a fat pad is creaky and prone to strain on any exertion. Dissection of the scar must be meticulous. The fat pad is a vascular structure, and unnecessary trauma leads to new adhesions. Postoperative treatment to prevent further hemorrhage and to promote absorption of reactionary swelling is vitally important. A Jones compression bandage for 10 days, followed by conscientious physiotherapy, is the course advised.

LESIONS OF THE ANTERIOR ENDS OF THE SEMILUNAR CARTILAGES

The medial or both anterior horns are commonly involved. The lateral semilunar cartilage seldom is injured by itself. The cartilage appears to be pushed back from its anterior attachments, and the anterior tip is embraced by the adjacent lobe of the fat pad in a bulky hard scar (Figs. 18-2; 19-4). If the lesion has been present for any

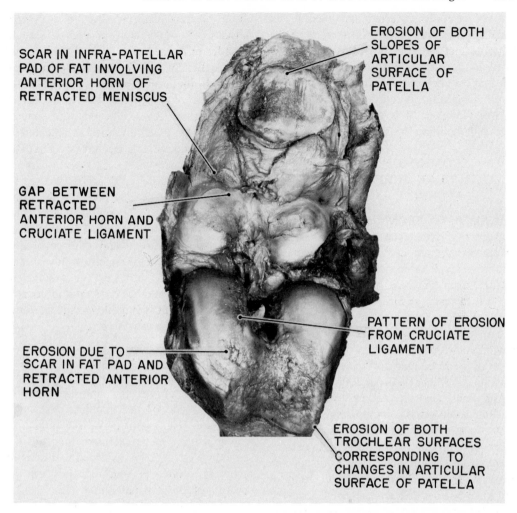

SCAR IN INFRA-PATELLAR PAD OF FAT INVOLVING ANTERIOR HORN OF RETRACTED MENISCUS

EROSION OF BOTH SLOPES OF ARTICULAR SURFACE OF PATELLA

GAP BETWEEN RETRACTED ANTERIOR HORN AND CRUCIATE LIGAMENT

PATTERN OF EROSION FROM CRUCIATE LIGAMENT

EROSION DUE TO SCAR IN FAT PAD AND RETRACTED ANTERIOR HORN

EROSION OF BOTH TROCHLEAR SURFACES CORRESPONDING TO CHANGES IN ARTICULAR SURFACE OF PATELLA

FIG. 18-2. Obviously this cadaveric knee was struck more to the inner than to the outer side. Though both surfaces of the patella are affected, the medial slope is much more so. There is a big hard scar in the medial side of the fat pad, and the scar involves the anterior horn of the medial meniscus which has been detached from the cruciate ligament. The fat pad and the retracted anterior horn have caused a rounded pattern of erosion on the medial femoral condyle. (Courtesy Royal College of Surgeons, England.)

length of time, a deep indentation is formed in the articular cartilage of the medial femoral condyle slightly more medially and anteriorly than the area of erosion from a retracted meniscus (Fig. 18-2). It may be possible to palpate the hard, tender lump in the anteromedial compartment of the knee. Rotation signs are present, and forced extension causes pain in this area. This is a troublesome knee that tends to become slowly but progressively worse—more so when the adjacent articular surface of the

femoral condyle has shared in the contusion. Recurring or persistent effusion and wasting of the quadriceps are adverse factors.

Treatment by manipulation of the knee under an anesthetic may be attempted but now fails to relieve symptoms. Therefore, the lesion is explored through the usual horizontal incision, which may be extended slightly further medially and upward. The mass of scar involving the retracted anterior horn of the cartilage is usually adherent to the tibia. The meniscus and the scar in the fat are carefully dissected and excised. In these cases it may be difficult to remove the quite normal posterior horn of the meniscus in its entirety through the anterior incision. As long as the residual fragment is not injured surgically, it may be left, without harm. However, it is always necessary to free and mobilize the whole of the fat pad.

CONTUSION OF THE ARTICULAR SURFACE OF THE FEMORAL CONDYLE

Again, it is usually the medial condyle that is involved. The blow falls on the anteromedial part of the articular surface of the condyle, or the damage may be secondary from pressure by the scar formed by the fat pad and the damaged anterior horn of the meniscus. The latter etches a progressive pattern of erosion which may be compared with that resulting from displacement of the semilunar cartilages. If the lesion lasts long enough, this knee follows a similar retrogressive course. Attacks of pain and swelling after activity increase in frequency and duration, the knee becomes more flexed, and eventually the patient feels he is walking on a stone in the knee. Excision of the cartilage and the scar and mobilization of the knee so that full extension is recovered may bring considerable relief. But on the whole these knees do not do as well after operation as do their counterparts with traumatic arthritis due to a deranged meniscus. Convalescence is more protracted, and the recovery of comfort, power and movement takes longer and is sometimes incomplete. There is no doubt that a badly damaged fat pad may be a lifelong hindrance.

This may be the fate, also, of the knee in which the articular cartilage of the femoral condyle has been directly and severely contused. The symptoms become progressively worse as in chondromalacia or articular cartilage damage from other causes. At first the area is tender and the knee joint irritable. The products of the degenerating cartilage provoke effusion, discomfort, limi-

tation of movement, wasting of the thigh muscles, etc. It is wise in such a case to consider prolonged protection of the affected area, at first by rest in bed, and bandaging, followed by crutches for walking until tenderness of the knee has disappeared. Aspiration of tense effusions, or hemarthrosis using local anesthesia, repeated if necessary, and possibly Healon (see Chap. 5) accelerate recovery.

Quadriceps drill may be started early, with non-weight-bearing movements when swelling permits. At operation, the articular cartilage shows all the signs of degeneration. The area loses luster and compressibility, fibrillates, and appears slightly yellowish and more opaque. If protected for a sufficient length of time, the knee does tend to become symptomless, but it is unlikely that the long-term prognosis is satisfactory.

THE PATELLA

Contusion of the patella leads to gradual degeneration of articular cartilage both of the patella and of the trochlear surface of the femur. The extent of cartilaginous erosion is usually more extensive than are the secondary effects of a displaced meniscus or recurring dislocation and depends on the severity of the original injury (Fig. 18-2). Symptoms, the assessment of disability, and treatment are discussed in Chapter 13.

It should be noted that although the dashboard may cause actual dislocation of the knee, a lesser injury may produce minor tears of capsule and ligament. These must be assessed carefully, for treatment for "dashboard injury" should never be delayed or casual in character. Every attempt must be made by conscientious therapy in the early days to prevent sequelae. As will be realized, disability from the four lesions described tends to become worse without, and lamentably, often in spite of, treatment.

REFERENCE

1. Hoffa, A.: The influence of the adipose tissue with regard to the pathology of the knee joint. J.A.M.A., *43*:795, 1904.

19

The Stiff Knee

Arthur J. Helfet, M.D.

In its broadest connotation, stiffness of the knee includes restriction of movement in one or more directions. It is a common sequel to injury of the knee joint itself, of the muscles of the thigh, or of fracture of the femur. It is an early symptom of arthritis, whether traumatic or rheumatoid or infective in origin.

The knee joint is activated by flexion-extension and rotator mechanisms. However, when movement is limited, it is usual orthopedic practice to place emphasis mainly on restrictions in the flexion-extension apparatus. Fixed limitations of movement are arbitrarily labeled as flexion or hyperextension deformities or "triple dislocation." But movement of the knee joint is a synchrony of flexion or extension with rotation, and, although one may be affected predominantly, limitation of range in any direction involves both. More often than not the rotator mechanism is primarily at fault.

Treatment of the stiff knee without diagnosis and exact localization of the structure which is the brake to movement is difficult and unsatisfactory. To distinguish the different conditions is not often easy, for several structures may be involved at the same time. Adherence of the quadriceps to the site of fracture of the femur is not always the cause of limitation of flexion of the knee joint. Adhesions between the menisci or the fat pad and the tibia may be at fault. Attempts to increase flexion of the knee by hingeing the joint under a general anesthetic or to correct flexion deformity by wedging a plaster cylinder posteriorly are unsatisfactory substitutes for removing obstacles to rotation of the menisci or to free movement of the fat pad.

ADHERENCE OF THE QUADRICEPS TO THE FEMUR

Stiffness after fractures of the shaft of the femur may be due to damage to and subsequent adherence of the quadriceps to the fractured area of the femur (Fig. 19-1). John Charnley[4] has recorded evidence that this rarely happens when the fracture unites in reasonable time but is liable to occur when union is delayed. Similar restriction of movement occurs when the thigh muscles are damaged without fracture of the femur. They adhere to the bone or to each other. Injury to the hamstrings may result in flexion contractures, the deformity being combined with internal or external rotation of the tibia, depending on whether the medial or the lateral muscles are predominantly affected.

Involvement of the muscle alone may be inferred if rotation of the knee joint remains comparatively free. Unless the muscles have become fixed with the knee in complete extension, passive limitation of flexion is not associated with a proportionate loss of passive rotation. But this is a rare state of affairs, for fracture of the femur or damage to thigh muscles is often associated with coincidental sprain or contusion of the knee; or the prolonged splinting necessary in treatment may lead to stiffness, especially in old people.

The site of muscle adherence is tender to deep pressure, and the patient usually is able to localize the area from the sensation of local tension when passive movement is forced. Forced flexion does not produce pain in the knee joint unless tension between the patella and the femur—or if the patella is fixed—on the patellar ligament, becomes excessive. Often the scar and the area of induration in the muscles are palpable.

The best preventive against adhesions after fracture of the femur is adequate reduction and splinting followed by conscientious quadriceps drill and hamstring drill, or what might more instructively be called "thigh drill," for exercise of the hamstrings is as important as of the extensors. After 3 or 4 weeks, if induration persists and the patient has difficulty in properly contracting the thigh muscles, judicious injection of a mixture of procaine and hydrocortisone is helpful. Manipulation under a general anesthetic may be attempted after the fracture has united soundly and consolidated but will succeed only if the adhesions are few and minor. Massive adhesions will not yield to manipulation. At a late stage, when

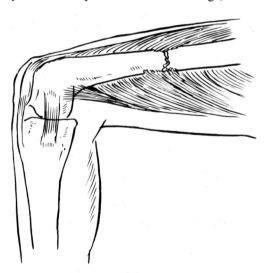

Fig. 19-1. Adherence of the thigh muscles to the shaft of the femur limits their excursion and therefore the range of movement of the knee joint.

exercise, physiotherapy, stretching, etc., no longer further improvement, gentle freeing of the muscles, or quadricepsplasty as described by T. Campbell Thompson,[6] or recession of the quadriceps tendon as devised by Bennett,[2,3] all give good results. The interposition of a membrane of fascia, nylon, or metal between the muscles and the femur is seldom necessary.

Recent experiments[1] showed that hyaluronic acid implanted into a wound in a dog prevented intraarticular inflammation in a joint and a decrease in granulation tissue reaction and fibrous tissue formation in subcutaneous wounds (see Chap. 5). This holds promise that dehydrated membranes of pure hyaluronic acid may be most useful in preventing new scar formation in this and other operations on joints and muscles.

MALUNITED SUPRACONDYLAR FRACTURE OF THE FEMUR

The influence of malunion of these fractures on movement of the knee joint is not always appreciated. The femur may have united in perfect anteroposterior and lateral alignment, but if rotation has not been corrected, full extension or flexion may be mechanically blocked. It would seem that if the lower fragment is rotated laterally, the tibia reaches the limit of internal rotation before the knee is fully flexed. The opposite would hold if the lower fragment is in malalignment in internal rotation. Recovery of movement is possible only after corrective osteotomy.

ADHERENCE OF THE CAPSULE OF THE KNEE JOINT

Adhesions may form between fibrous and synovial capsule or between fibrous capsule, synovium, and bone or may bind synovium to synovium as in the suprapatellar pouch. The adhesions follow sprain or contusion, as in the "dashboard knee," or hemarthrosis or infected effusions or wounds or ill-judged incisions.

In their formative or vascular stages these

adhesions are acutely sensitive to movement and tender on pressure. When the adhesion is established as fibrous avascular tissue, tenderness, less marked, is present only on deep pressure, while movement is painful only when forced.

Adequate treatment in the early days after injury is necessary to prevent these sequelae. While the adhesions are vascular, treatment is conservative—physiotherapy and local injections of procaine, hyalase, and hydrocortisone. Manipulation at this stage is accompanied by the unpleasant sensation of tearing tissue and produces reactionary bleeding and exudate. Painful swelling and increased restriction of movement results. When the adhesion is formed and avascular, manipulation is accomplished with a sharp snap, and movement is immediately free. There is little or no reaction afterward.

The knee is ready for manipulation when tenderness is localized and present on deep pressure only. Extensive adhesions do not respond well to manipulation and are usually associated with damage to other structures, such as meniscus and fat pad, as well. In that event surgical mobilization is necessary.

Reference has been made to the limitation of flexion that results from adhesions between the lateral ligament and the popliteus tendon or the lateral capsule (Fig. 19-2). Here, too, treatment to recover movement may require surgery.

ADHERENCE OF MENISCI AND FAT PAD TO THE TIBIA

This mechanism is responsible for stiffness of the knee joint after injuries associated with hemarthrosis (e.g., after rupture of the menisci from their vascular peripheral attachments) and after dashboard injuries. It is also a cause of stiffness after transient infection of the knee joint controlled by antibiotics. Adhesion of the menisci to the tibia is found in the knee in various stages of rheumatoid arthritis (Figs. 19-3 and 19-4).

This is true locking of the rotator mechanism. If the adhesions are firm and short, only hinge movement is possible. If the adhesions are lax, an arc of movement remains with synchrony of rotation approaching the normal. The condition is diagnosed either by the complete absence of passive rotation or by the relative restriction of rotation when compared with the extent of flexion or hinge movement present. Pain on forced movement depends on the firmness of the ankylosis present. Early vascular adhesions produce sharp pain on movement,

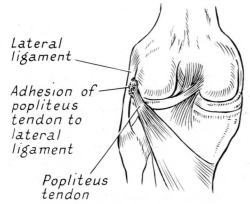

FIG. 19-2. If adhesions form in the tendon sheath of the popliteus or between the popliteus and the lateral ligament, movement of the knee joint is limited and painful.

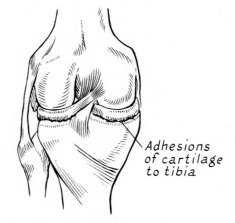

FIG. 19-3. Adhesion between menisci and tibia locks rotation and therefore limits flexion and extension.

whereas more force is needed to give the same discomfort when the adhesions are dry and firm. Tenderness follows suit. The site of adherence is the site of maximum tenderness—usually the anterior horn of the meniscus or the fat pad or both. As this condition often follows hemarthrosis, adherence of the menisci and the fat pad may be associated with adhesions of the capsule to the femur, and adhesions in the suprapatellar pouch. In this event, deep tenderness will be present over the femoral condyles, and thickening and tenderness may be palpable in the suprapatellar pouch.

The patient complains of limitation of movement with pain but usually adds a story of recurrent attacks of aching and effusion following undue activity of any kind. He may complain of "illusory giving-way." On certain movements or on irregular ground a sharp twinge of pain gives the impression of momentary instability. He tends to guard the knee and walk with trepidation.

Attempts to recover movement by forced flexion or hingeing are rarely successful. The arc of hingeing may be increased, but the gain is at the expense of the capsule and

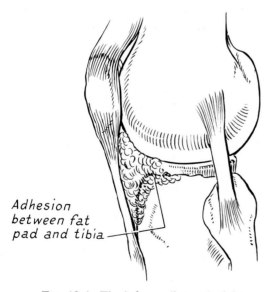

Adhesion between fat pad and tibia

Fig. 19-4. The infrapatellar pad of fat is a mobile structure. If it becomes fixed to the tibia and/or the meniscus, movement of the knee joint is affected.

in some instances includes stretching the cruciate ligament. The stretched capsule and cruciate ligaments are responsible for the anteroposterior laxity found in these otherwise stiff knees. However, this type of manipulation does sometimes free intracapsular adhesions. Recovery of rotation of the tibia on the femur is the maneuver to be practiced and is especially useful for mild adhesions between the fat pad and the anterior horn of the meniscus. The effect of regaining rotary movements may be demonstrated under general anesthesia. Without attempting flexion, gently manipulate the tibia on the femur in rotation. As rotation increases, flexion improves proportionately.

For mobilizing the really stiff knee, Sir Robert Jones described this method:

> In breaking down adhesions of the knee, I teach that the knee should first of all be fully flexed and fully extended. It then should be fully flexed and slowly extended, and during the whole of the last act the knee should be rotated inwards and outwards at least ten or fifteen times.[5]

Sir Robert was especially skilled in manipulation. In the author's experience it is easier to regain flexion and extension as rotation is freed. Attempts to flex should be accompanied by forced medial rotation of the tibia and extension with lateral rotation.

Some adhesions give suddenly with a dramatic increase in the range of knee movement. In others, improvement is limited, and one feels an elastic block to further movement. Now, open operation is indicated and holds good promise.

At operation one finds the anterior horn or the anterior half of the meniscus adherent to the tibia. The semilunar cartilage may show the yellowish stain of old hemorrhage. The coronary ligament is impregnated with or replaced by fibrous adhesions, and the usual easy mobility of the anterior half of the meniscus has been lost. Unfortunately, too, one usually finds that the anterior horn has been detached from the cruciate ligament and is consequently retracted and thickened. When the meniscus has been tied down for some length of time it feels hard. It has lost pliability and resilience. If retracted or adherent it should be excised.

The common areas of fixation of the fat pad are to the anterior horn of the meniscus and to the anterior surface and the anterosuperior border of the tibia. The adhesions should be divided gently and the fat pad mobilized. In some instances, lobes of the fat pad are adherent to each other, and these fibrous bands also should be freed. Further damage to the fat pad with the prospect of hemorrhage and new adhesions must be avoided. As soon as the adhesions have been divided, rotation of the knee joint as a whole recovers. With the leg flexed over the end of the table this is easily tested. The leg then should be straightened to make certain that full extension with rotation has been recovered. Flexion is usually immediately possible well beyond the right angle.

Intracapsular adhesions are usually demonstrated between the femur and the capsule in the recess of the joint above the medial cartilage. They may be freed by gentle dissection or may be snapped by manipulation after the cartilage has been excised and the fat pad mobilized.

The timing of the manipulation and/or operation are important. If performed while the granulation tissue and young adhesions are vascular, the resulting hemorrhage and exudate provide the basis for re-formation. When they are avascular, there is little tendency to recurrence. Choosing the right time is a clinical decision, the main criteria being localization of swelling and tenderness and minimal reaction to limited activity or physical provocation.

After-care is most important. Physical therapy and exercise after manipulation are designed to promote the absorption of any reactionary exudate and to maintain the range of movement gained. Excessive reaction denotes bad timing of the procedure. The knee should be rested and the manipulation repeated at a more suitable time. Postoperative care is the same as that after operation for the "dashboard knee."

The following case reveals some of these features: A boy of 17 taking a broad jump landed on the outer side of the right foot and injured his knee. He suffered a painful internal derangement and was unable to take weight on the knee which rapidly became distended. After admission to a hospital, the hemarthrosis was aspirated, but the surgeon was unable to reduce a "locked" knee. A few days later he performed an arthrotomy and reported a ruptured anterior cruciate ligament but no injury to the menisci. Postoperatively full extension of the knee was not recovered. The patient suffered continuous disability with intermittent exacerbations, when aspiration and splinting with no weight-bearing were necessary.

A year after the original accident a severe and painful swelling necessitated admission to another hospital. The knee was severely distended and after aspiration still showed 10 degrees limitation of extension. Flexion was possible through 50 degrees, i.e., from 170 to 120 degrees, but both lateral and medial rotation were completely fixed. All the "rotation signs" were positive. The anterior half of the medial meniscus was tender.

At operation it was evident that both the anterior cruciate and the medial meniscus had been disrupted from their attachments to the tibia and to each other. The meniscus had retracted, leaving a gap of ½ inch, and the anterior half had subsequently become adherent to the tibia. Immediately the meniscus was excised, full movement of the knee was possible. His convalescence was comfortable and benign, and he recovered a normally functioning knee.

This story illustrates dramatically the restriction of all movements when a point in the rotator mechanism of the knee is firmly tethered. As soon as the brake is released, both flexion and extension are recovered.

RHEUMATOID AND SEPTIC ARTHRITIS

All the components of the knee joint are involved in the inflammatory connective tissue reactions to rheumatoid and septic arthritis. As a consequence the synovium is fibrotic, the menisci and the fat pad become fixed to the tibia, and adhesions form between the articular surfaces.

It was common practice when the articular surfaces are destroyed to arthrodese the knee. A comfortable rigid limb was the result. When the inactive phase of the disease is reached, as the joint is relatively insensitive, and if destruction of joint surface is not gross, a more useful knee may be obtained after partial synovectomy, excision of both menisci, and freeing of the fat pad. Thirty to 60 degrees of comfortable movement has been recovered by this procedure. If the extremes of this range are not forced the patient walks with short steps but with confidence, especially after an effort is made to recover muscle power. As long as movement is painless this range, even though limited, has a distinct advantage over the arthrodesed joint and is especially worthwhile when the other knee is affected. It is easier to sit and dress, and the patients are content if able to walk to a car and to drive (see Chap. 14).

In recent years new techniques of arthroplasty have evolved, with increasing success. Following the progress in hip replacement, we have graduated from interposition of soft tissue and foreign materials through partial to total joint replacement. But special problems in the knee present more difficulties and a comparable level of success has not yet been achieved. However, as reported in Chapter 20, from the more advanced prostheses in experienced hands as much as 90 degrees of painless and stable movement may be expected. Instead of the stiff knee which in older patients is a serious handicap

there is promise of enough function to carry, to comfort, and to supplicate, if not yet to propel.

The perfect knee replacement device would have the following characteristics:

1. Replace normal movement or at least 120 degrees of flexion with approximately 13 degrees of synchronous rotation. It is not necessary to restore or replace the anatomy if a smaller and less cumbersome insert will reproduce normal function.

2. Have provision for joint stability inherent in its design and independent of the cruciate ligaments.

3. Be inserted with minimal removal of articular surface. This ensures that if it fails or loosens, it may be changed, or as a final resort the joint may be salvaged by arthrodesis.

4. Be of durable materials that articulate with minimal friction.

5. Be technically simple to insert.

6. Permit retention of the patella.

BIBLIOGRAPHY

1. Balazs, E. A., and Rydell, N. W.: Effect of hyaluronic acid on adhesion formation. (In press.)
2. Bennett, G. E.: Preliminary report of lengthening of the quadriceps tendon. J. Orthop. Surg., *1*:530, 1919.
3. ———: Lengthening of the quadriceps tendon. J. Bone Joint Surg., *4*:279, 1922.
4. Charnley, J.: The Closed Treatment of Common Fractures. London, Livingstone, 1957.
5. Jones, Sir Robert: Notes on Military Orthopaedics. London, Cassell, 1918.
6. Thompson, T. C.: Quadricepsplasty to improve knee function. J. Bone Joint Surg., *26*:366, 1944.

20

Engineering Principles of Knee Prostheses

Peter S. Walker, Ph.D.

Treating the arthritic knee so that there is relief of pain and restoration of function presents a difficult problem to the orthopedic surgeon. However, the variety of pathological conditions and the severity of the disease would indicate several different treatments. The major problem is often complete loss of cartilage in the femorotibial articulation, but in addition there can be instability due to bone and ligament destruction. Treatment of these problems by some type of prosthesis has been practiced for many years. Femoral molds have been used to present a smooth gliding surface to the tibia, but the results have been variable due in part to the difficulty of achieving geometric compatibility within the joint. The tibial plateau prostheses, such as the MacIntosh, have achieved some success, probably by providing a smooth tibial bearing surface and by increasing stability due to tightening of the joint. Various types of hinge prosthesis have been used to restore stability, particularly in cases of severe knee destruction. The hinges have not been without their problems however. Postoperatively, infection or delayed wound healing has occurred, and in the long run, there has been chronic

infection and symptomatic loosening of the prosthesis. Another feature of the hinges is that 3 or 4 cm. of bone usually have to be removed to permit their insertion, an obvious disadvantage if a revision operation becomes necessary. In recent years, new designs of total knee prostheses have been introduced that promise to improve on the previous designs. Firstly, there are the condylar replacement types which provide artificial bearing surfaces for the femoral and tibial condyles. A significant advantage of the condylar prostheses is that only about 2 cm. of bone is removed to insert them. In addition the components themselves are not bulky, and intermedullary stems are not used for fixation. On the other hand, the stability that the condylar replacements can provide is limited, so their main indication is for the treatment of arthritis without instability. To deal with the problem of instability, new concepts of hinge prostheses are emerging which seek to reduce the amount of bone removal needed and which allow more freedom of motion than is provided by a single axis fixed hinge.

Because of the emergence of new types of prosthesis, it is important to analyze the various factors of design. The device should be as small as possible, to reduce the amount of tissue removal and to minimize the volume of foreign material introduced. The shape is important for ease of surgery and for achieving natural function, particularly with the condylar replacement prostheses. The

Many of the studies relate to collaborative work at the Hospital for Special Surgery, in New York. The contributions of the following are particularly recognised: H. Shoji, M.D., C. Ranawat, M.D., J. N. Insall, M.D., M. J. Erkman, J. Behrens, B.S., and Y. Masse, M.D. (Hopital Cochin, Paris). Designers of knee prostheses are thanked for permission to publish information.

correct amount of stability should be provided and allowance made for motion in planes other than the lateral. For long-term success, there are several criteria. Highly stressed areas on the prosthesis must be avoided, because this could eventually result in a fatigue breakage. The forces should be transmitted to the bone as evenly as possible, avoiding any stress concentrations. Finally, wear of the components should be reduced as much as possible by the correct design and choice of materials. In order for a prothesis to satisfy these conditions, it must follow the mechanics of the normal knee. In the following sections, mechanical factors of the knee will be described,

and their implications to prosthesis design discussed.

MECHANICAL TERMINOLOGY AND CONCEPTS

Figure 20-1 illustrates basic mechanical concepts which are related to the knee joint. As a reference to describe the motion and the forces, orthogonal axes X, Y, and Z are drawn. Abduction and adduction occur about the X-axis, rotation about the Y-axis, and flexion-extension about the Z-axis. Anterior-posterior drawer is linear movement along the X-axis. In the lateral XY plane, if the femur flexes through a small

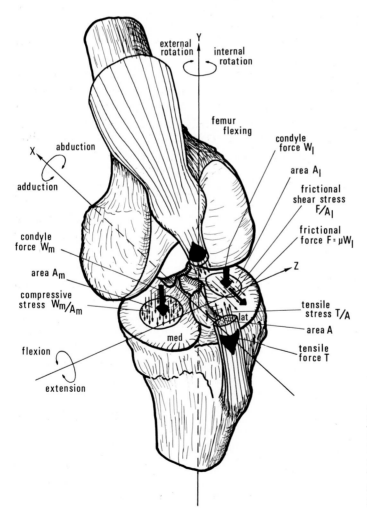

Fig. 20-1. Some mechanical principles of the knee joint. Orthogonal axes X, Y, and Z are drawn with respect to the tibia, and forces and motions described relative to these axes. Tensile, compressive, and shear stresses are illustrated.

angular range, then a point can be located about which the femur rotates relative to the tibia. This point is termed the instant center of rotation, and since the instant center will change constantly as the knee moves, the locus of its path can be used to describe the motion.

The forces and moments acting at the joint result in stresses on the various structures. The force (T) in the extensor tendon of area (A) sets up a tensile stress, T/A. The load on the condyles compresses the cartilage to form areas of contact A_m and A_l in the medial and lateral compartments, with compressive stresses of W_m/A_m and W_l/A_l. When there is sliding between the condyles, shear stresses are developed due to friction, their magnitude given by the frictional force (F) divided by area A. The force F itself is related to the vertical (normal) force by the coefficient of friction μ: $F = \mu W$. In human joints μ is very small, usually about 0.01, but it can be 0.05 to 0.15 in artificial joints.

Laxity in the knee is necessary for obtaining a free range of motion, but flexibility at the extremities is also important. Flexibility is related to tension or compression of the knee structures, the amount of flexibility

depending on Young's modulus of elasticity (E) of the materials concerned. E is defined as $\dfrac{\text{stress}}{\text{strain}}$, where strain is $\dfrac{\text{deflection}}{\text{original length}}$. Ligament, tendon, cartilage, and skin are strain stiffening, which means that E increases with strain, but cartilage is also strongly viscoelastic in that its deflection is very time-dependent.

MECHANICS OF THE NORMAL KNEE

The predominant rotational movement in the knee is in the lateral XY plane. A normal knee flexes to about 150 degrees although this facility is not extensively utilized. Assuming a sitting position in a chair normally requires about 110 degrees of flexion, unless the arms are used assistively. During level walking, maximum flexion is 70 degrees,[9,14] whilst in ascending or descending stairs, nearly 100 degrees of flexion can be realized.[14] Passive rotation of the femur on the tibia about the Y-axis (transverse rotation) increases as the flexion angle is increased, and although only a few degrees at full extension, it commonly reaches 30 degrees at mid-flexion. Walking is characterized by phasic internal and external

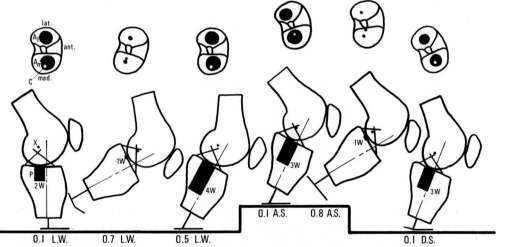

FIG. 20-2. The knee at various phases of level walking (*L.W.*) ascending stairs (*A.S.*) and descending stairs (*D.S.*). The stance phase is 0.0 to 0.6 of the full cycle and the swing phase is 0.6 to 1.0. Instant center of rotation in the lateral plane (*X*) and in the transverse plane (*C*); internal and external rotation; joint force (*P*) as a factor of body weight (*W*); and contact areas on the condyles (A_l and A_m) are shown.

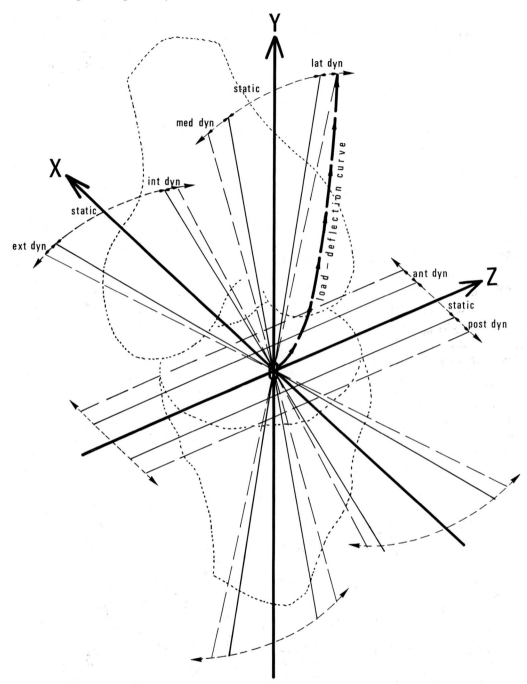

FIG. 20-3. Laxity and flexibility of the knee are expressed as static laxity and dynamic laxity. Lateral laxity, vertical transverse rotation, and anterior-posterior drawer are illustrated. The shape of the load deflection graph shows the tightening of the joint at an extremity.

rotation, averaging about 13 degrees for normal subjects.[9] In walking, one complete cycle is divided into two phases, the stance phase, which begins at heel-strike and ends at toe-off, and the swing phase, which begins at toe-off and ends at heel-strike. The stance phase is normally about 60 per cent of the cycle and the swing phase, 40 per cent. The highest vertical forces on the joint occur just after heel-strike, of 2 or 3 times body weight, and just before toe-off, of 3 to 4 times body weight.[11] Forces in ascending or descending stairs are 12 to 25 per cent higher than those for level walking. Figure 20-2 illustrates the forces in relation to flexion angle for the three activities discussed. In walking, the peak forces at 10 and 50 per cent of the cycle occur at about 25 degrees of flexion, whereas in ascending or descending stairs, there are force peaks at flexion angles up to about 80 degrees.[11,14] Also shown in Figure 20-2 are the contact areas on the articular cartilage surfaces. At

twice body weight, areas were measured in vitro to be 1.8 cm.[2] and 1.4 cm.[2] on the medial and lateral condyles respectively.[15] Extrapolation from this data using elasticity theory indicates areas of about 2.5 cm.[2] at the load peaks. The lateral views of Figure 20-2 show the positions of the instant centers of rotation. Although there is considerable variation of the instant center paths, the locus tends to move downwards and posteriorly as flexion proceeds. The average instant center coordinates with respect to the X and Y axes (Fig. 20-1) were X = 1.6 cm. and Y = 1.8 cm.[16] The location of the instant center for rotation about the Y-axis is uncertain, though it appears to be medial and to move towards the center as the knee is flexed.

Laxity and flexibility were mentioned earlier as being important features of normal knee function. Figure 20-3 illustrates these concepts in terms of static laxity and dynamic laxity. If a force is gradually applied

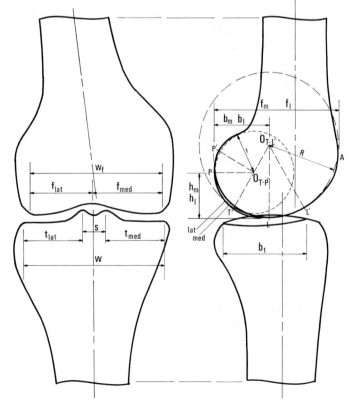

FIG. 20-4. A system for dimensionally describing the knee from radiographs. The dimensions marked on the anteroposterior view are self-explanatory. On the lateral view P, A, and L are at the posterior, anterior, and lower aspects, respectively; f_m and f_l denote the anterioposterior width from P to A for the medial and lateral condyles respectively; b_m and b_l denote the anterioposterior distance from P to L of the medial and lateral condyles respectively; h_m and h_l are the vertical height between L and P of the medial and lateral condyles. The lateral outline of the femoral condyles can be closely described by the arcs of two circles as shown. The two arcs sweep L' to T from 0° to 30° flexion, and T to P' from 30° to 120° flexion.

to the knee, there will a large initial displacement with little resistance, after which progressively higher forces will be needed for further displacement. The load-deflection graph of Figure 20-3 clarifies the behavior. The initial displacement is static laxity, and the further displacement in response to a defined maximum force is dynamic laxity. Measurements of laxity have been carried out in vitro under cyclic loading conditions at 0 degrees flexion. For example, at 0 degrees flexion, when static and dynamic moments of 6 and 150 kg./cm. were applied, the static rotation was 11.5 degrees, dynamic external rotation was 3.7 degrees, and dynamic internal rotation was 2.3 degrees.

Even in this brief discussion of knee mechanics, the variety of motions and forces and the complex kinematic and elastic response of the knee have become apparent. If a prosthesis only partially replaces the knee structures, as a condylar replacement does, then it must act in harmony with the existing structures. This was well illustrated by the abnormal mechanics of knees with meniscal injuries.[4] If the prosthesis is a radical replacement, such as a hinge, it must allow the musculature to function correctly and provide a good range of motion. The mechanical factors that specifically relate to prosthesis design will now be discussed in more detail.

SHAPE AND DIMENSIONS OF THE PROSTHESIS

Some dimensional description must be given to the knee to allow the rational choice of size and shape of a prosthesis. Figure 20-4 shows dimensions that can be obtained from radiographs, or from cadavers. If a large number of knees are measured, a given dimension typically shows a Gaussian distribution. In one study, the width of the femoral condyles was chosen as a reference, and other dimensions related to this.[12] Average dimensions obtained were approximately $w_f = 8.0$ cm. and $f_m = f_l = 7.1$ cm., whilst in another study at our laboratories, average dimensions were about 10 per cent lower

than these. Different knees were found to be reasonably proportional. It was interesting that the knee was symmetrical in some respects. For instance the following pairs of dimensions were closely equal: f_{lat} and f_{med}, f_m and f_l, h_m and h_l. Also, t_{lat} and b_m were only about 10 per cent greater than t_{med} and b_l respectively. In the design of condylar replacement prostheses the normal lateral outline of the femoral condyles should be closely reproduced to allow a full range of motion and to preserve the correct lengths of the cruciate and collateral ligaments. Of many geometrical descriptions possible, it is found that two circular arcs describe the shape almost exactly (Fig. 20-4) whilst a portion of an ellipse is also very accurate.

Another shape consideration for condylar prostheses is the curvature of the tibial spines with which the inner femoral condyles conform. The functional importance of this can be confirmed by studying the location of the areas of contact in load-bearing (Fig. 20-2).[15] The spines will control rotational laxity of the joint by distracting the joint as rotation occurs and by tightening the ligaments. Lateral subluxation will also be checked by a similar mechanism.

ROTATIONAL AXES

As discussed previously, the lateral instant center of the knee changes as the knee is flexed, but a normal pattern cannot be readily defined due to variations. In the case of condylar replacement prostheses, the knee will find its own rotational axis. However, a balance must be sought between how much the prosthesis allows the passive soft structures and the musculature to guide the motion, and how much the prosthesis actually guides the motion itself. Ideally, the prosthesis should act in the same way as the normal joint condyles themselves. However in a prosthesis designed to provide full stability, some axis of rotation must be inherent in the prosthesis itself. In the case of a simple hinge, the axis should be in the most advantageous position to approximate normal motion. Figure 20-5 shows the

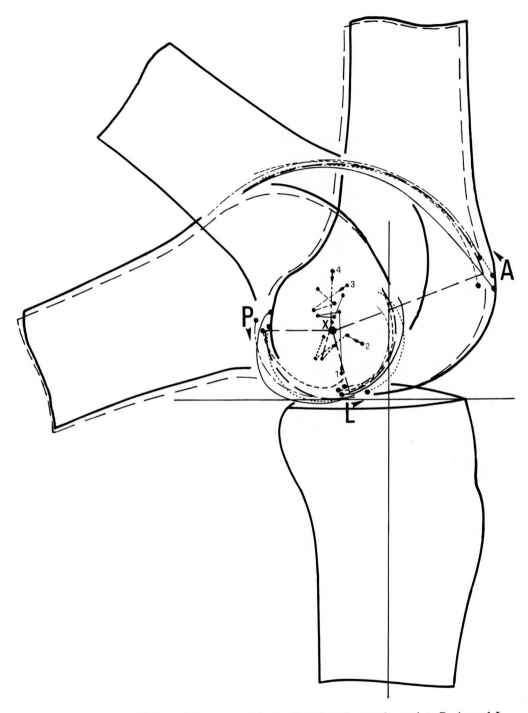

Fig. 20.5. The flexion of four normal knees described by tracing points P, A, and L on the femur relative to the tibia. The loci of the instant centers of rotation are plotted for each knee, and the differences are apparent. X is the 'average instant center' and if the paths of P, A, and L are traced about the fixed point X, the result is close to the normal.

motion of four normal knees, described by the motion of P, A, and L on the femur, and the instant centers of rotation. The paths of P, A, and L are close together, but the instant center loci deviate significantly. This paradox has been explained as the integrating effect of the motion of points in relation to the instant centers.[5] In consequence, if a point X is chosen at the center of the instant center loci, and the paths of P, A, and L are drawn with X as center, these paths are found to lie very close to the normal paths. This means that a fixed axis can provide accurate knee motion, but there is a stringent condition to this, illustrated by Figure 20-6. With respect to the ideal position for the fixed axis X, four other axes are selected deviating only 5 mm. in orthogonal directions. The heavy outlines of the femur are those of the normal knees

of Figure 20-5, and are compatible with the axis X. The four dashed outlines show the positions the femur would assume if it were correct in the 0-degree position and rotated to 90 degrees flexion about axes 1, 2, 3, or 4. Four types of abnormality of motion result: impingement of the posterior femoral condyles on the tibia; distraction of the femur from the tibia; anterior displacement of the femur; and posterior displacement of the femur. Each of the four axes display two of these abnormalities. The overall conclusion is that a fixed axis of rotation can produce normal motion in a lateral plane, but only if it is located very accurately.

Providing rotation about the vertical Y-axis is a difficult problem in prosthesis design. Two possibilities are to guide the motion by assuming some relation between flexion angle and rotational angle, and to

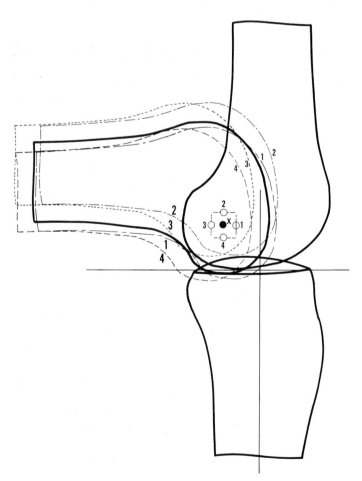

FIG. 20-6. If a fixed axis of rotation is chosen that deviates from X by only a few millimeters, significant distortions in motion occur. The femur is taken to be correct at 0°, and the outlines 1, 2, 3, and 4 are drawn at 90° flexion with respect to corresponding axes.

simply allow some static rotational laxity so that the knee can choose its own position. The difficulty of the former is that large variations occur depending upon the activity, so that a guided motion must at best be a compromise. However if there is no provision whatsoever for rotation, high torsional forces will be imposed on the prosthesis which could, in the long run, adversely affect fixation between the prosthesis and the bone.

FORCES ACTING ON THE PROSTHESIS

The magnitude of the forces imposed during normal activities has been described, and the prosthesis must withstand some or all of these forces. Ideally, the prosthesis should transmit the forces to the bone to restore the stresses that would occur normally. The condylar replacement types satisfy this to a large extent if the components are located against the condylar surfaces. However, the ability of the bone to withstand normal stresses may be impaired due to the disease. In normal joints, at three times body weight, with a contact area of 2 cm.^{2} on each condyle, the stresses on the bone will be about 50 kg./cm.^{2} This is transmitted by the underlying trabecular bone to the cortical walls. Normal trabecular bone is strong enough to accomplish this, but for diseased trabecular bone this may not be the case. Figure 20-7 shows three examples of trabecular pattern, one normal and two abnormal. The normal bone has a compressive strength of 140 kg./cm.^{2}, whilst the diseased trabecular structures have strengths of only 45 and 19 kg./cm.^{2} Therefore if a condylar prosthesis is to be used in joints with weak bone, the design must spread the load over a larger area than normal to prevent compressive failure of the bone. The situation should, of course, be alleviated in time by bone remodelling.

As well as being physiologically desirable, transmitting stresses to the bone in a nearly normal way can also reduce stresses on the prosthesis and on the fixation. For example when the tibial plateaus are supported flat

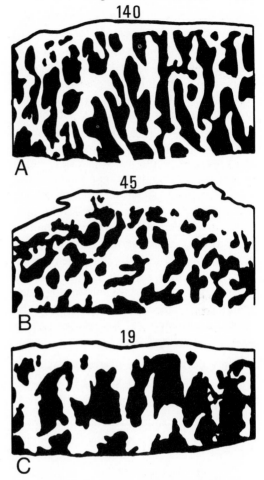

FIG. 20-7. The trabecular pattern of bone close to the surface of the condyles, showing the relative compressive strength in kg./cm.^{2}. (*A*) normal femoral condyles, (*B, C*) rheumatoid arthritis, tibial condyles.

on the underlying bone, they will carry mainly compressive stresses, and the same applies to securely attached artificial femoral condyles. However, in the hinge prostheses a great deal of reliance is placed on the intermedullary stems for stabilization, particularly when high loads occur at large flexion angles. In the latter case, the stem of the femoral component is subjected to a very high bending moment. This can perhaps be appreciated from Figure 20-8, which shows the forces in relation to their directions for the activities of walking, ascending, and descending stairs.

Data like those in Figure 20-8 should form the basis for a test program for any design of knee prosthesis. No matter how carefully a design may have been prepared, the complication of the prosthesis-bone system is such that realistic testing in vitro should precede human application. A suitable test might be carried out on a prosthesis that had been attached to a cadaver knee under mock surgical conditions. The testing should include the force and motion patterns shown, and strain gauges should be used to measure the stresses at strategic points on the prosthesis. In addition to normal forces, rotational forces occur,[11] which should be incorporated in the testing. The test environment should be at body temperature in a saline solution. By utilizing this system of testing, data would be obtained of the strength of the device, the strength of the fixation, and the wear of the components.

EXAMPLES OF PROSTHESES CURRENTLY USED

Condylar Replacement Types

The present condylar replacement prostheses use a femoral component of stainless steel or cobalt-chrome alloy and a plastic tibial component of ultra-high-molecular-weight polyethylene. In some designs there are separate parts for each condylar surface; in other designs, the femoral condyles and the tibial condyles are joined by anterior bridges. Greater versatility is provided by having separate pieces, but the surgery is slightly more involved. Other differences in the condylar prostheses are the amount of stability provided and the degree of conformity between femoral and tibial components. High conformity will decrease contact stresses, but may increase abrasive wear by retention of wear debris. Low conformity, on the other hand, will increase contact stresses, perhaps inducing fatigue wear, but abrasive wear will be reduced.

One of the first condylar prostheses used metal half-discs fitting into slots cut into the posterior femoral condyles and plastic runners fitting into slots in the upper tibia.[7] Replacement of only the surfaces over the load-bearing arcs of the femur and tibia was emphasized, and the design allowed a "polycentric" motion. The disadvantage of this prosthesis is that the parts are narrow so

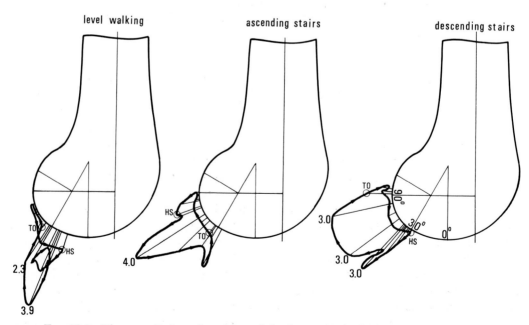

Fig. 20-8. The magnitude and position of the forces on the femur are shown for level walking, ascending stairs, and descending stairs. The force pattern for one walking cycle is visualized by starting at HS (heel strike), moving to TO (toe off), and returning to HS.

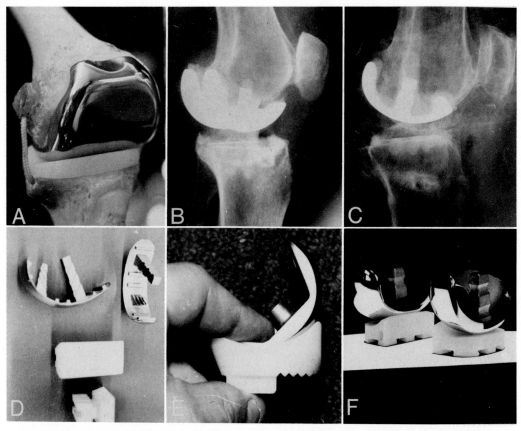

Fig. 20-9. Condylar replacement prostheses in current use: (*A*) Freeman-Swanson, (Imperial College, London); (*B*) geomedic (Howmedica, Inc.); (*C*) unicondylar (Hospital for Special Surgery); (*D*) Sledge[2]; (*E*) geomedic; and (*F*) Duocondylar (Hospital for Special Surgery).

that stresses are high and stability is reduced. More recent condylar designs have tended to increase the area of the components, as in the Sledge prosthesis (Fig. 20-9D).[2] Here the femoral component is cemented over the condyles, and the lateral outline of the femoral condyles has been reproduced. The plastic tibial plateaus are flat, which gives freedom of motion but provides no stability. The duo-condylar (Fig. 20-9F) and the uni-condylar (Fig. 20-9C) are, respectively, for the replacement of the bearing surfaces in both joint compartments or in one. As in the Sledge design, the shape of the femoral condyles is reproduced, but tibial spines are provided that match the inner curvature on the femoral component giving some rotational stability. The Geo-

medic design[1] (Figs. 20-9B and E) provides some anterior-posterior stability as well as rotational stability, and stability is reduced with flexion as in the normal knee joint. The robust construction of this prosthesis reduces contact stresses on the plastic, and reduces stresses in the device as a whole. Disadvantages are that the outline of the femoral condyles is a circular arc, and range of motion beyond 90 degrees flexion is not well provided for. All the prostheses described so far allow for preservation of the cruciate ligaments. The Freeman-Swanson prosthesis[3] (Fig. 20-9A) requires sacrifice of the cruciates but in return gives anterior-posterior and rotational stability. There are large bearing areas between the metal femoral component and the plastic tibial

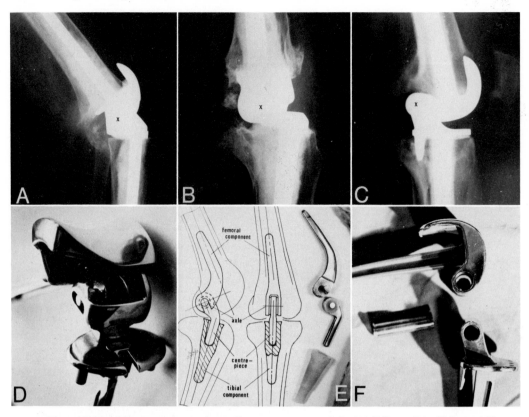

FIG. 20-10. Hinge-type prostheses in current use: (*A*) Walldius; (*B*) Shiers; (*C*) Guepar (Cochin, Paris); (*D*) Trillat-Bousquet (Lyons, France); (*E*) stabilizer (Hospital for Special Surgery, experimental only); (*F*) Guépar.

component which should minimize bearing stresses and also reduce the stresses on the underlying bone.

Experience will show which of the various features of the condylar prostheses is beneficial and more exact indications for this type of reconstruction. It is probable however that the condylar replacement principle will enjoy a very wide application, particularly in the treatment of arthritis with only mild instability.

Hinge Types

The earliest types of hinge have been in use for many years, the Walldius[17] (Fig. 20-10A) and the Shiers[13] (Fig. 20-10B) being perhaps the best known. The large amount of bone needed for their insertion is not only undesirable in the case of a revision operation, but is also a disadvantage

at the time of operation. This is because the geography of the joint is lost, and if the prosthesis is incorrectly placed, the mechanics of the knee will be distorted (Fig. 20-6). Also, the axes of the hinges have perhaps not been positioned to be consistent with a full range of motion and with a sufficient lever arm for the quadriceps muscle. A hinge prosthesis which has been introduced comparatively recently is the Guépar (Figs.) 20-10C and 20-10F). This does not require quite so much bone resection as the previous hinges, and the axis of rotation is placed close to the ideal axis position described in Figure 20-5. Also, the high forces imposed at large flexion angles are not transmitted entirely to the stem, owing to the partial containment of the distal femur by the prosthesis. An ingenious device that uses a cam arrangement to provide internal and external rotation has been designed by Trillat and Bousquet (Fig. 20-10D). The rotation is made to progressively increase with flexion angle as in the normal joint. The prosthesis is also preassembled, which simplifies the surgery. One disadvantage of the device, however, is that a large amount of bone is needed for its insertion. Several attempts have been made to resolve the bone resection problem by utilizing the intercondylar notch for location of the prosthesis. This is indeed feasible, because the ideal axis of rotation of the knee (Fig. 20-5) does in fact pass through this region. Lagrange and Letournel[10] use a plastic box about 4 cm. wide embedded in the femoral condyles, which is supported on a metal mallet, attached to a stem within the tibia. An even narrower device measuring only about 3 cm. in width was described by Herbert.[8] This device, like that of Trillat-Bousquet, allows rotational freedom with locking at full extension, which is achieved by an elegant geometrical arrangement of a ball in a cage. An experimental device called the stabilizer (Fig. 20-10E), again fitting in the intercondylar notch, has been shown to give very successful results in animals. Closely correct motion was achieved and full load-bearing was obtained. However, devices that remove the forces from the femoral and tibial condyles and transmit them to the cortical wall through intermedullary stems may be fundamentally incorrect. This, together with the points made earlier about stress transmission to the condyles, may, in the long run, be an important one. Remodelling of the bone due to an unnatural stress pattern, with attendant changes in blood supply, may result in eventual failure of fixation due to structural changes in the bone.

In conclusion, it could be said that there are encouraging trends in the design of prostheses to provide better treatments for the arthritic knee. This is certainly borne out by the short-term results obtained with the recent condylar and hinge designs, and within the next few years it is likely that the experience gained will show the desirable features of the different devices and the indications for each type. In addition, the long-term problems of fixation and of wear may well be ameliorated by the emergence of new materials.

REFERENCES

1. Coventry, M. B., Riley, L. H., Turner, R. H., and Upshaw, J. E.: The geomedic knee replacement: technique and preliminary results in 100 cases. Congres Annuel de la Societe Belge de Chirurgie Orthopedique et de Traumatologie, Brussels, April 1972. Proceedings, Acta Orthopedica Belgica, in press.
2. Englebrecht, E.: The sledge prosthesis, a partial prosthesis for destructions of the knee. Der Chirurg, *11*:510, 1971.
3. Freeman, M. A. R., and Swanson, S. A. V.: Total prosthetic replacement of the knee: design considerations and early results. Congres Annuel de la Societe Belge de Chirurgie Orthopedique et de Traumatologie, Brussels, 22-23 April, 1972.
4. Frankel, V. H., Burstein, A. H., and Brooks, D. B.: Biomechanics of internal derangement of the knee. J. Bone Joint Surg., *53A*:945, 1971.
5. Freudenstein, F., and Woo, L. S.: Kinematics of the human knee joint. Bull. Math. Biophys., *31*:215, 1969.
6. Girzadas, D. V., Geens, S., Clayton, M. L., and Leidholt, J. D.: Performance of a hinged metal knee prosthesis. J. Bone Joint Surg., *50A*:355, 1968.
7. Gunston, F.: Polycentric knee arthroplasty. J. Bone Joint Surg., *53B*:272, 1971.
8. Herbert, J. J.: Nouvelle prothese totale du genou a pivot axial. Congres Annuel de la Societe Belge de Chirurgie Orthopedique et de Traumatologie, Brussels, 22-23 April, 1972.
9. Kettelkamp, D. B., Johnson, R. J., Smidt, G. L., Chao, E. Y. S., and Walker, M.: An electrogoniometric study of knee motion in normal gait. J. Bone Joint Surg., *52A*:775, 1970.
10. Lagrange, J., and Letournel, E.: Arthroplastie total du genou avec un nouveau modile de prosthese. Annales Orthopediques du l'Ouest, *3*:43, 1971.
11. Morrison, J. B.: Function of the knee joint

in various activities. Biomed. Eng., *3*:573, Dec., 1969.

12. Seedhom, B. B., Longton, E. B., Wright, V., and Dowson, D.: Dimensions of the knee. Ann. Rheum. Dis., *31*:54, 1972.

13. Shiers, L. G. P.: Arthroplasty of the knee. J. Bone Joint Surg., *42B*:31, 1960.

14. University of California, Berkeley, College of Engineering. Report to Nat. Res. Council, Committee on Artificial Limbs, Washington, D.C. by H. D. Eberhart & Associates. Fundamental studies on human locomotion and other information relating to the design of artificial limbs. Part 1.

15. Walker, P. S., and Hajek, J. V.: The load-bearing area in the knee joint. J. Biomech., *5*:581, 1972.

16. Walker, P. S., Shoji, H., and Erkman, M. J.: The rotational axis of the knee and its significance to prosthesis design. Clin. Orthop. Rel. Res., *89*:160, 1972.

17. Walldius, B.: Arthroplasty of the knee using an endoprosthesis. Acta Orthop. Scandinav., *30*:137, 1960.

21

Osteochondral Fractures of the Articular Surfaces of the Knee

Joseph E. Milgram, M.D.

Compared with meniscal derangements, osteochondral fractures occur relatively infrequently. However, they are by no means rare, and diagnosis is not particularly difficult. Early recognition permits prompt and often complete repair.

Osteochondral fractures of the knee result from direct application of external forces (impact, crush; impact shear) or indirect application of muscular and gravitational forces.

FRACTURE BY DIRECT INJURY

There are, to be sure, fractures of the articular surfaces that are sustained through direct injury, as in the knee struck a violent blow. Such fractures are often severe, for a whole condyle may be separated or crushed (Plate 21-1). The roentgenogram will point to the mechanism of injury–direct impact or extreme leverage.

They benefit in most instances from open accurate reposition and substantial metallic fixation (Plates 21-2, 21-3). Motion is subsequently commenced in bed with the limb suspended in a snugly fitted, hinged, long-leg plaster cast. This second plaster is applied 4 to 5 weeks after operation. Weight bearing is delayed until revascularization of bone underlying articular surfaces is judged complete.

FRACTURE BY INDIRECT FORCES

Such forces expressed through excessive ligamentous tensions produced by motion, gravity, or muscular contraction are common in athletics.

Indirect Fracture by Avulsion

A typical avulsion of the anterior crucial ligament may carry off with it a large osteochondral portion of the articular surface of the tibia including the tibial spines. Such a segment when fastened back securely into its tibial defect by a long screw—or better by an encircling wire suture that passes through two drill channels from the anterior tibial cortex and with the leg subsequently adequately immobilized in a plaster cast, usually heals well. The bony cortex unites, and the narrow clefts fill with fibrocartilage, restoring both articular and ligamentous function.

Condyle–Tibial Spine Contact After Tibial Avulsion

Yet in just such a lesion in a 10-year-old boy, after accurate replacement and securely retained screw fixation of the articular segment and tibial spines, there developed, with growth, a gradual local enlargement of both tibial spines. Seven years later it was found that the enlarged medial tibial spine was now contacting the medial femoral condyle and had created a large condylar lesion containing a free body. Roentgenographic studies clearly revealed contact was made when the knee was in slight flexion and abduction of the leg or when the patient pivoted on the knee with the foot fixed on the ground (Plate 21-4). Normal adolescents may mani-

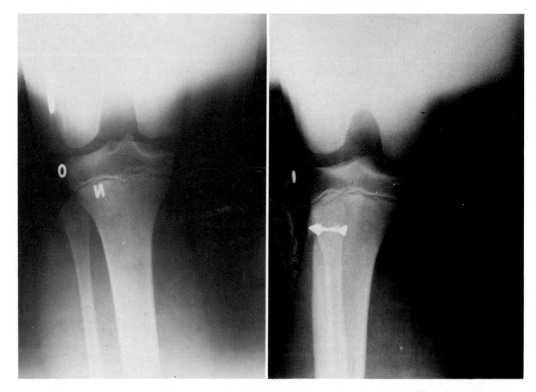

Fig. 21-1. An 11-year-old normal female seated, leg hanging over table edge with a curved cardboard cassette underneath knee and leg: (*left*) anteroposterior view. (*Right*) On passive external rotation of the leg, fibular position measures the degree of rotation of the leg on the fixed femur.

fest surprising rotational ranges (Fig. 21-1).

In a normal cadaver's knee, experimentally produced contact between tibial spine and lateral surface of the medial femoral condyle was demonstrated by implantation of a series of electrical contacts flush with these two areas and rotating the femur inward in slight flexion and abduction. When rotated the circuit was completed, and a light in the series circuit regularly flashed on contact (Fig. 21-2).

Condyle–spine contact is certainly the cause of so-called osteochondritis dissecans in some patients. It has been blamed repeatedly by older authors, and correctly so in certain cases, such as the special example related above. In six other osteochondritis dissecans lesions occurring in our patients with no similar gross enlargement of the tibial spines, contact was suggested on X-ray studies during rotatory knee motions.

Patellar Marginal Avulsions, Muscular or Tendinous

Avulsion lesions of the cortical margins of the patella may require oblique and tangential roentgenograms of both knees for diagnosis and may need local excision if immobilization fails to relieve pain. Occasionally avulsion includes portions of the articular cartilage. Then bony reduction and open fixation may offer a desirable reattachment of quadriceps or ligamentum patellae.

OSTEOCHONDRAL FRACTURES BY PATELLAR IMPACT

Osteochondral fractures of the knee are not uncommon and as a rule are sustained by adolescents or young adults. They are almost invariably the consequence of indirect injury, of apparently excessive forces devel-

Varieties of Indirect Osteochondral Fractures of the Knee

Fractures following spontaneous reduction of lateral dislocation of patella

1. Tangential osteochondral fracture of patella–acute.
2. Tangential chondral injury of patella and/or femoral groove for patella–recurrent.
3. Tangential osteochondral fracture of lateral femoral condyle–acute and recurrent.
4. Tangential compression fracture of lateral condylar wall–acute.

Fractures following tibiofemoral stresses

5. Cleft (or shell) osteochondral separation of femur (cartilage intact) initially–acute.
6. Osteochondral fracture (or erosion) (a) Following impingements of tibial spine, recurrent; some called "osteochondritis dissecans." (b) Meniscal lesion sequels.
7. Massive, pyramidal osteochondral fracture of medial femoral condyle–acute.
8. Posterior transcondylar fracture of medial femoral condyle–acute.
9. Posterior osteochondral fracture and irregular ossification of one or both femoral condyles.

Pathologic osteochondral fractures of known etiology

10. Osteochondral poststeroid fracture, medial femoral condyle.
11. Osteochondral poststeroid fracture, medial tibial condyle.
12. Osteochondral infraction, over subarticular area of cancellous weakening of many etiologies, local and general.

Pathologic osteochondral fractures of unknown etiology

13. Occasional varieties of osteochondritis dissecans in areas seemingly removed from likely trauma (cf. 6).

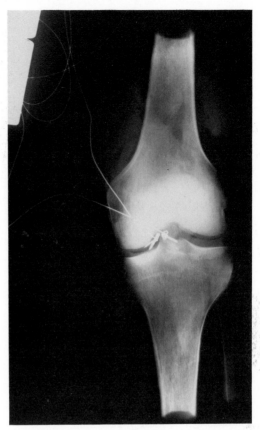

Fig. 21-2. Anatomic specimen in which electrical contacts installed flush with the surface of the medial tibial spine and adjacent condyle, repeatedly demonstrated that electrical contact was completed when tibia rotated and abducted in the position of slight flexion of the knee.

oped by a twist of the knee either in the erect or the flexed position, during the course of violent athletics or energetic dancing. Most of the patients are limber and supple but otherwise normal. Rarely does a history of either previous knee disability or substantial injury exist.

Kroner,[5] in 1904, reported the case of a 31-year-old woman who fell running and sustained a vertical frontal fracture of the patella.[5] The entire patella split into two frontal sections during a lateral dislocation. Subsequently, an "oyster shell fracture" was described by Villar in 1921.[14] "Verticofrontal fractures" were reported by Kleinberg[4] in 1923 and Lettloff in 1928.[6] Kleinberg suggested that a fall on the knee, forcing patella downward against femur could shove or scrape off part of the articular surface, and

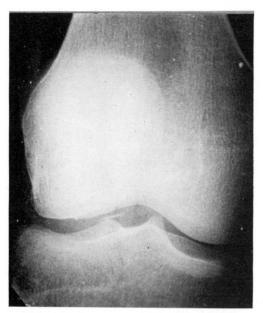

FIG. 21-3. Preoperative roentgenogram: a pencil line of fragment of cortex is visible at the tibial spine.

later he described a lateral dislocation of the patella without fracture in which the medial border of the patella remained caught for 5 days on the femoral condyle.

The term tangential osteochondral fracture of the patella was introduced by Milgram[7] in 1943 to describe the nature of the forces involved in the mechanism of production of patellofemoral articular injuries [8]

Tangential Mechanism of Fracture

As the knee is extended with the foot off the ground, the tibia rotates externally on the femur (see Chap. 1.). If the foot is fixed on the ground, the tibia is fixed and the femur rotates. It rotates internally as the knee extends, bringing the lateral condyle anteriorly. If at this moment the quadriceps has contracted, it holds the patella while the lateral condyle glides internally beneath the patella. In relaxed knees the lateral condyle passes completely medial to the patella. As the quadriceps continues to tighten, the medial edge of the patellar articular surface engages the lateral articular edge of the lat-

eral condyle of the femur. The patella is now momentarily fixed in the position of lateral dislocation. The exact area of engagement of the contiguous articular surfaces of the patella and the femoral condyle depends on the position of the knee in which the engagement has taken place.

As a rule, the accident occurs when the foot is fixed on the ground while the thigh twists or pivots medially on the fixed tibia. As the great quadriceps contracts, further extension of the knee is impeded by the fixed foot. Consequently, all of the quadriceps force is transformed into a medially directed force (tangential) that shoves the dislocated patella against the edge, the lateral wall, or the articular distal surface of the lateral condyle, depending on the degree of knee flexion.

The osteochondral separations result from this forcible impact of the dislocated patella on the lateral femoral condyle as the patella forcibly reduces itself from its lateral position. In other words, the patellar "hammer" may break in striking a glancing blow against the "anvil" of the lateral femoral condyle, thus creating a patellar osteochondral free body. In other cases the anvil is chipped or even crushed by the patellar hammer wielded by the powerful quadriceps.

Aside from these major and violent injuries, more subtle but also lasting damage may be inflicted on the patella and the lateral femoral condyle. The articular cartilage of the patella may be abraded, contused, split at the margins, or separated from its bony bed over a large area without becoming completely dislodged. Such loosened cartilaginous areas may not heal securely and later may undergo degeneration—so-called chondromalacia. Therefore, it may be difficult in later months or years to distinguish the changes that follow a single trauma from those of cumulative character due to innumerable traumata caused by imperfect kinesiologic construction, e.g., the consequences of abnormal motion of the patella in congenital or recurrent subluxation and dislocation, or in back-knee, knock-knee or ligamentous instability.

Fig. 21-4. A free body, avulsed from normal cartilage and bone is characterized by the appearance of "palisading" (columnar lines of split cartilage are seen). In addition the appearance of "the chef's hat" is early present (an adherent rim of the tangential layer avulsed from adjacent normal articular cartilage).

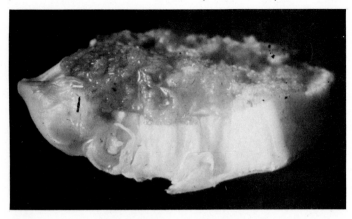

ACUTE LESIONS DUE TO PATELLOFEMORAL IMPACT

1. Tangential osteochondral fracture of patellar articular surface–free body comprising lower medial quadrant (Plate 21-5; Figs. 21-3, 4, 5, 6).

2. Chondral shredding (Fig. 21-5) or chondral separation from patella–small or giant blister (Fig. 21-5). "One-time" chondromalacia, Koenig. (See Fig. 21-18).

3. Tangential osteochondral fracture of lateral femoral condyle

    A. Large thin curved free body or bodies, much cartilage, usually little bone (Figs. 21-7, 8 to 21-14; Plate 21-6).

    B. Compression fracture of lateral condylar wall–depressed, extruding part of articular surface of the lateral condyle as a hinged osteochondral segment (Figs. 21-15 to 21-20).

4. Reciprocal injuries to articular cartilage and opposing bone in the form of contusions, abrasions, and intracartilaginous hematomata (knee joint blood trapped between the peripheral tangential and the deeper columnar layers of cells of the articular cartilage) producing blood-stained cartilage that cannot be wiped clean at operation. It should be kept in mind that injuries to avascular articular cartilage which do not extend deeply enough to reach the vascular layer of the cortex simply do not repair themselves. Only the cartilage cleft that reaches blood will fill with clot which repairs by fibrocartilage which in time may resemble hyaline cartilage. Superficial cartilage abrasions and tabs will gradually break free, leaving damaged gliding surfaces. The most superficial layers of normal cartilage are tangentially disposed to facilitate gliding.

The Manner of Production of Osteochondral Fractures of the Patella

The histories elicited from adolescents who have sustained osteochondral fracture of the patella indicate that dislocation and osteochondral fracture of the patella both occur in the phase of active extension of the knee —*viz.*:

1. A young female dancer doing a "split" slowly sank toward the floor with both knees in full extension when two "tears" took place, "a noise accompanying the second tearing pain." The knee swelled at once, and operation revealed both the typical medial inferior quadrant defect of the patella and the lateral condylar scrape.

2. A skater swinging into a turn on an extended knee slid the skate into a deep linear fissure in the ice and twisted on the fixed limb. Just before he fell, he felt a break and heard a loud breaking sound, with instant severe pain. Operation performed a few days later confirmed the osteochondral loss of the medial inferior quadrant of the patella and an abraded lateral condyle of the femur.

3. A lad trying to reach a shower wall-control above his head while standing with legs spread widely, twisted and sustained instant disabling pain followed by immediate swelling. Still standing, he was assisted from the shower stall. Operation 2 days later confirmed similar lesions.

4. Another lad engaged in "Indian wrestling" with a comrade. As both stood with arms engaged, legs fully extended with feet

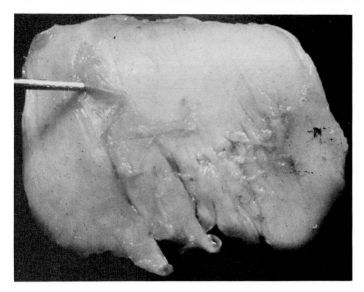

FIG. 21-5. Tangential forces have made glacial scratches in the body. The probe enters a cartilage blister.

widely separated, the patient twisted his knee forcibly, with instant disabling pain. Still standing, the knee extended, he was helped to a couch. The knee swelled rapidly, and operation soon after revealed the typical patellar loss and the condylar contusion.

As a rule, the patients suddenly stricken are flexible but not "double jointed" when surveyed later for evidence of joint hypermobility. Nor is there usually evidence of knock-knee or bowleg. Passive rotation of the flexed tibia on the femur seemed to be excessive in some patients but not in the majority.

Osteochondral Fractures in Recurrent Dislocation of Patella

Most instances of osteochondral fracture of the patella occurred in patients who had not suffered previous dislocation of the knee. However, three of our patients recorded a history of numerous painless subluxations or

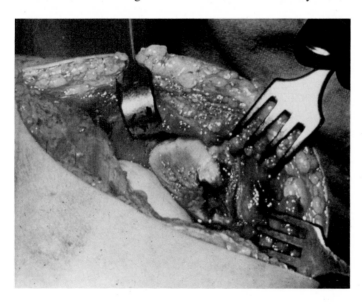

FIG. 21-6. Extensive acute tangential osteochondral fracture of the patella. Sole example in our series of a lesion so severe as to necessitate primary patellectomy.

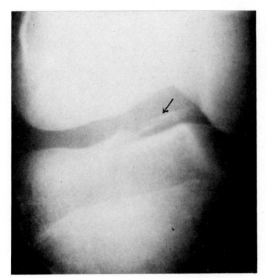

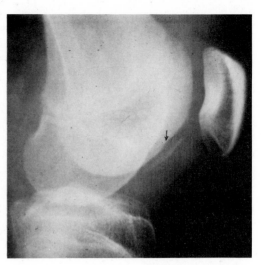

FIG. 21-7. This roentgenogram was made on admitting a patient with an osteochondral fracture of the lateral condyle made by impact of the patella. The double line of the fragment is visible on the anteroposterior view (*arrow*).

FIG. 21-8. Superficial defect is visible (*arrow*) on this lateral view of the lateral femoral condyle above a free fragment.

dislocations in the past. With these exceptions, no knee with fresh osteochondral fractures revealed at operation evidence of previous damage.

After recurrent dislocation of the patella, the lateral condyle of the femur and considerable areas of the patella may undergo degenerative changes characterized by softening and shredding (see Figs. 21-9 and 21-17).

Each of three adolescent females, after numerous lateral subluxations and dislocations during the course of many years, suddenly underwent a memorable episode in which very severe pain and a cracking sound accompanied the replacement of the dislocated patella. The knee at once distended with blood, and in two cases well-marked cutaneous linear hematomas which developed medial to the patella indicated medial capsule rupture. At the operations performed several months later, it was seen that osteochondral separation of the inferior quadrant of the medial surface of the patella had been sustained in each case. Also, the edge of the

lateral femoral condyle was fissured and abraded, the gliding condylar surface was lusterless, and the lateral synovia scarred. In each of the three the patellar loose body was removed. In two, medial capsular elongation of considerable degree was present. Subsequently, no pain or swelling was suffered, even though each patient resumed subluxation. Reparative reconstruction proferred later has not been accepted to date.

Case Histories of Tangential Osteochondral Fractures of the Lateral Femoral Condyle

Detailed histories of adolescents who sustained osteochondral fractures of the lateral femoral condyle indicate that possibly the patellar dislocation and certainly the femoral condylar fracture had occurred during the phase of considerable flexion of the knee, contrasting with the histories of fracture in extension obtained in cases of patellar tangential osteochondral fracture—*viz.*:

1. A 16-year-old boy was crouching in a football game when he was tackled as he lunged forward. He twisted his bent knee, sustained instant knee pain and disability

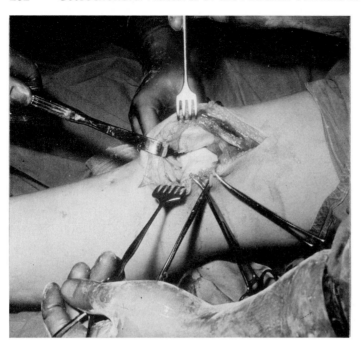

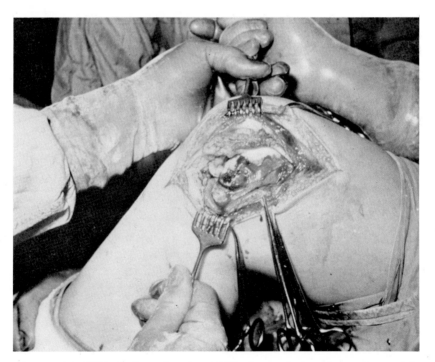

FIG. 21-10. With the knee flexed to 110° of extension as above, the condylar lesion is now visible (compare Fig. 21-9). Lateral condylar defect and free body lying anteriorly are seen. This indicates the degree of flexion needed for patella to contact femoral condyle in order to produce distal lateral condylar articular surface avulsion.

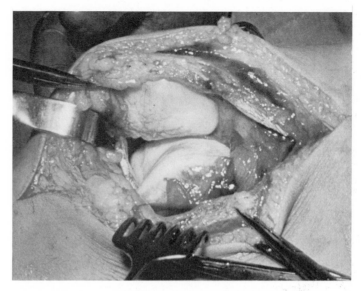

Fig. 21-11. A close-up view of the patella with the knee in extension reveals fresh, extensive loosening of normal cartilage from the bony bed. Hemorrhagic synovitis of the lateral condylar synovia is visible. The free body is seen tipped on edge at the left beneath the pole of the patella.

and remained with the knee bent until carried off the field for medical attention. A large fresh segment of the weight-bearing surface of the lateral femoral condyle lay free in the joint. The patella was badly abraded, contused and hemorrhagic.

2. An 18-year-old boy was squatting and leaning forward during a football game. As he projected himself forward forcibly, a player seized his ankle, fixing it to the ground. He twisted and felt instant "pain and tearing" in the knee. Disability was immediate. Operation 10 hours later revealed a fresh osteochondral fracture of the external femoral condyle. The patellar articular surface also was severely damaged, its cartilage having been loosened from its cortical bony attachment over a large area. The

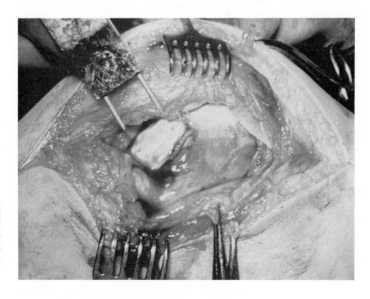

Fig. 21-12. A free fragment from a tangential osteochondral fracture is replaced and is stapled into the defect on the lateral condyle. Knee is in flexion.

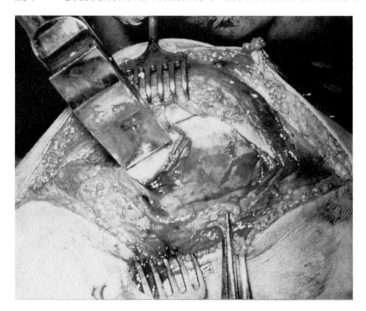

FIG. 21-13. The knee was immobilized in a noncontact position of flexion until staple was removed 8 wks. later. Firm precise union was achieved, and the knee continued to be symptomless 2 years later.

lateral condylar wall was the site of a depressed fracture (Figs. 21-14 to 21-20).

Diagnosis in Fresh Cases of Patellofemoral Injury

The history is suggestive, and, as a rule, diagnosis is not difficult. The knee is distended with blood, and the patient is usually unable to hold the knee actively extended or to activate the quadriceps strongly. The aspirated blood may contain fat droplets, particularly if an osteochondral body is visible on roentgenograms.

Roentgenographic Findings in Osteochondral Fractures

Roentgenographic study is helpful in most cases. Usually only anteroposterior, postero-

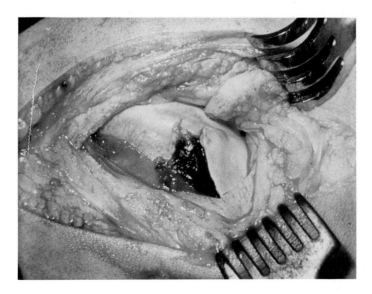

FIG. 21-14. Another variety of acute osteochondral fracture of the lateral femoral condyle is that wherein the lateral subchondral table or wall of the condyle is compressed and hence depressed by patellar impact, bursting the articular surface. A clot fills the depression of the compressed condyle.

FIG. 21-15. After the clot has been removed, the depressed lateral condylar wall visibly displaces the articular surface forward out of line, necessitating its reduction and fixation.

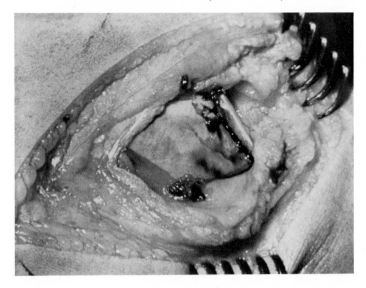

anterior, oblique and lateral views are possible, for the knee cannot be flexed without pain.

Patellar fragments, while occasionally based with a thick layer of bone (when they are easily seen on the lateral plate and when a corresponding defect is seen in the lower third of the patella in the lateral view), may be difficult to distinguish at first glance. However, if one studies the anteroposterior plate, one can usually see a "pencil line" of cortical bone ⅜ to ½ inch long lying in the joint space between the condyles. Then, checking back on the patellar cortex in the lateral view, one can make out a marginal cortical irregularity of ½ inch of the patellar articular surface matching the penciled line that marks the thick osteochondral body.

Femoral fragments are especially interesting because they usually arise from the

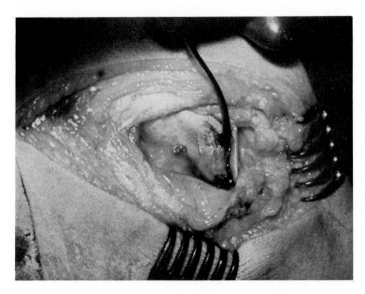

FIG. 21-16. Reduction of the articular surface: a skid levers out the depressed outer table of the femoral condyle to permit fitting the articular surface back in place.

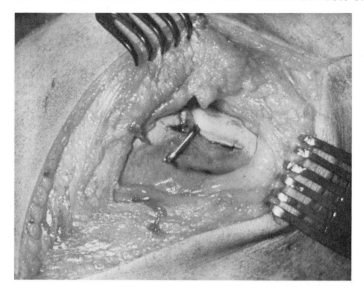

FIG. 21-17. Displaced articular segment is stapled back into accurate alignment. Immobilized for 8 weeks thereafter, when staple is removed.

curved distal end of the femur and consequently are curved and may include the groove for the lateral meniscus. The shadow of the body is projected as either a curved line (Fig. 21-21) or in the form of two lines with the ends overlapping (Fig. 21-12).

This type of shadow is pathognomonic of the lesion. Sometimes it is easier to distinguish the fragment on the anteroposterior than on the lateral view, although at times detection is impossible because of the minimal cortical avulsion which may accompany

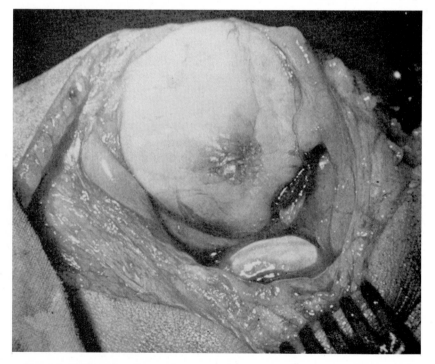

FIG. 21-18. Patella. Severe damage both centrally and at 5 o'clock is visible. Centrally articular cartilage has been loosened from its osseous attachment, and otherwise traumatized.

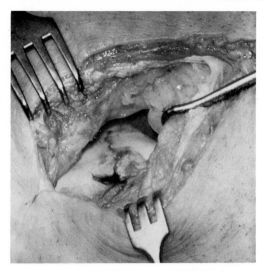

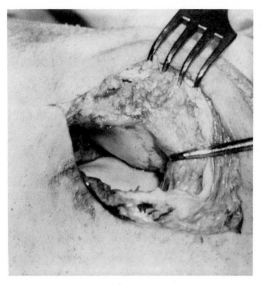

FIG. 21-19. Arthrotomy 8 weeks later. Staple is removed. Union of condylar fragments by fibrocartilage. A small subchondral defect persists—an indication to delay weight-bearing, until condylar reconstitution is demonstrable on X-ray studies. Otherwise the condyle may flatten subsequently.

FIG. 21-20. Appearance of patella (at right) 8 weeks later. Cartilage irregularities still are visible at the lower pole of the patella.

a thick cartilaginous fragment. When apparent, the defect in the cortical contour of the lateral femoral condyle also shows best on the anteroposterior view.

Depressed Fractures of Lateral Surface of Lateral Femoral Condyle Associated With Osteochondral Fracture of Articular Surface

Depressed fractures of the lateral condylar wall from the "hammer of the patella" are easily discerned in the anteroposterior view as depressions of the lateral wall of the condyle. The condylar articular surface may be undermined. Comparison with the normal knee makes the diagnosis clear. At operation the depressed segment needs to be elevated before the articular surface can be restored in contour. Delayed weight-bearing is desirable, since the cancellous structure must repair and consolidate if late flattening by such stressing is to be avoided (see Fig. 21-19).

Early Treatment of Osteochondral Fractures Due to Patellar Impact

Early and ideal treatment is possible only if the diagnosis is made promptly after injury.

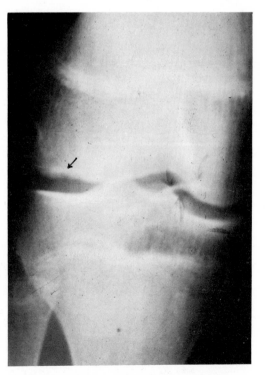

FIG. 21-21. A fresh osteochondral fracture of the lateral condyle. Curved free body (marked by arrows). Defect origin is visible in the lateral femoral condyle (small arrow).

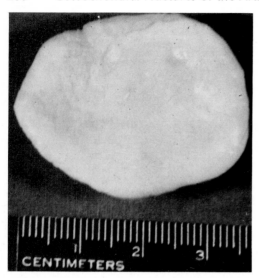

Fig. 21-22. An old osteochondral fracture (6 weeks) of the patellar body. Indistinguishable from osteochondritis dissecans of other than traumatic origin.

Patella. Usually the free body is small enough to discard without danger to the patellofemoral joint. The edges of the defect should be shaved slightly, and shreds should be trimmed if they threaten to become free bodies subsequently. Very rarely is patellectomy indicated, and then only in the case of virtually complete frontal plane decortication of the patella. Even then, in the young a trial of soft tissue flap covering might be considered. In an appropriate case the loose body, if not too thick to revascularize, may be fastened or stapled back into place. I have not replaced a patellar free body.

Femoral Condyle. A fairly large fresh osteochondral free body from the weight-bearing surface of the lateral femoral condyle carrying a layer of cortex should be replaced and secured in its original site. It should be protected for 3 months or more against contact or weight stresses by a cast applied in adequate flexion (checked by roentgenography if necessary). After union has been achieved, and any staple or nails removed, motion without weight bearing is commenced. To prevent late flattening by compression of the condyle at the site of reimplantation, walking on this limb should be forbidden for

3 months after removal of the splint. To be sure, a stainless steel staple requires removal later, but it provides maximal fixation, and the second arthrotomy for its removal permits one to judge the repair achieved and to decide whether or not the patient may safely commence weight bearing. The patella also may need minimal trimming of shreds arising from impact sites.

If the outer table of the femoral condyle is fractured and depressed, it must be levered out before the exploded hinged articular osteochondral segment can be pressed back into line with the rest of the articular surface (Fig. 21-14 to Fig. 21-20). A staple stabilizes the realigned table and the hinged articular segment while healing is progressing. The dead space beneath the once compressed and now elevated area must fill in before full bearing weight on the area will be tolerated without late compression (Fig. 21-19).

Late Treatment of Osteochondral Fractures With Separated Bodies

Fracture lesions of patella or lateral condyle diagnosed months late (Figs. 21-22 and 21-23) are treated by removing the free body, since body and bed have undergone alteration and revascularization, and firm reattachment in good alignment is not likely. Furthermore in fractures the site of the avulsed condylar segment is often surprisingly well repaired by slightly irregular fibrocartilaginous scar. Questionable lesions are those in which the area of loss is extensive, since the area usually corresponds to an area of condyle directly stressed in weight bearing. I have no personal information on the results of late operative reimplantation of freshened old lateral femoral osteochondral grafts. Unfortunately, both cartilage cells and bone of specimens 6 weeks and 3 months after traumatic separation have at times been found to be nonviable despite their continuous immersion in joint fluid. Yet, if the cartilage appears to be relatively good, a thin layer of bone is present, and the site of projected implantation is as yet poorly covered,

Plate 21-1. Knee crushed by impact.

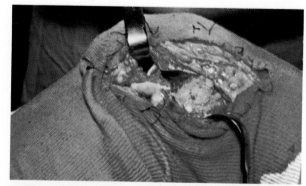

Plate 21-2. Test of condylar replacement and matching of articular segments.

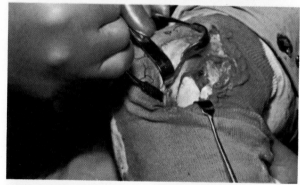

Plate 21-3. Multiple screw fixation (clipped short for subsequent removal by threaded pin extractor).

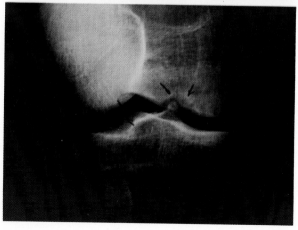

Plate 21-4. Condylar erosion and a free body arose from tibial spine-medial condyle contact.

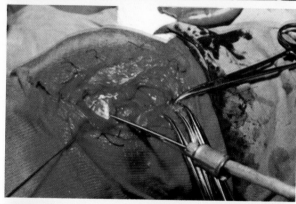

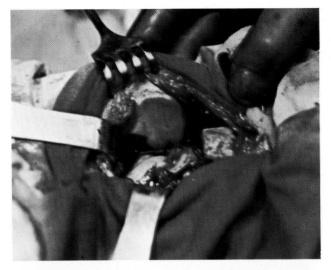

Plate 21-5. In this view of a tangential osteochondral fracture of the patella an inferior-medial quadrant defect is seen on the retracted patella. There is a free quadrangular body on the right. The external condyle is traumatized and hemorrhagic.

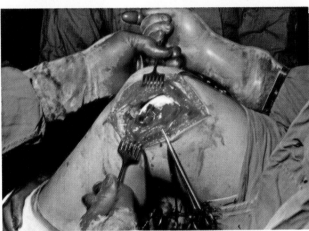

Plate 21-6. With the knee flexed the femoral lesion is exposed. (Compare exposure with Fig. 21-9) The patella is retracted. Indicates degree of flexion necessary for patella to contact femoral condyle to produce tangential fracture of lateral condylar articular surface.

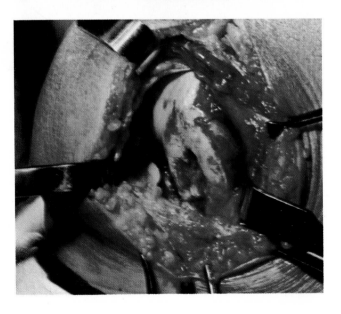

Plate 21-7. Cortisone Osteochondritis Dissicans of Femur. Typical appearance of ulceration of medial condyle. The cartilage lid lies partly visible to the left of the ulcer. Note ball like contents. Female age 67. History of bi-weekly intra-articular injections of steroids over a 4 month period administered for calcification of the menisci. Fairly comfortable and surprisingly mobile at time of exploratory 3 months later.

Fig. 21-23. A 9-month-old osteochondral fracture of the patella. Defect visible at site of origin on patella. "Osteochondritis dissecans" body lies above septum in opened suprapatellar pouch recess.

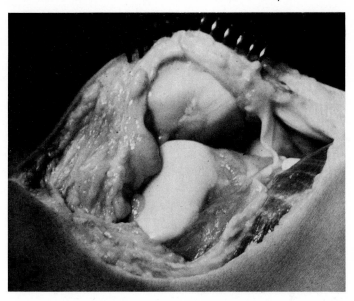

the experiment may be justified in special cases of fractures, particularly since freshening, drilling, and nail replacement have been successful in selected cases of osteochondritis dissecans of the medial condyle.[14]

OSTEOCHONDRAL LESIONS OF MEDIAL AND FEMORAL CONDYLES DUE TO TIBIOFEMORAL CONTACT

Other condylar injuries, rarer and less well understood, follow forceful twists or violent pivoting of the femoral condyle on the contiguous tibia. These lesions affect the middle and the more posterior surfaces of the condyles well away from possible patellar contact. The medial femoral condyle with a longer excursion than the lateral seems to be particularly vulnerable.

Osteochondral Cleft in the Medial Femoral Condyle

A singularly significant lesion—one which is probably of considerable clinical import and easily overlooked soon after injury—is the localized separation of the articular cartilage together with a thin bony subchondral plate as the result of a single twist of the knee. It is followed by ache but not effusion. Only x-ray evidence of a pencil line that de-

notes a subcortical ½-inch long cleft, with or without a tiny notch through the subchondral plate, enables the physician to recognize the site of a future osteochondral body (Figs. 21-24 and 21-25).

The cleft is localized on two lateral films, one made with the knee extended and the other in flexion. Localization not only helps in reconstructing the probable position of the knee at time of injury but suggests a position for immobilization in which further tibiofemur contact may be avoided. This is the very time when immediate institution of complete rest and freedom from tibial contact will offer the femur the opportunity of rapid and full repair. The well-vascularized cancellous bone cleft will anchor the articular cartilage securely if it is immobilized for a sufficiently long period of time. In other words, incomplete fractures are denoted by a narrow bone cleft paralleling the condylar contour. A niche indicates that a cortical break may have occurred as well.

This traumatic lesion is undoubtedly one mechanism responsible for the subsequent production of shell-like osteochondritis dissecans. A careful search for this lesion may reveal that it is less rare than our present experience indicates. We have seen this le-

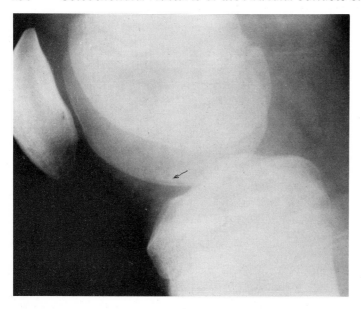

FIG. 21-24. Osteochondral cleft of the condyle was caused by sudden tibiofemoral crushing force of pivotal character (twist). Note the cleft (*arrow*) 10 hours after a dance injury (lateral view). Cleft must be sought. It is corroborated then on a flexion lateral view.

sion in three knees and in one ankle (lower tibia, bordering on upper surface of astragalus). In one knee a traumatic cleft lesion was not recognized, and the patient was treated with intraarticular steroids, whereupon a localized destruction lesion developed at the site necessitating arthrotomy which revealed a large, broken-down, ulcerated lesion of the femoral condyle.

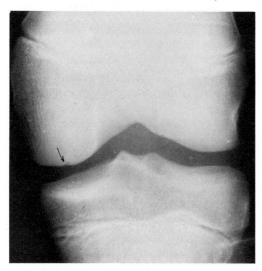

FIG. 21-25. Note notch in medial femoral condyle (*arrow*) (anteroposterior view).

Osteochondral Cleft in Medial Femoral Condyle Following a Violent "Twist"

A tall rangy lad of 12 years dancing "the twist" in August 1962 crouched and twisted violently on the flexed knee when "something moved in the knee, and I think the kneecap jumped sideways. It hurt a lot but it did not swell much. I've been limping the past 10 days since then." Roentgenograms revealed a tiny notch or infraction of the cortex of the medial femoral condyle and a ½-inch long subcortical cleft (Figs. 21-24, 25) indicative of incomplete localized avulsion of the cartilaginous surface of the condyle. The knee was placed in a plaster cast in considerable flexion, and he walked with crutches. The cleft filled with bone in 4 weeks, and clinically and roentgenologically the fragment reanchored. In 7 weeks the cancellous trabeculae regained normal configuration and retained this on follow-up roentgenograms.

An opportunity was afforded 11 years later to examine the site and appearance of his cleft healing when a bucket handle fracture of his medial meniscus necessitated meniscectomy. The cleft site was oval, roughly ½-inch long, and glistening. It was barely discernible, except for a slightly bluish tint in an otherwise glistening white medial femoral condyle.

Traumatic Massive Osteochondral Fractures of the Posterior Portion of the Medial Condyles

We have seen two patients in whom large thick pyramidal sections of the medial condyles separated after sudden severe trauma of pivotal type. In one the sharply punched-out fragment of fresh bone and articular cartilage was ⅜ inch thick, 1¼ inches long and ½ inch wide. It is hard to understand the mechanism capable of producing a fracture fragment of this shape and relatively large size. Pivotal forces could conceivably be responsible, but no conclusive evidence has been obtained.

An even larger fragment separated in a 15-year-old female. Her knee had been strapped into a reducing apparatus designed to produce automatic flexions and extensions of the knee by electrically stimulating the thigh muscles. Sudden excruciating knee pain occurred during a flexion motion, and when the repeatedly flexing knee was freed from the machine (and the patient revived) a large fresh fracture of almost the entire posterior portion of the medial femoral condyle was apparent. The fragment did not unite, and surgical removal of a body 1.25 x 0.5 x 0.7 inches has provided complete relief of pain. No signs of arthritis were present at follow-up 12 years after injury.

Kennedy[3] in 1966 reported the experimental production of several types of osteochondral fractures of each femoral condyle by combined rotation and compression forces in a "stress machine."

It seems reasonable to expect that if other more complex motions of the knee could be simulated and tested on the cadaver under various excessive stresses, we would gain increased insight into the pathologic physiology which produces other clinical varieties encountered. Some of these lesions have not been recognized as traumatic in the past.

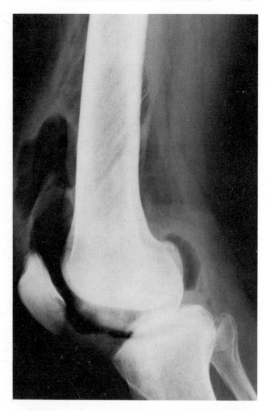

FIG. 21-26. Suprapatellar pouch, recess septum and communication. Pneumoarthrogram.

OSTEOCHONDRITIS DISSECANS

Osteochondritis dissecans is diagnosed when a segment of articular cartilage and underlying cortex of varying size and thickness separates from the host bone without apparent cause. Osteochondral fractures, particularly old ones, may be incorrectly so diagnosed, but as a rule the locality and the history differentiate the lesions. In others the history may implicate trauma (direct or indirect), but only occasionally conclusively, for example, when at operation tibial spine contact is demonstrable or a fragment from the medial femoral condyle attached to fibers of the posterior cruciate ligament is found. However, in most cases, traumatic etiology cannot be established. Infarction is a possible mechanism, but convincing proof is also lacking.

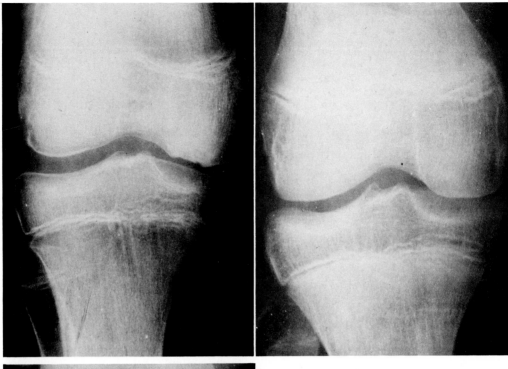

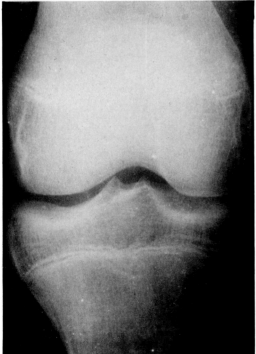

Fig. 21-27. (*Top, left*) Osteochondritis dissecans of medial femoral condyle; 12-year-old male; idiopathic; treated by brace immobilization in sufficient flexion to avoid contact with tibia; crutches. (*Top, right*) Complete repair followed 10 months' immobilization in brace. One year interval between this roentgenogram and that shown at *left*. (*Bottom*) Same knee after 21 months of active use. No retrogression.

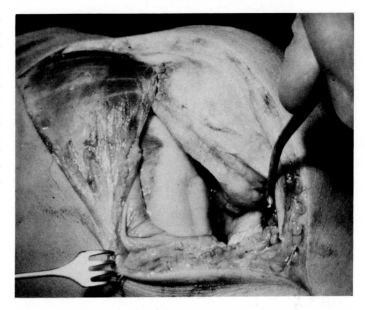

FIG. 21-28. Condylar prominence formed by displaced osteochondral fragment. Articular cartilage still intact. (See Fig. 21-29.) Knee joint was closed without surgical intervention and knee was immobilized. The fragment healed leaving a temporary condylar bony prominence which 2 years later had completely smoothed on x-ray. No functional or radiographic defect could be made out.

The lesion tends to occur in adolescents and is usually insidious. Discomfort may attract interest to the knee, or the first symptoms may be due to intermittent mechanical obstructions to motion due to a mobile free body. The patient may palpate "a bean" at times. During long intervals a loose body may remain lodged posteriorly or may come to lie anteriorly in a recess in the suprapatellar pouch separated from the joint by a valved septum (Figs. 21-23 and 21-26).

Other cases may be diagnosed roentgenographically before separation has developed. In most instances these cases heal with prolonged non-contact and non-weight bearing immobilization, and, consequently, diagnosis in this stage is most desirable (Fig. 21-27) (see also Chap. 8).

Not infrequently the lesion is bilateral and often symmetrically located. Consequently, both knees should always be surveyed.

Roentgenograms should be taken in numerous positions. Not only should anteroposterior and lateral views be obtained, but posteroanterior and tangential views may reveal sites of pathology not otherwise visible.

Since tibiofemoral and patellofemoral impact trauma should be considered among possible causes for the symptoms, ligamentous stability of the knee joint should be tested carefully at rest and when stressed as back knee. Elbow and wrists are also surveyed for laxity.

The appearance of osteochondritis dissecans in young children may also be produced by localized disturbances in condylar ossification. These have been observed to clear up spontaneously at times without treatment.[12] In general, however, in the presence of roentgenographic evidence of localized condylar fragmentation, treatment should be instituted, particularly in children past 10 years of age.

Lesions of the posterior portions of the condyles, best seen on anteroposterior views, have been seen to heal in 6 to 12 months, often with use of braces that restrict area contact on these condylar sites.

Often roentgenographic findings indicative of femoral subcortical osseous separation are associated with operative findings of intact articular cartilage. Consequently, it is not desirable to excise the osseous lesion. Prolonged immobilization in a position evading contact with the tibia has been rewarded in many cases by disappearance of the lesion (Fig. 21-27). This advice by Green[2] and Banks[2] and others has been confirmed by us repeatedly.

Even when the bone of the fragment has

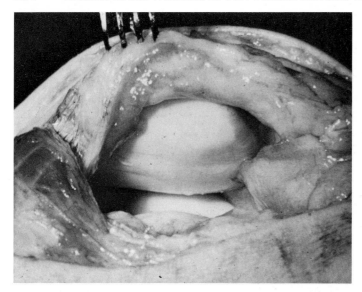

Fig. 21-29. Reciprocal longitudinal groove in articular surface of patella produced by abnormal excursion of patella over edge of femoral condyle. (See preceeding figure 21-28).

apparently been completely separated and appreciably displaced by the defect it may incorporate and heal back into place; in two instances it left as a sequel a bony prominence on the condyle. In one of these cases (Fig. 21-28) the condylar prominence was seen to displace the patella sufficiently so that by contact with the edge of the femoral condyle as the knee flexed and extended a reciprocal furrow had been gouged longitudinally in the articular cartilage of the patella extending from its upper to its lower pole (Fig. 21-29).

Such persistent local prominence on healing is rather conclusive evidence that the lesion was indeed a true separation and not merely an anomaly of ossification. That radiographic lesions, almost irrespective of age and state of epiphyseal maturity, so often respond to 4 to 12 months of immobilization by incorporation into the bony structure of the femoral condyles, is further evidence that healing is a response to the therapeutic program involved.

A plaster cast or a rigid-knee–long-leg brace with long-laced thigh and calf cuffs is provided in the position of flexion. The position of flexion is determined by roentgenograms showing that the lesion is not in

contact with the opposite articular surfaces. Fixation and crutches for 4 to 11 months has been successful in healing even advanced lesions.

However, if the body has separated and its condition on inspection is such as to offer little hope of its incorporation by stapling back into a freshened bed, it is discarded. The cartilaginous edges of a defect may be shaved or trimmed conservatively, using a bent segment of a flexible razor blade. At times we have drilled the exposed femoral bone bed, using a fine jeweler's drill, so that the clot that forms might promote development of fibrocartilage to fill the defect. It is difficult to judge whether drilling materially aided repair. Centrally located sites of patellar osteochondritis dissecans also have been drilled. In the common case of localized dislodgment of the inferior medial quadrant of the patella in tangential osteochondral fracture little subsequent disability is experienced after the loose fragment is discarded. We have not seen patellofemoral contact disturbances follow such removal, but they have been reported by others.

In several cases of threatened separation of an osteochondritic fragment of the femoral condyle, we have drilled the bed from without the joint under roentgenologic control. Preferably at open operation, the drill is passed through the medial wall of the medial condyle down to the bed of the lesion, care being taken not to perforate the articular cartilage. Unfortunately, only a few holes may be so drilled, but even so, it serves to stimulate vascularity for local repair. We have avoided drilling through intact cartilage from the joint side.

Patellectomy for indirect fractures or osteochondritis dissecans in childhood is rarely considered, and we have only once found it necessary in a complete tangential fracture.

Histologically, the loose bodies of osteochondritis dissecans are ultimately indistinguishable from fragments of old osteochondral fractures that have been in the joint long enough to show the effects of vascular separation from the host. A series of such loose bodies removed from patients at different and key intervals after injury reveal the progressive changes in the body that ultimately characterize specimens of osteochondritis dissecans. For obvious mechanical reasons, removal of all completely free bodies of whatever etiology is indicated, i.e., unless their recent origin and an adequate bone layer make the trial of reimplantation feasible.

The free body visible on roentgenograms may be difficult to find on opening the joint at operation. Occasionally it is posterior. Also, it may be found lodged in a compartment of the suprapatellar pouch. In some knees a complete septum with a semilunar-like valve is found through which the free body at long intervals finds its way into parts of the joint where it may interfere with joint motion (Fig. 21-23).

New bodies sometimes form and separate years after the initial arthrotomy for removal of a free osteochondritic loose body. Therefore, patients should be told before operation of the possibility of further operation if new areas separate at the margins of large condylar defects.

A not uncommon and rather unpleasant patellar lesion is osteochondritis dissecans of the middle third of the patella. It may be bilateral. Roentgenographic findings consist of subchondral cortical irregularity, or even crater formation. An arthrogram will at times be helpful. Pain on motion is not relieved by removal of one or more small bodies. Local curettage into bleeding bone and multiple drilling with a jeweler's drill followed by prolonged long-leg brace fixation in extension is advised. Patellectomy may ultimately be indicated. We have seen several unsuccessful metallic patellar implants.

Large condylar defects established in adolescence have produced evidence of degenerative changes in the third or the fourth decade, fortunately with few clinical complaints.

Cortisone Osteochondritis Dissecans

Since 1956 we have encountered the development of osteochondritis dissecans and cartilaginous free bodies in joints of patients who had been receiving steroid medication. Administration of the drug in a few earlier cases was oral, but in most patients the drug was instilled into the joint. No critical dose, particular steroid compound, or frequency of dosage could be ascertained. No age group was especially vulnerable, although most patients were 40 to 70. Oral dosage was followed by multiple or bilateral joint lesions. Intraarticular cortisone, in our measured opinion, incited characteristic and severe lesions in the joint injected and which came to surgery. Injections were usually lateral in knees, but lesions were almost uniformly of the medial femoral condyle (Plate 21-7).

From 1956 to 1973 we have encountered 37 patients with 47 sites of joint destruction in which, after study, this diagnosis was reached. Of these, 29 knees of 26 patients had gross radiologic lesions. In all but two patients the lesion was located in the stressed

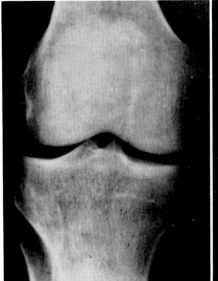
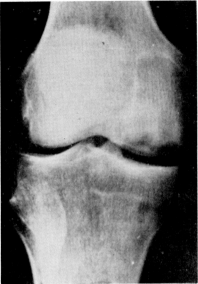

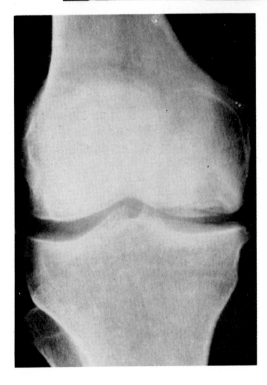

FIG. 21-30. (*Top, left*) Cortisone femoral osteochondritis dissecans in 68-year-old male who had received 8 to 10 intra-articular injections of hydrocortisone over a period of 3 months. No oral medication. Initial roentgenogram. Normal medial femoral condyle. (*Top, right*) Eight months later. A large decalcified zone has appeared in the medial femoral condyle. (*Bottom*) At 14 months. Collapse of decalcified zone with large free osteochondral fragment now visible beneath the medial femoral condyle.

Decalcified areas of cancellous bone are visible at 8 months deep in both femoral condyles, outlined faintly by scalloped sclerotic margins. Likewise both tibial condyles contain subchondral cancellous areas of decalcification. Pivotal stress concentration produces the osteochondral fracture exposing the "ulcer," which is the subchondral defect "with the lid off."

FIG. 21-31. (*Left*) Cortisone tibial osteochondritis dissecans. Female, age 62. Anteroposterior view. Large fragment separated from the medial condyle of the tibia. Confirmed at operation. Followed 6 months of oral administration of cortisone. A decalcified lesion also appeared beneath the articular surface of the tibia in the ankle joint. (*Right*) Lateral view of same knee.

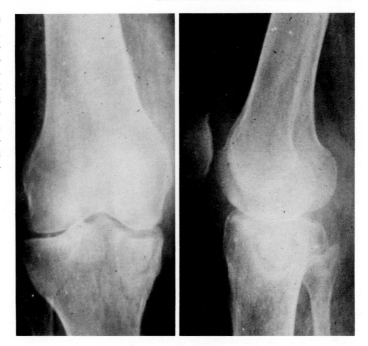

prominence of the medial femoral condyle. In the two exceptions (who had taken oral steroids) medial tibial condyle areas were involved (Fig. 21-31).

The sequence of events in the knee joint appears to be as follows: Some months after commencing use of the drug, either intraarticularly or orally, the affected condyle presents an area of subchondral bone atrophy. Of particular interest are other deeper areas in the cancellous bone of both femoral and tibial condyles, where loss of trabeculation is discerned, often far removed from the later subchondral condylar lesion (Fig. 21-30).

Preceding the breakdown in the medial femoral condyle, bubblelike areas of absorption are apparent locally in the subcortical cancellous tissues. It is best seen in the early stage in the lateral view.

Next the sclerotic cortical plate undergoes linear fracture or infarction and subsequently flattens. Separation of a cortical osteochondral body in the pivotal zone of the medial condyle follows. Pain is usually moderate and motion is commonly surprisingly free for so severe a radiological area of pathology.

At operation, cartilage necrosis and separation of cartilage from subcortical bone are exposed, often with deep dirty appearing ulceration in the medial condyle (Plate 21-7). Loose large cartilage fragments are often present. Cartilage destruction, subchondral defects, and aseptic necrosis of subchondral bone are confirmed at operation and are usually extensive.

In one instructive instance the steroid lesion developed in the medial femoral condyle at the site of a previous purely traumatic subchondral cleft lesion in an active man. On elevation (at operation) of the cleft—pedicled flap a nest of loose balls of necrotic, white-grey, poorly staining tissue was exposed, tightly packed in a deep medial condylar ulcer. The balls had been prevented from falling out into the joint by the persistence of one segment of the cartilage flap and were therefore visible in situ.

The mode of chemical action of the drug on articular cartilage has been intensively studied by Mankin.[7] To date there is no similar data available of the action of steroids on cortical and cancellous bone and marrow. It seems remarkable that following intraarticular injections such widespread, profound, deeply located lesions should develop.

The direct trauma of the concentrated stresses of weight bearing, we believe, is the factor which fractures the locally atrophied subchondral cortex left unsupported by absorption of cancellous trabeculae, most often in this medial femoral zone. We believe that the chance distribution of atrophic zones is the reason it does not occur more frequently at the site of stress in the knee joint.

Three roentgenographically similar lesions have been seen in patients with osteoporosis who never received steroids. Two of these healed well with continued bracing and general measures aimed at improving the osteoporosis. As these knees were not opened, we are unable to report on their actual appearance.

We are not aware that similar major destructive and ulcerated lesions were reported prior to the introduction of steroids.

We distinctly do not believe that general use of steroids in knees is worth the unpredictable hazards instanced and have long dispensed with intraarticular administration.

The mechanism of action of the drug whereby these joint lesions are produced is not yet understood. Theories currently vary from loss of pain sensation and cessation of normal reparative processes in articular cartilage to vascular occlusions. It seems unlikely that direct trauma would involve normal subcondylar bone as deeply as the changes seen in these cases would postulate. Our views are outlined above.

Ultimately, in the hip joint, the progressive disintegration resembles the classic picture of a Charcot joint. Two cases have had both hips affected. In one young adult oral administration of moderate dosage for an atopic dermatitis of the forearm was followed after some months by hip disturbance that occasioned the discovery of the osteochondral lesions, which developed first in one hip and, after an interval of months, in the other. No critical dosage could be ascertained. Stopping cortisone therapy did not stop breakdown in the hips observed.

Spontaneous efforts at repair have been followed with interest in three severely unstable cases not subjected to surgical intervention. The knees in three patients treated by abstinance from steroids and continuous (day and night) use of a long-leg brace of the Goldenberg type, in which the axes of joint motion including rotation are controlled with special care, improved very significantly in the course of a year. The area of destruction visible on roentgenographs, compacted, regained contours and then filled in, even if it did not return to normal. The associated instability of the joints was very materially improved. The patients have continued with the brace in comfort for several years after the onset of conservative observation. Fusion was early refused by one particularly severely involved patient, and the alternative of a prosthesis was not tendered.

REFERENCES

1. Freiberger, R.: Aseptic necrosis of the femoral heads after high dosage. Corticosteroid therapy. N.Y. State. J. Med., *65*:127, 1965.
2. Green, W. T. and Banks, H. H.: Osteochondritis dissecans in children. J. Bone Joint Surg., *35A*:26, 1953.
3. Kennedy, J. C.: Osteochondral fractures of the femoral condyles. J. Bone Joint Surg., *48B*:436, 1966.
4. Kleinberg, S.: Vertical fracture of the articular surface of the patella. J.A.M.A., *81*: 1205, 1923.
5. Kroner, M.: Ein fall von Flachenfractur und Luxation der Patella. Deut. Med. Wochenschr., *31*:996, 1905.
6. Lettloff, D.: Der verticofrontale Bruch der kniescheike, Austernschalenbruch. Arch f. Klin. Chir. *153*:808, 1928.
7. Mankin, H. J. *et al.*: The acute effects of intra-articular hydrocortisone on articular cartilage. J. Bone Joint Surg., *48A*:1083, 1966.
8. Milgram, J. E.: Tangential osteochondral fracture of the patella. J. Bone Joint Surg., *35*:271, 1943.
9. ————: Osteochondral fractures of the knee joint. Mechanism of Production. IX

Congress Int. de. Chir. Orth. et da trauma. Transactions Bruxelles p. 760-762, 1964.

10. ———: Mechanism of production of patellar and femoral free bodies in the knee joint. J. Bone Joint Surg., *46B*:787, 1964.

11. ———: Osteochondral lesions of the knee joint. Experimental tibial spine–femoral condyle contact. J. Bone Joint Surg., *48B*:392, 1966.

12. Sledenstein, H.: Osteochondritis dissecans of the knee with spontaneous healing in children. Bull. Hosp. Joint Dis., *28*:123, 1957.

13. Smillie, I. E.: Osteochondritis dissecans. Edinburgh, E. & S. Livingston Ltd., 1964.

14. Villar, R.: Fracture vertico-frontale dite "en coquilles de Huitre de la Rotule." J. Med. Bordeaux, *48*:121, 1921.

22

The Principles and Practice of Stable Internal Fixation in the Treatment of Fractures Involving the Knee Joint

M. E. Müller, M.D.; J. Goldsmith, M.D.;
J. Schatzker, M.D., B.Sc. (Med.)

Conservative treatment of fractures involving the knee joint has frequently led to unsatisfactory results with the knee joint remaining unstable, stiff, and painful. Open reduction and internal fixation in the past has similarly led to poor results. The choice between operative and conservative treatment of these fractures requires experience and judgement.

Since 1958, the AO group in Switzerland has devoted a great deal of time to the study of the many problems present in the treatment of fractures of the knee joint. From these studies have evolved techniques that are now standard. They permit anatomical reduction and rigid stable internal fixation so that plaster fixation can be abandoned and active painless mobilization of the joint and of the injured extremity can begin within a few days of surgery.

The best way to fix bony fragments accurately is by means of interfragmentary compression achieved with lag screws, tension band wire, or the so-called compression plate, or a combination of any of the three. The main principle of all these compression systems is to bring as large a fracture surface as possible under compression with the implant under tension. If the bony surfaces that are compressed are not large enough to permit rigid fixation, an autogenous cancellous bone graft must be employed.

The techniques that the Swiss AO Group found best shall be discussed with particular regard to the type of fracture, operative exposures, biomechanical principles, and postoperative treatment.[4]

FRACTURES OF THE PATELLA

In fractures of the patella the following factors are important: mechanism of injury, number of fragments, damage to the articular cartilage, and rupture of the extensor apparatus.

Loss of the patella leads to degenerative changes in the femoral condyles and, on occasion, extensor lag of 10 to 15 degrees may be present. Weakness during the last 10 to 15 degrees of extension is the rule. For these reasons patellectomy will be exceptional. If the patella, as a result of direct trauma, is markedly comminuted, an accurate reduction is often impossible and patellectomy is frequently indicated. If the extensor apparatus is intact, then only patellectomy is performed. If not, the quadriceps and patella tendon are sutured together, and a triangular segment from the extensor apparatus is excised in order to shorten longitudinally the expansion of the retinaculae patellae.

In all the other cases we make every attempt to maintain the integrity of the patella.

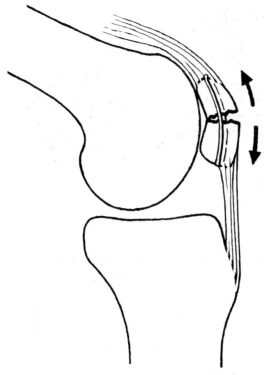

FIG. 22-1: After conventional cerclage wiring with the wire running around the middle of the patella, the fragments invariably come apart on the anterior surface when the knee is flexed. Therefore this procedure is not advisable.

If late degenerative changes do occur, a patella prosthesis may be the best solution in preference to a late patellectomy.

In longitundinal fractures of the patella displacement of fragments usually does not occur. The extensor apparatus is intact, and no operative intervention is necessary. If the fragments separate, then stable fixation can be easily achieved after accurate reduction with one or two lag screws.

Transverse fractures or avulsions of the distal pole of the patella are usually the result of indirect trauma. These fractures are usually the result of a sudden powerful contraction of the quadriceps when the knee is flexed. This causes the patella to be forced against the femur which then acts as a fulcrum. Separation of the fragments is the rule, and in most cases the lateral expansion of the quadriceps mechanism is ruptured.

Treatment of Simple Transverse Fractures

Wire fixation of simple transverse patellar fractures is not new. If circumferential wiring is employed, displacement of both fragments with a separation anteriorly is almost inevitable (Fig. 22-1). Pauwels has shown that if a circumferential wire is placed posterior to the center of axis of the patella, the fragments open anteriorly.[5] If, on the other hand, the wire is placed anterior to the center of axis, tensile stresses that previously caused the displacement and separation of fragments are converted into compressive forces and serve to maintain the reduction and apposition of fragments.

We expose such a fracture through a transverse incision centered over the patella and examine both femoral condyles. Prior to reduction the tendon fibers are scraped back from the fracture line for a distance of 2 to 3 mm. An accurate reduction is then obtained and maintained with two towel clips. Two wires are used to secure fixation. The first is placed deep to the insertion of the quadriceps and patellar tendon. The second wire is placed more superficially and passes through the Sharpey's fibers (Fig. 22-2). The fracture is slightly overcorrected, and the wires are then tightened and tied. When the knee joint is flexed, the overcorrection vanishes, and the fracture surfaces are squeezed together with compression. The quadriceps expansion is then repaired, suction drains are inserted, and the wound is closed.

Comminuted Fractures

Comminuted fractures of the patella are exposed in the same manner as is a transverse fracture of the patella, but the fixation has to be supplemented with two longitudinal K-wires to stabilize the small fragments. The fixation is then completed with two tension band wires as illustrated in Figure 22-3.

Avulsion Fractures

Avulsion fractures of the lower pole of the patella cannot be stabilized with the

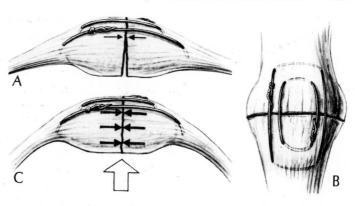

FIG. 22-2. The principle of tension band wiring of the patella: (*A, B*) The wire is passed around the insertion of the ligamentum patellae and the quadriceps in front of the patella. This wire is tightened until the fracture is slightly overcorrected. A second wire is passed more superficially. (*C*) As the knee is flexed and the quadriceps contracted, the pressure of the condyles against the patella compresses the bony fragments together.

tension band wire alone; the distal fragment tilts in toward the joint. A small distal fragment must therefore be stabilized with a small AO cancellous screw before the tension band wire is applied (Fig. 22-4). Only in the case of many small distal fragments that cannot be secured by means of screws is the excision of the lower pole the method of choice.

Rupture of the Patellar Tendon from the Patella

In the case of rupture of the patellar tendon from the patella, the disruption of the tendon is repaired, but the suture line must be protected from tension. This is achieved by means of a figure-of-eight tension band wire placed proximally around the quadriceps tendon and distally around a cortical screw inserted transversely just distal to the tibial tubercle (Fig. 22-5). The wire and screw are removed after 6 months.

Postoperative Care

Postoperative splinting and positioning is extremely important. Fractures of the patella are immobilized in a compression bandage for 48 hours and protected during the postoperative period on a Braun frame, which maintains the knee in 45 degrees of flexion. The foot is somewhat higher than the knee and the ankle is at 90 degrees with

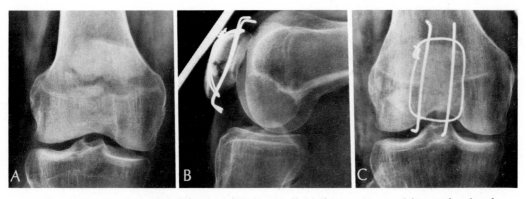

FIG. 22-3. A comminuted fracture of the patella (*A*) was managed by tension band wiring with Kirschner wires. (*B, C*) The Kirschner wires were first introduced longitudinally to stabilize the small fragments.

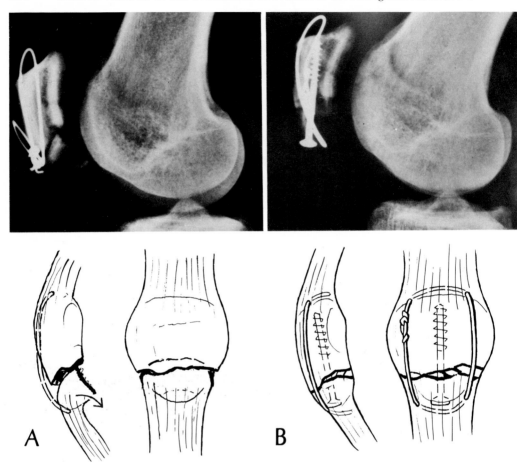

FIG. 22-4. (*A*) In avulsion fractures of the lower tip of the patella, tension band wiring alone tips the distal fragment. (*B*) The lower fragment must therefore be stabilized with a small cancellous screw before the tension band wire is applied.

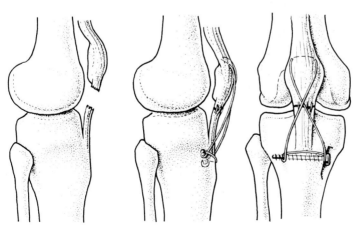

FIG. 22-5. Repair of a ruptured patellar tendon. The suture line is protected with a figure-of-eight tension band wire passed proximally around the quadriceps insertion and distally around the transverse screw inserted in the tibia just distal to the attachment of the patellar tendon. Immediate movement can begin without fear of disrupting the repair. The wire and screw are removed after 6 months.

the foot supported, so it will not drift into equinus (Fig. 22-6). Quadriceps exercises are begun early with the help of a physiotherapist. Early flexion of the knee joint is most desirable because in extension the patella does not articulate with the femur. In flexion, on the other hand, the articular surface of the patella lies against the articular surface of the femur. Normally the patient with a fracture of the patella rigidly fixed will bend his knee joint approximately 70 to 90 degrees after 1 week. It is necessary to walk with two canes thereafter for an 8-week period.

FRACTURES OF THE LOWER FEMUR

Supracondylar and condylar fractures of the femur usually occur as the result of severe trauma since the distal femur is structurally very strong.

The reduction of these fractures and maintenance of the reduction by conservative means is difficult. It is important to note that in intercondylar fractures both the patellofemoral and tibiofemoral joints must be reestablished to prevent posttraumatic arthritis. After conservative treatment a perfect functional result is the exception rather than the rule. Early motion is not possible in these cases, and stiffness of the knee joint ensues. Stiffness occurs because of incomplete reduction with shortening of the femur and formation of adhesions between the quadriceps and the fracture site with resultant loss of the suprapatellar gliding mechanism.

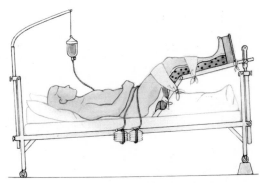

FIG. 22-6. Postoperative positioning of patients with patellar or tibial fractures.

In order to avoid these complications, an anatomical open reduction followed by rigid internal fixation is recommended. Where severe bony comminution is present, autogenous cancellous bone grafting must be performed. Postoperatively the knee is maintained at 90 degrees of flexion, and active mobilization of the extremity begins on the day following surgery.

Fractures of one condyle have, as a rule, no ligamentous disruption associated with them for the ligament remains attached to the condyle. In a young person with strong cancellous bone such a fracture can be rigidly stabilized with one or two cancellous bone screws. These screws act as lag screws and therefore, as in all lag screws, the thread must not cross the fracture line (Fig. 22-7).

In compound fractures minimal internal fixation should be carried out. For young patients with compound fractures, debridement and simple screw fixation may be suffi-

FIG. 22-7. A fracture of one condyle in an elderly person with osteoporotic bone is repaired with a combination of buttress plate and lag screws.

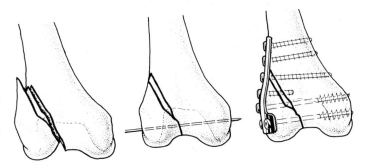

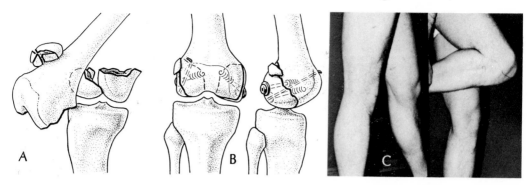

FIG. 22-8. A compound fracture of both femoral condyles (*A*) was reduced and stabilized with two cancellous lag screws. (*B*) Note that threads must not cross the fracture line. Movement was begun immediately. (*C*) Eight years after the operation the patient has full range of motion and no residual arthritis.

cient. Figure 22-8 illustrates a compound fracture of both condyles in a young patient with an excellent postoperative result.

Transverse supracondylar fractures are stabilized under axial compression by means of a tension band plate. If such a fracture is associated with bone loss medially, then this is filled primarily with autogenous cancellous bone at the time of the internal fixation. If such fractures are comminuted and have two, three, or four fragments, then reduction begins by reducing each fragment in turn and wherever possible securing interfragmentary compression by means of lag screws. Once the reduction is complete, the fractures are neutralized by a neutralization plate applied to the lateral cortex. For proximal supracondylar fractures a straight plate can be used that is slightly curved between the middle and the distal third of the femur. More distally a condylar blade plate is used. Any bone defects are filled with autogenous cancellous bone.

Supra- and intracondylar fractures are stabilized by means of the AO 95 degree condylar blade plate. Fixation is again supplemented by autogenous cancellous bone whenever bone loss is present. In reduction and fixation of these fractures one always begins with the intraarticular fracture lines. Once the intraarticular fracture is solidly fixed, the supracondylar component is dealt with. The condyles are rarely involved in comminution. But if such is present and results in bone loss, then again autogenous cancellous bone graft from the ilium must be employed. When the condylar blade plate is used, the axis of the frontal plane will remain physiological as long as the blade of the plate is parallel to the articular surface of the knee.

The condylar blade plate as created by the Swiss AO in 1959 is a one-piece device with a fixed angle of 95 degrees. The blade portion in profile is shaped like a U. The blade of this blade plate is always inserted parallel to the articular surface of the condyles which subtends an angle of 81 degrees with the anatomical axis of the femur (Fig. 22-9). As long as there are no anatomical abnormalities and the blade is inserted parallel to the articular surface, the plate portion will come to lie along the lateral cortex of the femur. Care must be taken, however, to direct the device properly in the sagittal plane for malposition such as recurvatum might ensue when the blade plate is improperly oriented. The standard condylar blade plate has two holes for cancellous screws of 6.5 mm. diameter and three holes for cortical screws of 4.5 mm. diameter.

The special feature of the AO angled plate is that the channel for the blade of the plate must be cut by means of a special seating chisel on which a guide for securing the

Fig. 22-9. (*A*) The standard condylar blade plate has two distal holes for cancellous screws and three holes for cortex screws. Condylar plates of longer shaft lengths for comminuted fractures are provided with seven, nine, or twelve holes. (*B*) The condylar plate guide is shaped like a mold for the shaft portion of the condylar plate. (*C*) The physiological axis of tibia and femur showing the angles they form with the knee joint itself.

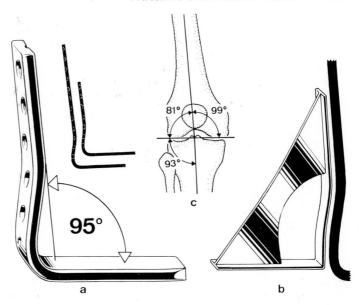

orientation in the sagittal plane is adjustable (Fig. 22-10).

Internal Fixation of Intraarticular Fracture of the Distal Femur

Surgical Exposure. The lateral approach is used. The skin and the investing fascia are incised, and the incision is carried to the level of the tibial tubercle. If the joint is to be widely exposed, the lateral half of the infrapatellar tendon is reflected; a medial parapatellar incision is seldom necessary (Fig. 22-11). The vastus lateralis is retracted anteriorly and reflected from the intermuscular septum. The perforating vessels, wherever encountered, are ligated and cut.

When complete, the exposure includes the lateral surface of the femur from the linea aspera forward, to and including the joint.

Technic. After the joint is exposed, the fracture lines are reduced under direct vision and temporarily stabilized by means of Kirschner wires (Fig. 22-12). Sometimes, especially in comminuted fractures of the condyles, the reduction is much easier if the knee joint is flexed 120 degrees or more in order to relax all the flexors of the knee. The vertical component of the T- or Y-fracture should now be fixed under compression with one or more cancellous lag screws placed anteriorly and posteriorly to the projected position of the blade plate and 3 to 4 cm.

Fig. 22-10. This special seating chisel is made for inserting condylar blade plates. (*A*) To cut the channel for the blade it has a profile indentical to that of the blade of the plate. During insertion it is held with the slotted hammer to prevent rotation. The hammer also serves as an extractor. (*B*) The standard U-section of the blade. (*C*) The chisel guide helps to establish the sagittal plane.

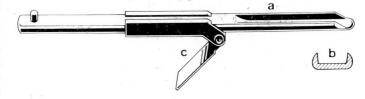

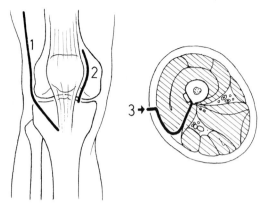

FIG. 22-11. (*1, 3*) The so-called mail-box approach for distal femoral fractures. Very seldom the knee joint must be inspected through a counter incision (*2*).

above the joint. Then the supracondylar fracture lines are reduced and temporarily fixed by means of bone clamps or Kirschner wires. One Kirschner wire is inserted transversely through the knee joint parallel to the articular surface of the femoral condyle. A second Kirschner wire is placed under the patella. The third Kirschner wire is inserted through the femoral condyle as low as possi-

ble—about 1 cm. above the articular surface. It is inserted parallel to the first and second Kirschner wires respectively and serves then as the guide wire for the introduction of the seating chisel. The position of the third Kirschner wire, the guide wire, is now checked with the condylar positioning plate. The guide wire should be parallel to it.

The special seating chisel with its guide set parallel to the long axis of the femur is now hammered in making sure that the chisel blade is parallel to the third or directional K-wire. This allows the blade plate to be correctly aligned in both the sagittal and coronal planes, no matter what the supracondylar comminution. The chisel is removed and the plate inserted. One or two cancellous screws are inserted not only in the distal part of the plate but also into the distal fragment of the fracture to increase the fixation of the blade plate. These cancellous screws, as they engage the medial cortex, increase the interfragmentary compression on the intracondylar fracture surfaces. The reduction of the supracondylar fracture is checked, and accurate axial com-

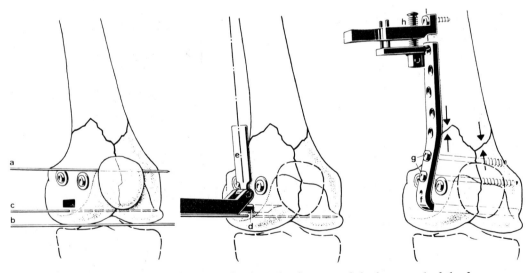

FIG. 22-12. Technique of internal fixation of a fracture of the lower end of the femur. One Kirschner wire is placed beneath the patella (*a*) and another in the joint parallel to the articular surface (*b*). The guide wire (*c*) is inserted into the bone 1 cm. above the joint surface and parallel to the other Kirschner wires. The special seating chisel (*d*) is introduced parallel to the guide wire and its aiming device (*e*) lies parallel to the femoral shaft. Two cancellous screws (*g*) are inserted into the distal fragment through the blade plate (*f*) before the tension device is attached proximally.

pression is now obtained by securing the tension device to the femoral shaft and placing the plate portion under tension. Reduction should be perfect and the fixation rigid. If there is any loss of bony continuity medially, it must be reconstituted at the time of fixation with autogenous cancellous bone graft. The bone graft will serve in due time as a physiological bone bar medially and will prevent bending forces from fatiguing the plate.

Postoperative Care

Once internal fixation is completed, the extremity is immobilized on a special splint with the hip and knee flexed to 90 degrees (Fig. 22-13). Assisted active movements are begun in 48 hours. After 6 days the splint is discarded, and the patient is encouraged to sit with his leg over the edge of the bed and to begin active unassisted

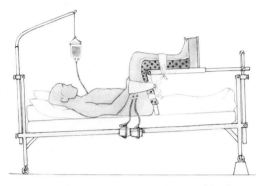

FIG. 22-13. Postoperative positioning for fractures of mid- and distal femur.

movements. With this postoperative regimen flexion has never been a problem. On the eighth postoperative day the patient is allowed out of bed. Full weight bearing is not allowed for 2 to 3 months. In the interim partial weight bearing not exceeding

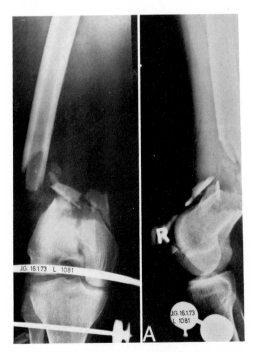
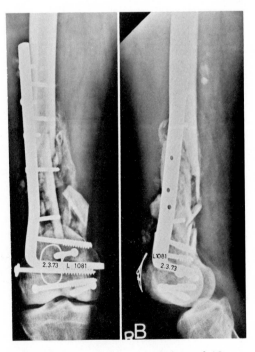

FIG. 22-14. (*A*) Comminuted compound fracture of the right femur with loss of 10 cm. of bone. (*B*) After reduction of the joint surfaces and fixation of the fragments by means of four lag screws, the blade plate was inserted. The defect was filled with cancellous bone grafts and a bone fragment found in the patient's car after the accident. After 2 weeks the patient was able to walk with two crutches, and after 6 weeks he was able to bend his knee joint to 90 degrees.

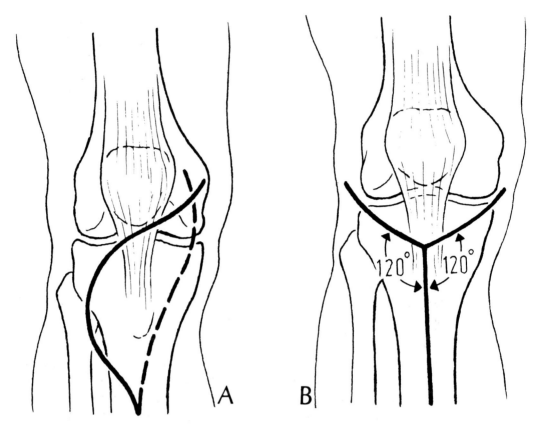

Fig. 22-15. (*A*) Incisions for the medial or lateral parts of the tibial plateau are centered over the medial or lateral condyle respectively. (*B*) The arms of an incision to expose both parts of the tibial plateau must form 120-degree angles. This incision allows repair of both condyles and any associated ligamentous damage at the same time. If greater exposure is needed, the patellar tendon is elevated by Z-plasty.

10 to 15 kg. (measured with the patient standing on a scale) is allowed. The patient uses two crutches. Plates are removed after 18 months. Before any metal is removed, however, the internal architecture of the cortex must have become homogeneous throughout as seen radiographically. The removal of these implants is necessary after bony union because these implants are rigid, provide too much stress protection and prevent the bone from responding to normal physiological stimuli. There is also the possibility of metallic corrosion. Figure 22-14 gives an example of a severe femoral fracture treated by means of lag screws, condylar plate, and bone plasty.

FRACTURES OF THE TIBIAL PLATEAU

The metaphyseal portion of the tibia in its expanded cancellous proximal end is especially vulnerable to injury. The proximal tibia overhangs the shaft posteriorly and is not supported by diaphyseal cortical bone below. For these reasons fractures of the tibial plateau are more frequent than of the femoral condyles.

An associated medial ligamentous rupture may occur when the joint is mainly subjected to a valgus stress. If this stress is resisted by the lateral plateau, a tension build-up results in the medial ligament with its eventual rupture. If the plateau ruptures,

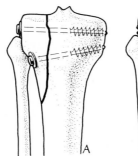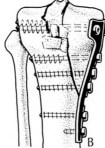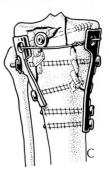

Fig. 22-16. The three classical tibial plateau fractures and their treatment: (*A*) Cleavage fracture–two lag screws are sufficient only in young patients. (*B*) Depressed fracture–after elevation of the depression, a cancellous bone plasty is necessary. Fixation by means of lag screws and T-plate. (*C*) Comminuted fracture treated by means of a circumferential wire and two T-plates–cancellous bone plasty is almost always necessary.

no tension is generated medially and the ligament remains intact. If further valgus force is applied, however, with further depression of the plateau, the medial part of the lateral femoral condyle may come into contact with the lateral tubercle of the intercondylar eminence, transfix it, shifting the fulcrum medially and thus causing further tension to be applied to the medial compartment. This tension, if great enough, will rupture the medial ligament. Thus, a medial ligament rupture may occur with an intact or a depressed tibial plateau.

We do not routinely explore the ligaments as does Courvoisier.[2] We rely on the clinical findings of medial discoloration, swelling, pain, instability, and stress X-rays in order to establish our criteria for ligamentous exploration.

Choice of Treatment

Böhler and others have shown that most of the tibial plateau fractures treated conservatively may achieve good to excellent results and that the only absolute indication for an open reduction is an irreducible intra-articular fracture.[1] Before a conservative or a surgical course in undertaken, careful consideration must be given to all problems at hand, for a conservative approach may prejudice any subsequent surgery. Smillie has stated categorically that it is a mistake to attempt closed reduction using skeletal

traction and powerful traction only to decide subsequently that the reduction is unsatisfactory.[6] The hazard of infection is greatly enhanced with the introduction of the Steinmann pin by the contusion of the underlying tissues and skin.

Surgical Approaches to the Head of the Tibia. An incision is chosen such that the final scar does not lie over the metal implant. Thus the position of the plate must be decided before the incision is made.

Surgical Approaches to Medial or Lateral Part of the Tibial Plateau. We employ either a medial parapatellar incision or a curvilinear incision centered on the lateral plateau (Fig. 22-15A). The joint is reduced under direct vision and provisionally stabilized with K-wires. Final fixation is carried out with lag screws or with lag screws in combination with a buttress plate.

Surgical Approach to Both Parts of the Tibial Plateau. A triradiate incision with 120 degrees between its arcs gives good access to both medial and lateral parts of the tibial plateau simultaneously (Fig. 22-15B). The incisions meet not over the tibial tubercle but over the middle of the patellar tendon. To expose the articular surfaces the meniscotibial ligaments are incised and the menisci are elevated. To gain better exposure in very comminuted fractures it is necessary to elevate the patellar tendon. At the end of the procedure the meniscotibial

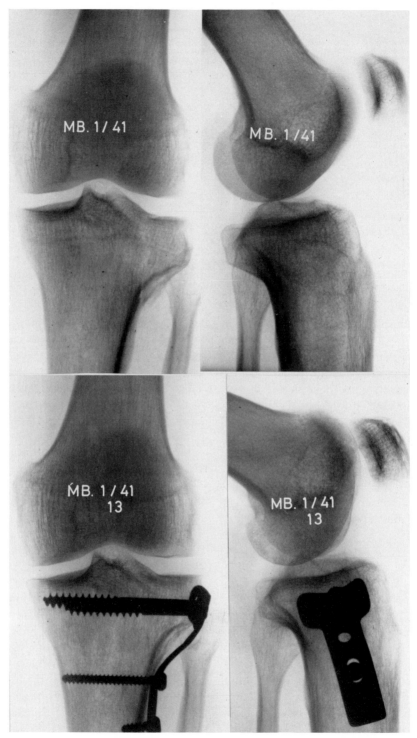

FIG. 22-17. (*Top*) Depressed fracture of the lateral tibial plateau treated by means of a T-plate and cancellous bone plasty. (*Bottom*) Result after 13 weeks. The patient was bearing full weight and had a normal range of movement.

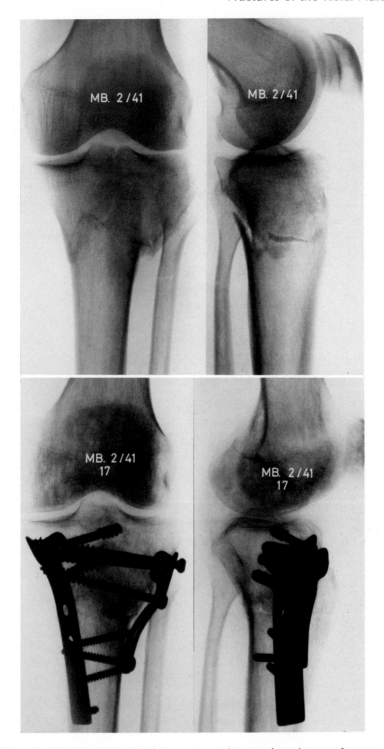

FIG. 22-18. (*Top*) Two T-plates were used to repair a cleavage fracture of both tibial plateaus. (*Bottom*) After 17 weeks there was no difference between the movements in the right and left knees, and the patient could bear full weight without pain.

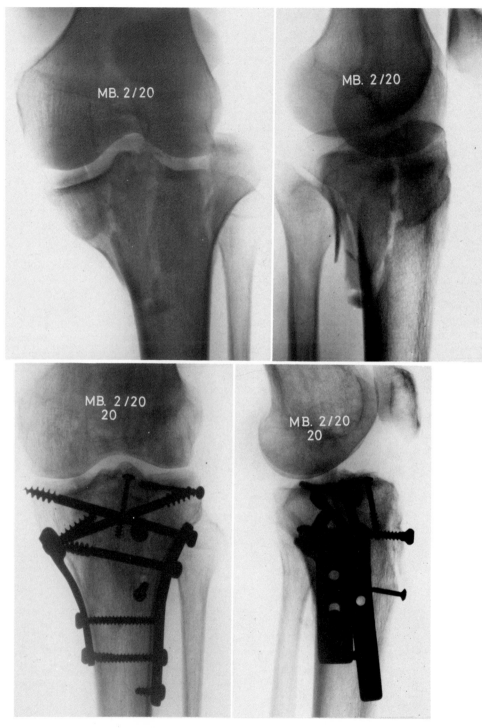

Fig. 22-19. A comminuted fracture of both parts of the tibial plateau required difficult internal fixation and rebuilding with cancellous bone. The tibial tuberosity was osteotomized during the operation in order to get an adequate view into the joint. The torn medial meniscus was excised. Twenty-two weeks after surgery the patient had 100 degrees of flexion and could bear full weight.

ligaments are resutured. If a medial ligamentous disruption is also present, it can be repaired through the same incision.

Operative Techniques

We distinguish three types of tibial plateau fractures (Fig. 22-16):

Cleavage Fractures (Fig. 22-16A). Cancellous screws with washers alone are adequate only in young patients with strong cancellous bone and no osteoporosis. In all other patients a buttress plate is combined with the lag screws to prevent redisplacement.

Depressed Fractures. Depressed fractures should be elevated by upward pressure from below. It is sometimes desirable to drill a large hole 5 to 6 cm. below the joint line of the tibia and thus distal to the fracture. Then with a bone punch, introduced through the hole, elevate the depressed fracture. The fracture is overreduced slightly, and the resultant defect deep to the fracture is filled with autogenous cancellous bone. Fixation is then carried out as shown in Figure 22-16B.

Comminuted Fractures (Fig. 22-16C). To repair a comminuted fracture it may be necessary to expose the whole plateau. For better visualization the meniscotibial ligaments may have to be divided as well as the patellar tendon. Sometimes reduction is only possible after a cerclage wire has been passed circumferentially around the upper tibia. Great caution is exercised so that the wire does not injure the posterior vessels and nerves. If a cerclage is used, fixation is supplemented with two T-plates. Extensive cancellous bone grafting is carried out to fill any ensuing defect, and wherever possible interfragmentary compression is achieved with lag screws. In these comminuted fractures we stress five points: (1) The joint under the meniscus must be restored. If the meniscus is torn in its substance, it is excised. If it is only peripherally detached, it should be resutured. (2) The reduction must be perfect. (3) Cancellous bone graft-

ing must be employed. (4) The fixation must be stable. (5) Associated ligamentous tears must be repaired.

Postoperative positioning as well as postoperative care is identical with that for fractures of the patella (Fig. 22-6).

SUMMARY

Fractures about the knee pose many technical, biomechanical and biological problems. They are no longer unsolved problems, and the patient is no longer committed to life-long disability by the fracture. Full recovery is possible, but it requires careful preoperative assessment, meticulous surgery with no compromise in biological or biomechanical principles, and careful functional after-care.

In conclusion we can only reiterate the opening remarks of the AO Manual: "Open treatment of fractures is a valuable but difficult method which involves much responsibility. We cannot advise too strongly against internal fixation if it is carried out by an inadequately trained surgeon, and in the absence of full equipment and sterile operating room conditions. Using our method, enthusiasts who lack self criticism are much more dangerous than skeptics or outright opponents."

REFERENCES

1. Böhler, L.: Die Technik der Knochenbruchbehandlung. Wien: Maudrich, 1957.
2. Courvoisier
3. Müller, M. E.: Fractures basses du fémur. Acta Orthop. Belg., *36*:566, 1970.
4. Müller, M. E., Allgöwer, M., and Willenegger, H.: Manual of Internal Fixation. Technique recommended by the AO-Group. Berlin-Heidelberg-New York: Springer, 1970.
5. Pauwels, F.: Gesammelte Abhandlungen zur funktionellen Anatomie des Bewegungsapparates. Berlin-Heidelberg-New York: Springer, 1965.
6. Smillie, I. S.: Injuries of the Knee Joint. Edinburgh-London: Livingstone, 1970.

23

Rehabilitation of the Knee in Athletes

James A. Nicholas, M.D.

The athlete who has had a knee injury poses a rather special problem in that total rehabilitation is the goal. One might suggest that if rehabilitation of an athlete to a high level of performance is possible, why should these goals not be extended to the general population. The author regards this as a practical and proper approach.

1. To rehabilitate the knee, one should determine whether the defect is in motion, power, or stability, or in all three components. If there is loss of motion one should know whether it is intraarticular or extraarticular (Fig. 23-1). Extraarticular loss of movement results from contracture of the anterior quadriceps and thigh muscles, which limits patellar excursion, whereas lack of extension may be due to calf or hamstring contraction. The basic rehabilitative effort in anterior or posterior thigh contracture is to stretch muscles to increase excursion.

2. Lack of power is the most common result of knee injury and is often underestimated. Too frequently only the quadriceps are considered, and one fails to realize that all other muscles of the thigh are involved in knee strength. Knee joint control is a function of all the muscles that span the hip to the knee. For this reason, abductor and adductor power, particularly abductor power, is always lost after knee injury. No matter how intensively quadriceps drill is performed it will not restore loss of power of the abductors or hip flexors. Such loss of power can produce symptomatic synovitis.

Finally, stability of the knee may be impaired by previous injury, or the patient may be loose-jointed and have a rather lax knee. In rehabilitating such knees, power is reacquired more slowly although the restoration of motion is easier. The acquisition of maximum strength in a loose knee is imperative, else reinjury in sport is inevitable. Knees with intraarticular block to motion should be rehabilitated not through the joint, but only by relieving contracture. The loss of motion in such cases may require surgery.

3. Loss of power can be tested manually in the sitting patient by pushing down as hard as possible on the top of the patella or thigh. If there is no pain, weakness in flexion can be measured in terms of hand or finger resistance when compared with the opposite side. With the weight suspended over the foot, while sitting and actively flexing the hip the average person can lift about ten per cent of the body weight 25 times (Fig. *4* 23-2). Loss of power may not be recognized unless one watches the person perform athletic activities, such as running and jumping, when a slight abductor limp or hip flexor limp will be demonstrated. Abductor power should be checked, as should thigh flexion, knee flexion, and extensor power in both straight leg raising and from a flexed position. Abductor power should be checked by abduction with the knee straight, weight being transmitted across the lower leg. It is important in rehabilitation to recognize such weakness.

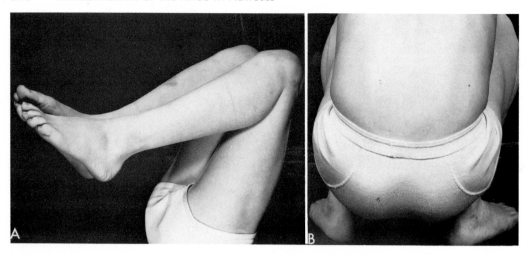

Fig. 23-1. Flexion of the knee may be measured by heel-to-buttock distance comparing one knee to the other. Flexion should be performed from both prone and supine positions.

✱Loose-jointed individuals may have a mild patella alta and a rather significant degree of tibiofibular rotation. The leg may have an increase in external or internal rotation of perhaps 30 degrees or more, in which case in the sitting knee the patellar tubercle passes lateral to the lateral line of the patella, or medial to it, in internal rotation. With instability of a developmental type, it is essential to recover as much power as possible. ✝With loss of stability due to injury, restoration of power plus the use of an adequate brace, such as the Lenox Hill Derotation Brace may permit participation in sports without resort to surgery.

Any loss of movement or power that cannot be recovered is a severe drain on the stability of the knee. The author feels that one should compare one leg with the other and insist on obtaining equal power in both legs in all components. This has to be achieved by full discussion of the objectives with the patient, careful measurement, and the use of active resistive exercises. Both legs should be strengthened to their *maximum* possible.

PROCEDURES FOR RESTORATION OF MOTION

Loss of movement in the knee can occur from two sources, within the joint and without. Often it is due to a combination of both. Frequently, a knee after hemarthrosis from injury to the patella, heals, but lack of excursion may develop in the quadriceps and upper thigh muscles. Since squatting is painful and not permissible, the patient does not squat. However, if the hip and knee joints are normal, it is possible to obtain such movement by extending the hip, grasping the ankle behind, and bringing it toward the ceiling as one stands (Fig. 23-3). This will stretch the anterior thigh musculature and produce increased excursion of the quadriceps. The same exercise can be done with the foot on a chair behind one; then one stands bending the opposite leg while the hip on the affected side is extended. Active forceful flexion should not be attempted until the anterior thigh musculature has been stretched. Hip flexion contracture can be stretched out in the same manner.

Myostatic contracture of the hamstrings frequently causes limitation of extension of the knee and will produce tightening of the quadriceps mechanism along the patellofemoral ligaments. It is important to rid athletic individuals of such contractures. An excellent exercise is wall stretching of the heel or calf muscles on an inclined plane (Fig. 23-4). The heel cord and calf muscles are stretched as the patient stands about 16

FIG. 23-2. Active power of the quadriceps can be developed by lifting weight with knee flexed. The patella is not stressed as it is when the knee is extended from flexion. This is quite useful when there is patellofemoral pain.

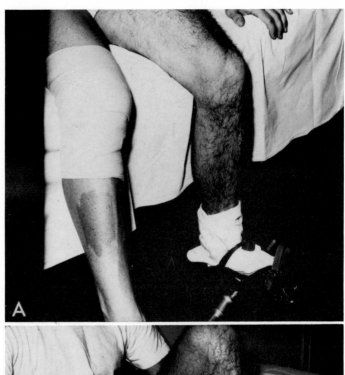

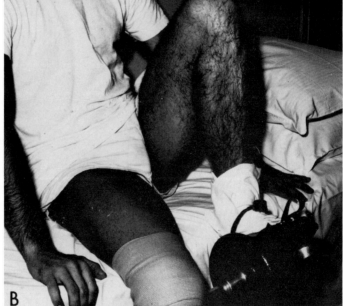

inches from the wall, with the heels placed square on the ground: the chest is moved to and against the wall while the knee remains extended.

To stretch the upper thigh, the foot is placed on a chair while the opposite knee is bent until the affected leg is parallel to the floor (Fig. 23-5). Usually this tends to flex the knee on the affected side. The patient forces the knee into extension so far as possible, keeping the foot dorsiflexed by bending the opposite knee. By these means hamstring and calf may be stretched to a considerable degree. If the spine is now flexed, all the muscles from spine to feet are stretched.

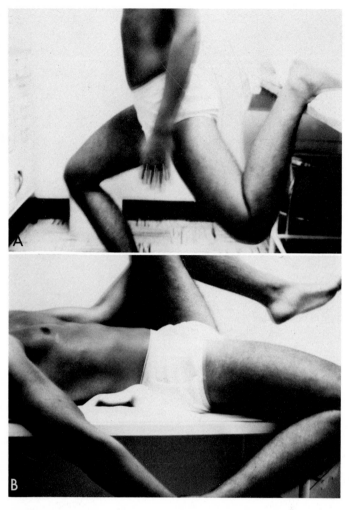

FIG. 23-3. The quadriceps stretch, an important test and treatment for anterior thigh contracture, which can limit knee movement.

The abductors may be stretched in the manner described by Ober or by bending forward with the legs crossed, bending first to one side, then to the other. Lateral bending of the spine with legs crossed, while standing erect, is another way to produce upper lateral thigh stretch.

It should be recognized that myostatic contracture entails loss of power in the lost segment of motion. Rehabilitation of the athlete's knee is not complete unless full power is recovered over the whole range of motion.

POSTMENISCECTOMY
REHABILITATION

After meniscectomy the first exercises are straight leg raises and quadriceps setting until motion gradually reaches 90 degrees of flexion. At that point, rather than knee extension which may irritate the joint, the author institutes sitting hip flexion with weight on the foot. This is based on the premise that the quadriceps muscles span the hip joint as well as the knee joint, and are associated by their fascial connections with the iliopsoas and lower abdominal muscles, all contributing accessory power to the knee in athletic stress. In this way, power is developed in the quadriceps by transferring resistance to its upper end. The weight is suspended over the foot, the knee is lifted off the ground, perhaps 6 inches, while the patient sits over a table supporting himself. Twenty-five repetitions of this are done with that amount of weight which the patient can lift without pain. The opposite leg is tested as a control. The aim is to

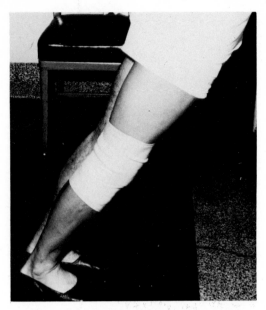

FIG. 23-4. Heel cord stretching helps eliminate hamstring and heel cord contracture.

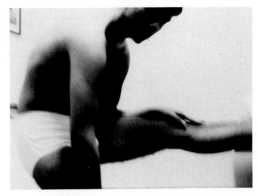

FIG. 23-5. The standing hamstring stretch is an excellent method to remove upper thigh contracture without hurting the back.

develop equal power in both legs. Once this is accomplished, the patient is encouraged to achieve maximum "liftability." Many individuals can lift up to 40 or 50 pounds, after having started with only 5 or 10 pounds. This is extremely important in preventing reinjury. Knee extension against resistance, if not painful, is then instituted, as well as active resistive abduction.

Abduction Exercises—Straight Leg Raising

The patient should lie on his side and lift sideways with weight over the ankle, beginning with ten repetitions that he can perform without pain. The weight the weakened leg can lift is actually very little, and it should not cause pain. The first target is the unaffected leg. When the two are equal, both legs should be strengthened. The weight the patient lifts sideways is in no way related to the amount he can lift while sitting.

After recovery of power in abduction and thigh flexion, knee extension exercises to obtain terminal vastus medialis power are performed often with greater effect than by the conventional system described by de Lorme, whose system, if tolerated, is also

used. Where indicated additional exercises are also useful.

The author does not advise discarding the weights once maximum power is reached. Weight lifting should be resumed every quarter of the year, to see whether there has been a dropback. After injury there usually is, especially in hip flexion-abduction. The leg does tend to lose power in different seasons of the year because of the differing demands on it. If there is a drop-off, the patient should be encouraged to retrain the leg to play tennis in spring or golf in the summer, or ski in the winter. Symmetrical leg power is extremely important, for even slight loss of power in a "transfer weight" type of sport will cause increased load on the knee joint.

No weight lifting should be done if it causes pain or swelling, nor should one try to force weights if there is discomfort. Active resistive exercises in limited cycles of perhaps 25 knee lifts, ten in knee extension and ten side lifts, repeated two or three times after a few minutes rest once a day are usually adequate unless there are special weight loading machines available.

Persistent Stretching

Continuous stretching while weight lifting is important, and stretching periodically as a warm-up is important in a tight-muscled individual. Tight-muscled individuals tend

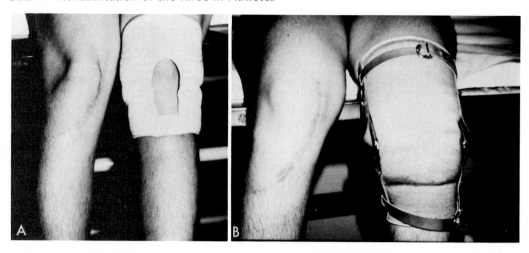

FIG. 23-6. This support is used by the author to restrain the patella.

to be unable to touch their toes with their hands and must do hamstring stretching, as previously outlined, daily if they are to play games in which a tight hamstring endangers the knee. The loose-jointed can put their palms to the floor, have recurvatum of the knee, and can toe out the entire extremity as much as 180 degrees. To such people stretching exercises are useless for there is no contracture, but weight-lifting exercises are desirable, for they may have considerable lack of power.

Many systems of rehabilitation are available after knee injuries and should be applied at all ages. Even a 70-year-old with a broken hip who recovers from the fracture and walks well may have residual thigh flexion and abductor weakness as well as contracture. Though the hamstrings and calf may be strong with ability to walk, there is usually contracture of these muscles while the antigravity muscles, such as the thigh flexors, are not strong. The system outlined by the author has been valuable in recovering symmetrical strength even in older people.

The use of a swimming pool is an excellent means for recovery of thigh muscle power. Repetitive abductor exercises and walking in water with the level up to the groin will produce considerable upper thigh and abdominal abductor power. For good swimmers treading water, 200 to 300 times

in the deep part of the pool is also an effective way to develop upper thigh power. Goose stepping in the water, with the knees fully extended, is another way to strengthen the quadriceps. Flutter kicking in the water sometimes results in pain in the patella, a warning sign that the exercises should be modified.

REHABILITATION IN YOUNG ADULTS WITH CHONDROMALACIA

It is difficult to rehabilitate a weak knee that has patellar pain. Patellar pain may be due to "subluxability" of the patella; it can be associated with chondromalacia or with patellar tendinitis. Knee extension exercises produce pain. Even straight leg raising without any resistance can produce pain. This can be a most vexing situation for if the patient cannot recover power, the symptoms may be worsened. The best way to deal with this, I think, is to use some type of patellar restraining support for the knee. This can be a horseshoe of felt wrapped around the knee, the open part distally secured with an Ace (crepe) bandage. This protects the patella from excessive movement. A hinged knee brace that envelops a foam rubber support in the shape of a horseshoe has been very useful in the author's hands (Fig. 23-6). This protects particularly patients with patella alta. Rehabilitation starts with sitting thigh flexion. Such exercises, as they lift the knee with the weight over the foot, will cause no pain, whereas trying to extend the knee from the flexed position will cause pain in chondromalacia, as will straight leg raising. By gradually increasing the exercises, one can build up considerable power and then substitute more conventional quadriceps exercises. A second method is to see if the patient, sitting, can straight leg raise without pain. If so, the sitting patient can bend the knee from a raised straight leg position to the point where pain begins, usually at about 30 degrees. By flexing and extending in this painless range, considerable power can develop before ultimately reaching the full range of motion.

RESTORATION OF FUNCTION IN THE UNSTABLE KNEE AFTER SURGERY

As much as a year may be required to recover maximum motion, power, and stability after reconstructive surgery for ligamentous tears. It is important to protect the repaired ligaments for at least 6 weeks in plaster and perhaps another 6 or 8 weeks in the corrected position to prevent stretching. In other words, when anteromedial instability is repaired, the knee should be turned in with the tibia rotated internally and the leg in varus. The use of a brace that will hold this position, such as the derotation brace, will permit restoration of motion in this plane while preventing external rotation or valgus stress, as can occur even while turning over in bed. Patients who come out of plaster should be placed in such braces or a support that controls motion in this position for several weeks. Such braces should be worn night and day, or at least as much as can be tolerated, so that the ligaments are not stretched until they become strong. *The aim of rehabilitation is to restore movement of the knee to 90 degrees gradually and to recover full extension.* This can be done by passively and actively flexing and extending the knee slowly, using whirlpool or warm baths as a supplement and never turning the leg into a position detrimental to the repair.

Appropriate and converse manoeuvers are used for posterolateral instability after reconstruction restored anteromedial rotation.

As the knee reaches a right angle, and often with a brace for support, the author starts gentle flexing exercises. One might argue that this stretches the ligaments but actually, if the load is small and within the limits of tolerance, it will develop muscle, ligament, and tendon strength. Ligaments can remodel to such an extent that they will increase in strength as has been reported by R.J. Larsen and Stan James of Eugene, Oregon.

Abduction exercises with the leg straight are done next. As thigh flexion increases, knee extension and other exercises can be started. It may take 3 months to achieve power equal to the opposite side. Since contractures are common after ligament surgery, it is wise to stretch the posterior capsule gently in individuals with anterior instability or the anterior capsule in individuals with posterior instability.

SUMMARY

Rehabilitation of the injured knee requires close teamwork between the surgeon, his paramedical aides, and the patient. Restoration of motion, followed by restoration of power, with protection from instability by bracing, supportive bandages, and shoe corrections or restriction from sport until the knee is capable of standing up are the essential measures whereby individuals after knee injury can be returned to full function. Restoration of motion is essential, for any fixation of the patella will lead to compressive changes on the articular surface. To restore extension and flexion it may be necessary to stretch the hamstrings and to increase quadriceps excursion by stretching the muscles in front of the thigh. Active resistive movements can be accomplished in many ways, using hydrotherapy, pool or weights, as have been described. Although ligaments which have been torn may have healed in a weaker or slacker form, accessory rehabilitation of all the thigh to calf muscles to the peak of their performance can control many an unstable knee.

Index

Numerals in italics indicate an illustration.